Nutritional and Herbal Therapies for Children and Adolescents

A Handbook for Mental Health Clinicians

Nutritional and Herbal Therapies for Children and Adolescents

A Handbook for Mental Health Clinicians

George M. Kapalka
Associate Professor, Monmouth University
West Long Branch, NJ
and
Director, Center for Behavior Modification
Brick, NJ

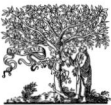

AMSTERDAM • BOSTON • HEIDELBERG • LONDON
NEW YORK • OXFORD • PARIS • SAN DIEGO
SAN FRANCISCO • SINGAPORE • SYDNEY • TOKYO

Academic Press is an imprint of Elsevier

ELSEVIER

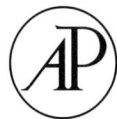

Academic Press is an imprint of Elsevier
32 Jamestown Road, London NW1 7BY, UK
30 Corporate Drive, Suite 400, Burlington, MA 01803, USA
525 B Street, Suite 1900, San Diego, CA 92101-4495, USA

Notice
No responsibility is assumed by the publisher for any injury and/or damage to persons or
property as a matter of products liability, negligence or otherwise, or from any use or operation
of any methods, products, instructions or ideas contained in the material herein. Because of rapid
advances in the medical sciences, in particular, independent verification of diagnoses and drug
dosages should be made

British Library Cataloguing-in-Publication Data
A catalogue record for this book is available from the British Library

Library of Congress Cataloging-in-Publication Data
A catalog record for this book is available from the Library of Congress

ISBN : 978-0-12-374927-7

For information on all Academic Press publications
visit our website at www.elsevierdirect.com

Typeset by Macmillan Publishing Solutions
www.macmillansolutions.com

Printed and bound in the United States of America

10 11 12 13 14 15   10 9 8 7 6 5 4 3 2 1

Working together to grow
libraries in developing countries

www.elsevier.com | www.bookaid.org | www.sabre.org

ELSEVIER   BOOK AID
             International   Sabre Foundation

Contents

Preface

Many years ago, when symptoms of most psychological disorders were just beginning to be identified, the prevailing belief was that these symptoms were the result of deeply embedded psychogenic conflicts that required psychoanalysis to work through. Over the past five decades, however, a plethora of research revealed that many individuals with these disorders exhibit structural and functional differences in their brains. According to our current knowledge of the neuropsychiatric aspects of psychological disorders, attention deficit hyperactivity disorder (ADHD), Tourette's disorder, obsessive compulsive disorder (OCD), panic disorder, depression, bipolar disorder, and schizophrenia are characterized by significant changes in the brain. Moreover, the earlier the onset of the symptoms, the more significant those brain differences appear to be.

Since brain changes are likely to be reflected in feelings and behaviors, psychopharmacological approaches were developed to try to address some of the biological factors that may be responsible, at least in part, for the symptoms. Indeed, many of these have proven effective in reducing (and, sometimes, eliminating) the symptoms of some psychological disorders, and intervening pharmacologically may be beneficial, and in some cases is indispensable, since without medications some symptoms (for example, psychosis) are not likely to resolve.

As advances in psychopharmacology continued, a biopsychosocial approach developed and aimed to conceptualize effective mental health treatment as falling across three dimensions – biological (use of medications), psychological (counseling and psychotherapy), and social (group and family counseling, development of social supports). Over time, medicine (especially, psychiatry) began to favor the biological aspects and pharmacological interventions. However, the biopsychosocial approach was developed to balance the three aspects of mental health care, and many mental health professionals continue to approach psychological care from the biopsychosocial perspective, utilizing pharmacological approaches in conjunction with psychosocial treatment, especially when treating individuals with disorders that are known to be associated with significant changes in the brain.

BIOLOGICAL VS. PSYCHOSOCIAL TREATMENT

When treating disorders with known biological etiology, many non-medical mental health professionals seek to minimize pharmacological approaches and initially try psychosocial treatment. This is a reasonable approach, especially with children. However, many factors may contribute to the decision to utilize pharmacological approaches, in conjunction with or instead of psychotherapy.

Type of Symptoms

Some symptoms may lend themselves well to psychotherapy. For example, depression or generalized anxiety generally respond well to psychosocial treatment, and results of numerous research studies reveal that individuals who undergo psychotherapeutic treatment for such symptoms exhibit statistically significant improvement (for example, see Beck, 1995). Of course, improvement does not necessarily mean the elimination of symptoms, so in many cases conjoint psychopharmacological treatment may offer additional benefits.

Conversely, some symptoms do not seem to respond well to psychotherapy. For example, delusions, hallucinations, racing thoughts, and other symptoms associated with severe psychopathology do not tend to significantly diminish with psychosocial interventions. True, concurrent psychotherapy may help the patient's overall adjustment, but the core symptoms are not likely to resolve without the use of at least some pharmacological interventions.

Severity of Symptoms

Even those symptoms that may often be manageable without medications may sometimes require a pharmacological approach. For example, milder forms of depression, impulsivity, anxiety, or agitation may respond well to psychotherapy. However, severe variants of these symptoms may be difficult to treat with talk therapies, and intense symptoms are likely to require psychopharmacological treatment. For example, it may be very difficult to communicate with a severely depressed or agitated patient, and a severely anxious patient may have difficulties coming in for psychotherapy. Thus, most clinicians find that symptoms that are very impairing usually require an approach that includes pharmacological treatment.

Onset of Relief

When psychotherapy is effective, progression of improvement is gradual and requires several sessions to become evident. Even those variants that are called 'brief therapy' generally require 8–15 sessions before significant improvement is expected. When the patient is very uncomfortable, and when the symptoms debilitate the patient and significantly interfere with normal functioning, waiting this long for improvement may not be prudent.

Although this is not always the case, many pharmacological treatments produce at least some improvement within days of the onset of treatment, although a few weeks (in some cases, 4–6) may be needed for more comprehensive response. However, this is still faster than psychotherapy, and the amount of improvement seen with medications may be greater than the improvement seen with psychotherapy over the same period of time. Especially when symptoms are severe, it may be more appropriate to initiate pharmacological treatment immediately, perhaps conjointly with psychosocial interventions. Relief is likely to be faster when such a strategy is utilized.

Time and Effort

When pharmacological and non-pharmacological approaches are likely to be equally effective, as is the case with pharmacological or psychotherapeutic treatment of depression, non-medical mental health professionals prefer to utilize non-medical treatments, and pharmacological interventions are seen as a 'last resort' when therapy does not seem to produce sufficient relief. While this may be reasonable in some situations, professionals need to be sensitive to other reasons that may drive the use of pharmacological interventions.

In order for psychotherapy to be effective, patients need to attend sessions regularly. If rapid progress is needed, sessions need to be scheduled at least weekly. However, driving to the therapist's office once per week, and spending an hour in the office, may be difficult for some patients (or families) with significant time obligations. When the patient is a child or adolescent, psychotherapy must be done outside of school hours, since missing school 1 day per week to attend psychotherapy is neither practical for the family nor beneficial to the student. However, it may be difficult to find therapists with significant amount of evening hours to accommodate the patient's schedule, especially when weekly treatment is needed.

In addition, geographic considerations also affect the decision to enter psychotherapy. In urban or suburban areas, child and adolescent psychotherapists may be prevalent. In rural areas, however, this situation is much more likely to be problematic, and patients may not live in reasonable proximity of qualified and competent pediatric mental health professionals. Thus, even when a family may prefer to try psychotherapy instead of pharmacy, their ability to get to the therapist's office may be limited.

Cost of Care

The cost of weekly psychotherapy for 8–15 weeks is likely to constitute a significant expense for many families, and few are able to cover such costs out of pocket. In the United States, most children and adolescents who have health care coverage are covered by private plans, usually purchased through the parent's employer. The quality of this coverage varies widely. Unfortunately, mental health care is often considered to be the 'step-child' of the health care industry, and levels of coverage for mental health treatment are often much lower than they are for medical care. Although laws on the federal and state levels have been passed to close that gap, many exclusions exist and the disparity between medical and mental health coverage continues.

Limiting the patient's access to care is one common method of containing health care costs. Many individuals with managed health care coverage have benefits that primarily are evident 'on paper' and virtually disappear when the insured seeks treatment. Gatekeepers are assigned that review the need for care, and these reviews delay sessions and interrupt the continuity of care. Usually, four to six sessions may initially be authorized, and additional reviews are needed for each subsequent block. It is up to the discretion of the gatekeeper to authorize further treatment, and when the gatekeeper feels that sufficient progress was attained, or that sufficient progress is not evident, further authorization may not be issued. Although every insurer has appeals procedures that may be utilized, these appeals are internal to the insurer, and usually no external review exists that may be invoked if the insurer continues to refuse to authorize care. To make matters worse, appeals often take months, and meanwhile the patient is getting no care.

In addition, millions of children and adolescents in the US have no health care coverage. While federal and state authorities are striving to close this gap, there continues to be a significant portion of our society that cannot afford mental health care and has no insurance coverage. Various agencies exist that may service these individuals, including networks of community mental health centers (CMHCs) that provide care to those who need it, sometimes without (or with minimal) cost. However, in many states, CMHCs are overextended and long wait times are necessary (in some cases, up to 8 weeks) before the agency is able to provide care. Meanwhile, patients are suffering and are receiving no treatment. In addition, in rural states, the nearest CMHC may be quite a distance away.

For all of the reasons reviewed above, patients and/or their families may choose to utilize psychopharmacological treatment either instead of, or in addition to, psychosocial interventions.

MEDICATIONS VS. NUTRITIONAL AND HERBAL SUPPLEMENTS

When patients decide to use pharmacological interventions, they must consider whether to use prescription medications or over-the-counter compounds. Once again, patients are likely to consider many factors when making such a decision. Many patients are skeptical about the use of prescription drugs. There are complex reasons for this perception, some of which are more legitimate than others. It is important for mental health professionals to understand the reasons that drive these perceptions, and help their clients separate truth from fiction when considering naturopathic interventions.

Distrust in Pharmaceutical Companies

One reason for skepticism about prescription drugs is the availability of information that continues to come to light about the influence of the drug industry on studies that investigate the effectiveness of medications. The process of bringing a medication to market is more convoluted in the US than in the vast majority of countries around the world. Overtly, this may imply that medications marketed in the US are safer than those marketed elsewhere, and the Federal Drug Administration (FDA) seeks a greater amount of safety data before the drug is approved. In practice, however, drug manufacturers have a significant amount of influence over various portions of this process. Although the FDA requires three stages of studies to investigate the safety and efficacy of medications, there are no requirements that compel drug manufacturers to report *all* research findings to the FDA, and it is becoming increasingly evident that drug manufacturers perform many studies and only choose to release to the FDA the findings of those studies that support the drug's safety and efficacy. Consequently, the public is losing confidence in widely publicized claims of effectiveness, and drug manufacturers have lost a lot of creditability with the American public.

As a result, people are turning to nutritional and herbal supplements. Often, these are perceived as viable alternatives that have been around for thousands of years, and have been used for various purposes in many cultures through many centuries. Thus, they must be effective. However, this assumption is often inaccurate. Although the efficacy of medications *must* be established through empirical studies, no such requirement is placed on nutritional and herbal supplements, unless they are being specifically marketed to treat an existing illness or disorder. Since nutritional and herbal supplements are not usually marketed in this way, they are exempt from this requirement, and the vast majority of supplements have undergone a miniscule amount of research. Thus, frequently, the efficacy of a naturopathic compound is presumed, rather than established. A major goal for this book is to help readers determine which supplements have been shown to be effective, and which are only presumed or expected to be (with little research support).

Marketing

Medications can only be advertised to treat the specific condition for which they are FDA approved (the so-called 'on-label' use). Although medications are brought to market to treat a specific condition, in subsequent research they are sometimes shown to be effective for another disorder. Because of the staggering cost involved in filing another application with the FDA, most drug manufacturers do not do so, knowing that any prescriber can potentially prescribe any medication to treat any disorder so long as in the prescriber's professional opinion there is good likelihood that the medication will be effective. This 'off-label' use is usually based on the availability of research studies that support the use of the medication for a specific purpose, even though the original FDA approval was issued to treat a different disorder.

The situation is different with nutritional and herbal supplements. While these compounds cannot be marketed to, for example, 'treat symptoms of ADHD' without submitting evidence of efficacy to treat this disorder, they can be advertised to 'improve attention' or provide other similar benefits, as long as no specific claim is being made to treat ADHD. This is exemplified by the marketing practices of Focus Factor, a vitamin compound that lacks any objective efficacy in treating symptoms of ADHD, and yet it is commonly sold to 'improve attention.' Obviously, this loophole in current regulations is successfully exploited by the manufacturers of nutritional and herbal supplements, and clients must understand that they have to be even more skeptical about claims of efficacy of nutritional compounds than about similar claims made regarding medications, for which advertising practices are more tightly regulated.

Regulation

The manufacturing and sale of prescription (as well as over-the-counter) medications are tightly regulated, and manufacturers are mandated to assure that each pill contains the exact amount of the compound that is being listed. For example, 20 mg of methylphenidate must contain very close to 20 mg of the active compound. Similar control is exercised over the other ingredients. Every medication (as well as supplement) contains active and inactive compounds. The inactive compounds include the coating of the pill as well as the binder that holds the active compound together. In the case of prescription drugs, the binder is also researched to make sure that it is inert psychologically but behaves predictably when the tablet dissolves, delivering the active compound in an expected manner. In addition, when the formulation is patented, the entire contents are fixed. Thus, when a medication is sold, both the active and inactive compounds behave predictably and exist in the pill in the exact amounts specified on the label (within very tight tolerances).

Unfortunately, in the United States, there is an almost complete lack of oversight over the manufacture and sale of nutritional and herbal supplements. Since the supplement market is left to self-regulate, consumers have no way of assuring that a 200 mg capsule of SAM-e really contains 200 mg of that compound or, for that matter, *any* amount of that specific compound. In addition, since the formulations being sold usually are not patented, different forms of the active compound may be used by different manufacturers (and different binders are likely to be utilized), and therefore identical doses of the same compound from various manufacturers are likely to dissolve differently and have different bioavailability. This makes the use of supplements very unpredictable.

Dosage and Effects

Prescription medications are extensively refined and most contain a single active compound that is carefully isolated and studied, its pharmacokinetics and pharmacodynamics are established, and patients have a lot of information available about how much they need to take, how long it will take before improvement can be expected, potential adverse reactions, etc. By contrast, supplements are unrefined and often contain dozens of active compounds, all of which have different pharmacokinetic and pharmacodynamic properties. This makes supplements much more unpredictable and difficult to study, since separate active components are not isolated and individually examined. Generally, clients who take supplements can expect a much broader spectrum of effect, and changes may be observed not only in behaviors targeted by the supplement (like symptoms of ADHD), but many other, unrelated reactions.

Because supplements have not undergone much research, pragmatics of their use are often poorly established. For this reason, it is hard to determine the effective dose, the manner in which the dose needs to be titrated, the onset of effect, and the duration of action of the substance. While some studies have addressed those issues, most have not. In addition, the limited research that has been performed was usually done with adults, rather than children or adolescents. Thus, clinicians that plan to use supplements with children or teens must generally extrapolate from adult data.

Perception of Danger

Patients often have concerns about the safety of prescription medications. This is especially the case with some classes of medications, like psychostimulants and antidepressants. Stimulants have been portrayed as 'dangerous drugs' in much of the media coverage. They have been likened to cocaine and amphetamines, and exaggerated fears have been propagated about the addictiveness of these compounds. In some media coverage, levels of side effects seen with the abuse of cocaine and crystal meth have been extrapolated to also be relevant to Ritalin and related medications. This distorted view of the danger of stimulants has resulted in widespread fear of these medications.

This apprehension has been exploited by makers of other drugs and manufacturers of naturopathic supplements. For example, atomoxetine is marketed to be an alternative to stimulants with the presumption that the 'dangerous' side effects associated with stimulants are not a risk with this medication. As is often the case, the truth is different than the presumption – for example, atomoxetine is associated with more significant side effects than any of the psychostimulants, and a careful review of any comprehensive reference (for example, Bezchlibnyk-Butler & Jeffries, 2007) reveals that psychostimulants, as a group, present with less frequent and less dangerous side effects than any other category of psychotropic medications. Clinicians and clients need to be aware that media coverage is based, at least in part, on the sensationalism of the tale. It does not make an interesting story to say that stimulants are safe and effective and have helped millions of patients with ADHD. It makes for a more interesting story to film a segment on *48 Hours* about the dangers of stimulants ('Out of control,' November 9, 2001), and the viewership for such a show is likely to increase, even if the message within it is greatly distorted.

Similar problems are evident in the public perceptions of other medications. For example, antidepressants have been linked to suicidality, and a black box warning has been mandated for all antidepressants and related drugs (like atomoxetine). The perception that most people have is that anyone taking an antidepressant is more likely to commit suicide. However, this perception is inaccurate and highly skewed. No completed suicides, connected to the use of these medications, have been reported thus far (Bezchlibnyk-Butler & Jeffries, 2007). What seems to be evident is that within the first 2 weeks of initiating treatment, a small percentage of patients may have some transient thoughts about suicide. It is apparent that no one acts on these thoughts, and these thoughts dissipate after the first 2 weeks, and further increases in the medication, if needed, are not associated with this risk. The same findings have been reported for children and adolescents (Bezchlibnyk-Butler & Virani, 2004). Still, this is not commonly known by the public, and therefore the perception of antidepressants as 'dangerous drugs' is propagated.

Because of these exaggerated fears, naturopathic compounds are often expected to be safer. After all, these are extracts of plants or other naturally occurring elements, and anything that comes from nature is presumed to be safe. Clinicians must dispel this misperception. Naturopathic compounds, on the whole, are not any safer than medications. In fact, some of the deadliest compounds occur naturally – radon, strychnine, gyromitrin (deadly toxin commonly found in wild mushrooms), etc. Mistakenly assuming that something is safe just because it occurs naturally can be lethal. Of course, supplements available for sale generally are not as toxic, but still sometimes carry risks similar to some prescription medications. For example, use of kava kava, a relaxant sometimes taken to treat symptoms of anxiety, may result in liver damage (Bezchlibnyk-Butler & Jeffries, 2007).

ORGANIZATION OF THIS HANDBOOK

This book is intended as a reference for those clinicians who wish to learn more about the potential benefits of the use of nutritional and herbal supplements with children and adolescents. The book focuses on psychological disorders that commonly occur in the pediatric population, and coverage is primarily aimed at those disorders usually treated with medications, where patients and/or clinicians may wish to attempt to avoid prescription drugs and try supplements instead.

The book is divided into two parts. The first part covers conceptual issues to give clinicians appropriate background necessary to understand the action of psychoactive supplements. Chapter 1 covers a discussion of the aspects that must be considered when making a decision about whether the use of a medication or a supplement is appropriate. Clinicians are encouraged to consider all the categories outlined in that chapter and thoroughly discuss these with the patients in order to help them make an informed decision about which direction to take in treatment.

The next three chapters provide an introduction to the medical concepts that are necessary to master in order to understand the action of specific compounds. Chapter 2 outlines pharmacokinetics – the processes in which the body acts on an ingested substance and changes its effects. Chapter 3 discusses pharmacodynamics – specific mechanisms in which ingested compounds may act on the brain and exert some effect. Chapter 4 reviews neurotransmitters and other molecules that are commonly associated with psychogenic effects.

The remainder of the book provides a discussion of disorders that may be treated with the use of nutritional and herbal supplements. In each chapter, compounds are reviewed for which efficacy in treating symptoms of the disorders has been investigated or presumed. Results of available studies are reviewed, and guidelines about using the supplements with children and teens are provided.

Based on the amount of supporting research evidence, the supplements are divided into four categories.

- Supplements with Established Efficacy. Compounds that have been researched in placebo-controlled, randomized trials, and have consistently been shown to improve symptoms. The use of these supplements is most likely to result in clinical improvement and clinicians are encouraged to begin treatment by utilizing these compounds.
- Supplements with Likely Efficacy. Compounds that have been researched through placebo-controlled, randomized trials that have mostly (but not entirely) revealed improvement in symptoms, or those supplements that have primarily been researched through open-label studies that consistently reveal symptom improvement. The use of these supplements may be beneficial and clinicians may consider these supplements when no supplements with established efficacy are available, or when supplements with established efficacy did not sufficiently reduce symptoms.
- Supplements with Possible Efficacy. Compounds that exhibit sound rationale for their use and preliminary research reveal promising results. The use of these supplements is considered experimental, and clinicians are advised to utilize these compounds only as a last resort.

- Supplements Not Likely to be Effective. Compounds that lack sound rationale for their use, lack evidence in human trials, and/or present dangers that outweigh any potential benefits. Despite marketing claims to the contrary, the use of these compounds is not likely to result in any benefits and may be associated with unnecessary risk of harm. Clinicians are advised against the use of these supplements.

To further guide clinicians in selecting compounds that are appropriate given the specific cluster of symptoms evident in each patient, each chapter concludes with an algorithm that takes into account the amount of research support available for each compound, as well as the specific mechanism of action of each supplement and its applicability to the treatment of various categories of symptoms.

Chapter 1

Deciding Between Medications and Supplements

To medicate or not to medicate: that is the question that millions of parents ask themselves when faced with significant psychological or behavioral symptoms their child or teen exhibits. Parents who decide that a trial of prescription medications is a reasonable course of action usually see a medical professional (for example, a pediatrician or a pediatric psychiatrist). Those who want to avoid prescription medications seek non-medical mental health treatment. Many of these parents contact psychologists, professional counselors, marriage and family therapists, or social workers to try to address the symptoms through psychotherapy and behavioral interventions. At the onset of treatment, both medical and non-medical mental health professionals need to decide whether psychotherapy and behavioral interventions are likely to be sufficient to address the symptoms, or pharmacological interventions may also be needed.

When a patient comes in for mental health treatment, the clinician initially needs to assess the symptoms and their progression. Various factors must be considered, including symptom severity, onset, precipitating factors, associated features, and patient's functioning in various settings – at home, in school or at work, and with peers. Proper history must also be gathered in order to understand the course of the symptoms.

Before a treatment plan is developed, an appropriate diagnosis should be made. The importance of a diagnosis lies in its ability to provide direction for treatment. Because various syndromes sometimes present with similar symptoms, differentiating them is needed, since each syndrome, despite apparent similarities, may need to be treated differently. Clinicians whose work is grounded in a knowledge base obtained from results of scientific studies understand that, for example, treatment of panic disorder must be different than treatment of generalized anxiety disorder, and treatment of major depression is not the same as treatment of dysthymia.

After a diagnosis is assigned, clinicians draw upon their expertise and experience in order to review various treatment options available to address the symptoms. Those who follow the biopsychosocial approach consider the contributions that each of its three constituents can make to the overall improvement, and discuss with the patient (and/or the family) how to implement interventions that address changes within each component.

Many of the disorders diagnosed in children and adolescents are candidates for biopsychosocial treatment. Following the diathesis-stress model (Zubin & Spring, 1977), most clinicians accept that when symptoms of a disorder become evident, those symptoms are the result of two factors – underlying biological vulnerability, and environmental factors that may have enacted upon it. Moreover, both occur on a continuum – in some cases, the underlying biological vulnerability is so significant that very little (or no) environmental stress is needed to produce symptoms, while in other cases the biological vulnerability is minimal and will only become enacted upon when stress or trauma are very significant.

Many disorders have been shown to be associated with biological changes in the brain. These include attention deficit hyperactivity disorder (ADHD), Tourette's disorder, obsessive compulsive disorder (OCD), major depression, bipolar disorder, and schizophrenia. When a patient is diagnosed with one of those disorders, the first decision that faces the clinician is whether to suggest a psychosocial treatment, a psychopharmacological treatment, or a combination of both.

In some cases, when symptoms do not appear to be notably severe, a psychosocial approach may be more appropriate. As discussed in the Preface to this handbook, various factors need to be assessed when a decision is made whether or not to treat symptoms through psychotherapy. These include not only the severity of symptoms, but additional considerations such as the accessibility of psychological care, the family's resources, and the availability of mental health insurance coverage. Clinicians need to remember that even if psychological treatment may be expected to reasonably alleviate the symptoms, factors pertaining to affordability and availability of care may still indicate that pharmacological treatment may be more practical.

When symptoms are more severe, psychological treatments may be insufficient. Psychosis, mania, and other forms of serious psychopathology often do not respond well to psychological care. In those cases, psychopharmacological approaches are likely to be needed.

When the decision has been made that pharmacological approaches will be utilized, whether as monotherapy or in addition to psychosocial treatments, the next question that needs to be considered is whether to use prescription medications or naturopathic supplements. As discussed in the Preface, misperceptions may drive this decision-making process, and clinicians need to be vigilant about dispelling misconceptions about medications and nutritional/herbal supplements. On the other hand, there are legitimate and well-founded reasons to consider, and these are discussed in this chapter.

WHEN TO USE MEDICATIONS

The decision to use medications or naturopathic supplements should be made after reviewing several crucial aspects of the effectiveness and accessibility of various compounds. The ideal situation exists when a method that is most likely to be effective in treating the symptoms is available and accessible, and the patient and/or family are receptive to the recommendations and supportive of such an approach. Clinicians should strive to maximize the likelihood that such a combination of factors exists in all cases.

Type of Symptoms

Some symptom groups are not likely to respond to non-medical treatments. Hallucinations, delusions, flight of ideas, pressured speech, and similar symptoms of more severe disorders (like schizophrenia or bipolar disorder) are less likely to diminish with naturopathic supplements. Although this book includes chapters about naturopathic treatment of these groups of symptoms, it is assumed that supplements in those cases may be utilized as an adjunct to other treatments, or when those symptoms are present in a mild variant, as an associated feature of another disorder. For example, it is not likely that naturopathic supplements will be sufficient to successfully treat symptoms of schizophrenia. However, milder psychosis that occasionally occurs with another disorder (for example, major depression) may be attempted to be controlled through the use of an appropriate naturopathic supplements.

Severity of Symptoms

The severity of symptoms should also be a top priority when a decision about whether to use medications or supplements is made. For most supplements, no head-to-head comparisons between the use of supplements and corresponding medications have been done. A few supplements have been researched in this manner, and those studies generally revealed that the supplement was better than placebo, but not as good as treatment with prescription medications (Lake & Spiegel, 2007). Consequently, when symptoms are severe, any improvement that is likely to be evident when supplements are administered will probably be minimal.

Patients need to consider this factor especially in light of data that suggests that even prescription medications are less effective when symptoms are severe. For example, mild or moderate symptoms of depression or ADHD tend to respond well to medications and mono-therapy with a single compound may be sufficient. However, when symptoms are severe, a single drug is less likely to be effective and several medications may be needed to control the symptoms (Barkley, 2006). Thus, symptoms of some disorders, in milder variants, may respond well to psychosocial and naturopathic interventions, but the same disorders in more severe versions, when symptoms are more debil-itating, are not likely to respond to nutritional and herbal supplements.

Expectation of Efficacy

As discussed above, few head-to-head comparisons of medications and supplements have been performed, and those that have been done often reported that supplements are not as effective as medications. Clinicians, patients, and family members need to take this into consider-ation when attempting treatment with naturopathic supplements. When it is desirable to manage the symptoms as effectively as possible, and as quickly as possible, use of medications, rather than supplements, should be preferred.

Conversely, for symptoms that are mild-to-moderate and may have already responded to psychosocial interventions, at least in part, supple-mentation with nutrients or herbal extracts may be reasonable. Although expectation of improvement will be less dramatic, it may be sufficient, especially given the fact that another treatment is being utilized that will help maximize the overall improvement.

Cost

Almost all naturopathic and herbal supplements are available over the counter, rather than by prescription, and the vast majority of insur-ance plans do not cover treatment with such compounds. Consequently, patients who desire treatment with these supplements must pay the costs out of pocket. In some cases, the cost may be significant. For example, some preparations of herbal extracts and nutritional supplements cost several dollars per tablet, and at least one tablet per day must be administered. This means that a monthly supply may cost 30 dollars or more, especially if several pills per day must be taken. Many families may find this cost to be prohibitive.

Conversely, those families with good medical insurance are likely to be able to obtain prescription drugs at a cheaper price. This is especially true when generic preparations of the prescription compound are available. In those cases, a monthly supply of the medication may only cost a few dollars. Interestingly, although mental health care coverage is scant in many insurance policies (especially those where managed health care approaches are utilized), most plans do not have significant restrictions on prescription medications, especially those available in generic forms. Since all categories of psychotropic medications now have many generic compounds within them, treating a disorder with these medications, rather than naturopathic supplements, may often be less expensive.

Access to Medical Professionals

When a child or an adolescent is diagnosed with a psychological disorder, and a decision is made to utilize a psychopharmacological approach, it is necessary to locate medical professionals who will be able to prescribe the medications and monitor the response. Traditionally, this has been done by pediatric psychiatrists. However, in the United States, there is a nationwide shortage of psychiatrists (Goldman, 2001) that is especially evident among pediatric psychiatrists (Thomas & Holzer, 2006), and therefore psychiatrists often refuse new patients and require several months' wait time for the initial appointment. Other medical professionals try to fill this gap. Throughout the country, nurse practitioners prescribe medications and some accept children and adolescents on their case loads. In some states, other medical professionals also prescribe, such as medical psychologists and doctoral-level pharmacists, and access has improved. However, in most other states, the availability of prescribers is insufficient, especially in rural settings.

This problem is compounded by managed health care practices that severely restrict the availability of medical specialists. In managed plans, pediatricians are established as primary medical practitioners for children and adolescents, and must approve all specialist care. In their day-to-day practice, pediatricians encounter a vast array of medical problems that may require specialized care. However, managed health care plans keep track of specialist referrals and often penalize those pediatricians who, in the opinion of gatekeepers employed by the insurer, overutilize specialist care. Thus, pediatricians must carefully weigh each referral and consider that, for example, each child referred to a specialist for a psychotropic medication may deprive another patient from the ability to receive needed cardiac care. Not surprisingly, research findings reveal that nowadays most psychotropic medications are prescribed to children by their pediatricians (for example, Olfson *et al.*, 2002).

In sum, access to care may be a determinant of whether prescription medications or naturopathic supplements may be utilized. Those patients who need a psychopharmacological intervention and have access to a pediatric psychiatrist, and/or are treated by a pediatrician who is willing to prescribe medications to treat psychological disorders may be better off utilizing this option. However, those patients who have limited access to medical treatment and/or exhibit symptoms that lend themselves well to management with naturopathic stimulants may be good candidates for such treatment.

WHEN TO USE NATUROPATHIC SUPPLEMENTS

While in some cases it may be preferred to attempt a trial of medications, in other situations it is reasonable to try a naturopathic supplement and carefully monitor patient's progress. The likelihood of a positive response is determined by many factors, some of which are discussed below. When a decision is made by considering these aspects, clients are selected that are more likely to exhibit a positive response, and a subsequent trial with a supplement is more apt to produce positive results.

Type of Symptoms

Generally speaking, symptoms that are likely to respond to psychosocial interventions, at least to some degree, are good candidates for naturopathic treatment. This means that symptoms of depression, anxiety, distractibility, impulsivity, or agitation may be good candidates for treatment with herbal and nutritional supplements. As discussed below, this may especially be the case with milder variants of these symptoms.

Conversely, when the above symptoms are accompanied by manic of psychotic features, naturopathic supplements are less likely to be effective. While some supplements have been shown to occasionally be effective in lessening such symptoms, response rates are inconsistent. When these symptoms are present, naturopathic supplements should only be utilized as a last resort (when other treatment approaches are not available), and a positive response to naturopathic supplements is more likely when level of severity is low and those symptoms constitute associated, rather than core, features of the disorder. For example, supplements are less likely to control psychosis that is a core symptom of schizophrenia than psychotic symptoms that are associated features of major depression.

Severity of Symptoms

The severity of symptoms should also be a top priority when a decision about whether to use medications or supplements is made. Mild or moderate symptoms are generally good targets for naturopathic supplements. In accordance with the diathesis-stress model, milder symptoms generally indicate a lesser degree of underlying biological vulnerability, and therefore biological disturbances in the function of various brain parts are likely to be less pronounced. In those cases, where dramatic changes in brain functions are not sought, an approach that utilizes nutritional and herbal supplements instead of medications seems appropriate. Of course, if the supplements do not prove effective and further interventions are needed to manage the symptoms, use of medications may still need to be considered.

Cost

Although families with medical insurance may be able to obtain prescription drugs at an affordable price (especially when generic formulations are prescribed), millions of Americans have no health insurance. For them, the out-of-pocket costs of prescription drugs may be higher than they can afford. Although generic preparations are cheaper, a 1 month supply of the medication may still cost about the same as a 1 month supply of a naturopathic supplement, and in some cases, vitamins or other nutrients may be cheaper.

Another factor must also be considered in the cost. Since naturopathic and herbal supplements are available over the counter, no prescription is needed. Thus, when supplements are utilized, the only associated cost is the price of the pills, whereas the price of prescription drugs (even if generics are used) must also include the cost of a doctor's visit. For individuals with no health care coverage, this may be a tipping point that will turn them toward a naturopathic substance.

Access to Medical Professionals

As discussed above, most areas in the US experience a significant shortage of child psychiatrists. Although some other prescribers may be available, major portions of the country have limited access to pediatric prescribers. Consequently, pediatricians have now become the primary medical practitioners that prescribe psychotropic medications.

However, although highly knowledgeable about medicine and medications in general, most physicians complete only 6 weeks of exposure to psychiatry during medical training (Serby *et al.*, 2002) and receive no further required training in psychiatry during pediatric residency (Kersten *et al.*, 2003). Thus, pediatricians often limit the type of medications they are willing to prescribe. While most pediatricians are familiar with psychostimulants and some antidepressants, many are reluctant to utilize other classes of psychotropics. Thus, a family of a child or adolescent who suffers symptoms of a disorder that requires another class of drugs (for example, an anxiolytic) may have difficulties locating a prescriber who can write an appropriate prescription.

Nutritional and herbal supplements do not require a prescription. They are easily available at local pharmacies and herb stores, and may be purchased on-line at a significant discount. Those patients who reside in areas where access to pediatric mental health prescribers is limited will be able to quickly initiate treatment because they can easily find a naturopathic supplement in a local pharmacy (or on-line), and they will not need to negotiate a quagmire of problems commonly associated with seeking medical mental health care, including long wait times, significant distance to the prescriber's office, higher costs of care, or the frustration of dealing with managed health care plans that aim to increase profit by minimizing access to care.

Patient Refuses Medications

Many mental health professionals encounter patients and clients who are not receptive to medications. This is especially evident with parents of children and adolescents. Sometimes, parents overtly state, at the onset of treatment, that they are opposed to medications. At other times, they may not volunteer this information at the start, but when any mention is made of the use of medications, parents are reluctant to accept the recommendation. In some cases, parents may seem receptive, but delay making an appointment, lose the referral given by the clinician, or use other passive means to resist the recommendation.

Reasons behind such behaviors are complex. Admitting that their children need to take medications to control psychological symptoms may invoke protective feelings about their children. Considering the use of medications may make parents feel like there is something wrong with their offspring, since most children do not have to take drugs to be 'normal.' These feelings are common, especially when the disorder is a 'psychological' one, rather than a condition perceived as mostly 'medical' (like thyroid dysfunction or diabetes).

Some parents, especially fathers, may feel that any condition that involves psychological feelings and behaviors results from inadequate inner strength to control these problems. This is especially evident in disorders like depression, anxiety, or ADHD. Parents often feel that treatment should be able to help children and adolescents exercise sufficient mental control to stop the symptoms and go about their life. Ultimately, this may be the goal of most psychosocial treatment, since building coping skills, changing cognitions, and learning to stop and think before performing a behavior involves building the ability to exert mental control over the symptoms. Parents, however, may not realize that, in some cases, working with the child or adolescent directly may not be sufficient. When symptoms are significantly severe, it may be truly difficult, if not impossible, for the client to become able to increase control over them in any way. Clinicians need to help parents recognize that, in those cases, trying to work without utilizing some form of psychopharmacology is akin to 'fighting biology' and 'shoveling against the tide.'

In those situations, parents often find it easier to accept a recommendation for a naturopathic intervention, like a nutritional or herbal supplement. Because these compounds are perceived to be 'natural,' parents do not feel that their child or adolescent is taking a 'drug.' Consequently, most parents do not feel the sort of feelings described above, or are likely to feel them less intensely. In the end, they are more likely to follow through on a recommendation for a naturopathic supplement, whereas they may not follow through on a referral for medications.

When considering the feelings described herein, clinicians must not only think about the parents' attitudes and feelings toward medications, but also have to deliberate the reaction of the patient himself or herself. While some children may not recognize the difference between a medication and a supplement, teenagers are likely to do so. When the topic of medications is broached, many teenagers experience the same feelings as their parents and are likely to oppose the medications. Those same adolescents are often more receptive to the use of naturopathic supplements.

Limited Response to Psychosocial Treatment

At times, a decision may initially have been made to treat symptoms through a psychosocial approach, but the progress may have been slow, inconsistent, or limited. Many factors may account for such a situation. Generally, at least some verbal skills are necessary to meaningfully participate in psychotherapy. However, young children may have poorly developed verbal skills and their ability to comprehend cognitive interventions may be limited. Although play therapy approaches have been developed, they generally are less effective than traditional 'talk therapies' to treat symptoms of ADHD, depression, anxiety, or other psychological disorders commonly seen in children (Nathan & Gorman, 2002). Thus, when children find it hard to participate in 'talk therapy,' the utility of psychosocial interventions may be limited to parent training approaches. Although these are usually effective in reducing symptoms to some extent, especially with disruptive disorders (such as ADHD), they rarely produce a complete symptom resolution. Thus, children who initially have been treated with a psychosocial approach but have made limited progress may be good candidates for a trial of a naturopathic supplement.

Adolescent males may especially be likely to find it hard to engage in counseling. The socialization of males in our culture includes powerful codes that define appropriate and inappropriate behaviors. Since early in life, boys are taught to suppress vulnerable emotions (Robertson & Shepard, 2008). This is done through modeling (for example, boys do not commonly see their fathers express tender or vulnerable feelings, especially not to them directly), as well as reinforcement (boys are usually rewarded for suppressing the expression of pain, sadness, or similar feelings). Consequently, many boys do not develop the language that is needed to express a wide range of emotions, and are likely to be uncomfortable in a setting that focuses on expressing those emotions (for example, in a therapist's office). Although therapists that are competent and experienced in working with this population utilize a variety of techniques to work through this problem, the fact remains that some adolescents do not completely engage in treatment and exhibit limited progress with counseling interventions. These teens may be good candidates for a trial of a naturopathic supplement.

CHOOSING A SUPPLEMENT

When clinicians follow the above criteria to select candidates for naturopathic treatment, it is more likely that those clients will benefit from treatment. Once the decision is made that a trial of a nutritional or herbal supplement will be initiated, professionals need to subsequently decide which compound will be recommended as the first-line treatment. The discussion in each subsequent chapter of this handbook that reviews specific disorders will guide clinicians when making such a decision.

When a compound is administered, it should undergo an adequate trial. This is defined as a trial that lasts for a time period that has been shown in research to be sufficient to usually produce a response, and during this period the dose and frequency of administration must fall within a range expected for clinical response. If research has not identified the specific time period, adequate trial should consist of a 4–6 week administration at the frequency and dose expected for clinical response.

Most compounds will not be initialed at a clinical dose. Instead, the lowest available dose is usually started, and the daily dose is gradually titrated upward, at specific intervals (discussed for each compound), until dosage within the therapeutic range is obtained. Once this occurs, a formal trial period begins and should last for a minimally sufficient amount of time to produce a response (as described above). Of course, such a trial should only continue when adverse effects are not evident or seem minimal and are easily tolerated.

Generally, mental health professionals should start with those supplements that have established efficacy. If no such compounds are available for the specific disorder that is being treated, supplements with likely efficacy should be considered. Similarly, if an adequate trial was attempted with a compound that has established efficacy and no significant improvement is evident, clinicians may switch to or add another supplement within the same category, or if no others are available within the same category, try one from the next lower classification. Clinicians should avoid compounds classified as not likely to be effective.

Mental health professionals should also consider what to do if a partial response is evident, or when the patient exhibits symptoms from various categories that cannot adequately be treated by a single compound. When medications are utilized, combinations of drugs are sometimes prescribed. This is predicated on data that reveals that those medications that are used together do not produce adverse interactions (as discussed in the next chapter). Unfortunately, such data is rarely available for naturopathic supplements.

If the concurrent use of two or more supplements is considered, clinicians should proceed very cautiously and initially perform an adequate clinical trial for one compound, aimed at those symptoms that produce the most discomfort and impairment. After one compound has been introduced and seems to be well tolerated, another compound may carefully be added, titrating it more slowly and carefully monitoring clinical response as well as adverse effects. Clinicians should consider each supplement's pharmacokinetics before attempting polypharmacy. If any attempted compound exerts any effects on the liver, it is likely that this compound may not be able to be safely used with other supplements, or with any medications (sold over the counter or by prescription).

Chapter 2

Pharmacokinetics

Psychopharmacology is the study of the mechanisms, effects, and use of substances that act on the brain and subsequently change behavior. Substances that act on the brain are often referred to as being psychoactive, and sometimes they are called psychotropic, since they are administered to result in some type of change in the psychological status of a person. In this book, the psychotropic effects of many nutritional and herbal supplements are explored.

When substances act on the brain and changes become evident, these changes manifest in many aspects of behavior. Psychoactive substances may change the way a person acts (reducing behavioral compulsions, psychomotor agitation, hyperactivity, or restlessness), feels (reducing depression or anxiety), and thinks (reducing mental obsessions or depressive ruminations). Thus, when psychotropic substances are used, broad effects evident in thoughts, feelings, and overt behaviors are sought.

When a psychoactive compound is administered, it is presumed that the substance will enter the brain and affect its electrochemical function. For example, many compounds are thought to change the rates of neuronal firing associated with various brain pathways. Therefore, psychoactive substances are those compounds that cause changes in cognition, behavior, emotion, etc. by changing the function of the brain.

However, when a substance is administered into the body, it must find its way into the brain in order to exert its effect. Along the way, the compound will encounter digestive processes (if administered orally), circulatory effects, metabolism, and excretion. After all of those processes have transformed the substance, that which still remains in the circulatory system may then find its way into the brain. Consequently, when studying psychopharmacology, it is common to consider two aspects separately – those of pharmacokinetics and pharmacodynamics. Pharmacokinetics are those processes that involve the action of the body on the drug, and pharmacodynamics are those actions that the drug is able to exert on the body (especially including the brain).

Pharmacokinetics are discussed in this chapter, and pharmacodynamics are introduced in the next chapter.

When considering pharmacokinetics, it is customary to discuss its various stages, including absorption, distribution, metabolism, and excretion. These processes affect the drugs sequentially, and many aspects of each of those stages may alter the drug's ability to reach the target of interest (the brain). Each stage will separately be discussed, with particular attention given to the aspects of each of those processes that specifically pertain to naturopathic psychotropics.

When various properties of pharmacokinetics are considered, most of what is known about these processes comes from studies with adults. While some of that knowledge is directly applicable to children and adolescents, there are aspects of pharmacokinetics that differ between children, adolescents, and adults. The discussion in this book will punctuate such differences whenever these have been established from results of prior research.

ABSORPTION

In order for a substance to enter circulation, it must be absorbed. To be absorbed, the substance must be introduced into a portion of the body that allows absorption. Various routes of administration are available, and each method affects the manner in which the substance will subsequently be absorbed. Consequently, each method presents benefits and drawbacks, especially when a substance has to be given to a child.

Routes of Administration

As outlined in Table 2.1, various routes of administration are utilized when compounds are introduced into the body. Generally, these can be classified as enteral and parenteral, and each category has within it several methods commonly used to deliver an active substance.

Enteral

Enteral administration delivers the compound into the body through the gastrointestinal (GI) tract. Both ends of the GI tract can be utilized – the mouth and the anus. Administering medications and other compounds by ingesting them orally is, by far, the most common route of administration for medications and supplements. Usually, a pill is swallowed, thus ingesting the substance into the stomach. Prescribers commonly refer to this method of administration as 'by mouth' or PO (from Latin 'per os'). Usually, oral administration is most convenient because it is least invasive.

Substances prepared for oral administration may be available in a variety of pills, including tablets, capsules, and caplets. Tablets are

TABLE 2.1 Common routes of administration

Enteral (through GI tract)
Oral (per os, PO)
Intrarectal (PR)
Parenteral (outside GI tract)
Pulmonary
Surface absorption
Transdermal
Sublingual
Transmucosal
Injections
Intravenous (IV)
Intramuscular (IM)
Subcutaneous (SC)
Intrathecal
Intracerebroventricular
Intraperitoneal

commonly round, and are sometimes coated so that they do not easily dissolve in the mouth. Capsules are oblong and may contain granules of the active compound that release as the outer coating is dissolved in the stomach. Caplets are a cross between the two, and usually are oblong tablets that are softer than traditional round tablets and may dissolve more easily (for example, geltabs). Either way, the substance is introduced into the body when the outer coating dissolves in the stomach and the contents become available for absorption.

Although they offer a convenient way to ingest a substance, pills are problematic for some populations. Children and the elderly may have difficulties swallowing pills, and may resist taking them. It is especially common for children to dislike taking pills. Very young children may have their mouth and throat incompletely formed, limiting the ability to swallow a solid pill. Similarly, children with significant developmental delays may not have formed adequate muscle tone and nerve control to allow sufficient ability to swallow a pill. Generally speaking, those children who have difficulties speaking, and/or cannot swallow a moderate mouthful of water without it dripping out of their mouth, may exhibit immature muscle and nerve development and may not have adequately formed the swallowing reflex to swallow pills.

Some children also dislike pills for psychological reasons. They may be afraid that the pill will be hard to swallow, may hurt while passing through the throat, or may choke them. They may also associate pills with unpleasant medical experiences, like invasive examinations or giving a blood sample. Some children and adolescents may also fear that the compound will change their personality or cause unpleasant side effects. For many teenagers, taking the substance may be a part of a larger power struggle, where accepting the pill may symbolically be seen as succumbing to the parents' wishes and giving up control. The pill may communicate to the teens that something is presumably wrong with them and they are given this compound to get 'fixed.' In these instances teens may refuse to swallow the substance.

Instead of pills, using other means of oral administration may sometimes be preferred. Some capsules may be opened, 'sprinkled,' and mixed into food. Generally, a strong-tasting, acidic food provides a convenient base. For example, it is common for parents to sprinkle some medications into a spoonful of apple sauce, mix it in, and have the child swallow this mixture. In addition, some medications are available in liquid form (as oral solution or syrup) that can be swallowed directly and/or mixed into other liquids if needed.

Herbal and nutritional supplements are primarily available in a variety of pill forms. Most are capsules that contain the active compound, but traditional tablets sometimes are also produced. When a child or adolescent has difficulties swallowing the pill, some capsules can be opened, allowing the contents to be mixed into a food base. However, many of the supplements have a strong taste, and therefore the base may not sufficiently hide the flavor, thus resulting in a horribly tasting concoction. Trial and error will be needed in those cases.

Some supplements can also be brewed into a tincture. This method, however, requires careful control of the strength, and if preparation is inconsistent, doses of various strengths will result and the compound will be administered unpredictably. This is likely to adversely affect efficacy. Thus, whenever possible, parents are advised to administer supplements in pill form, and if tincture preparation is needed, directions must carefully be followed each and every time it is prepared.

Administering a substance by mouth (PO), either in pill or liquid form, presents additional pharmacologic challenges. When the compound is swallowed, it travels down the esophagus, passes the lower esophageal sphincter, and enters the stomach. No absorption takes place in the stomach. Instead, the main functions of the stomach are to eliminate undesired bacteria that may have been ingested with the foodstuff, break down the food into a semi-liquid mass that allows distribution over a larger surface area for easier digestion, and release contents into the small intestine. The breakdown of the food is attained by various gastric acids that are quite caustic. While many (but not all) nutrients ingested during meals generally survive this environment, some supplements may not. For this reason, some pills are covered with a coating that resists the stomach acids and allows the contents to pass into the small intestine, where absorption begins. However, liquid preparations obviously do not allow for such a mechanism, so any tincture that is ingested must survive the stomach environment in order to be available for absorption in the small intestine.

Ingesting substances by mouth has another major disadvantage. As mentioned above, no absorption takes place in the stomach, and absorption begins when contents of the stomach are released into the duodenum (the first portion of the small intestine). The stomach is preprogrammed to release its contents into the duodenum at a controlled rate, allowing the small intestine sufficient time for chemical digestion and absorption to take place. This means that there is a time delay between the ingestion of a substance (like a pill) and its release into the small intestine. When a compound is taken on an empty stomach, it is passed into the duodenum more quickly. Since it becomes absorbed right after it enters the small intestine, the action of effect may be seen in about 15–20 minutes. This is generally the fastest onset that can be expected with any orally administered compound, and usually the delay is more significant. Factors like the contents of the stomach when the compound is ingested, the solubility of the compound (discussed in the next section), and the metabolic processes (addressed later in the chapter) significantly affect the rate of absorption, and, generally speaking, most substances ingested orally take between 30 and 60 minutes before absorption begins (sometimes much longer). Consequently, oral ingestion is among the slowest routes of administration.

When it is necessary to deliver an active compound into the body as soon as it is possible, and injections are not possible or practical, the substance may be introduced into the body via the rectum. This is commonly used in emergency settings – for example, some seizure medications are available in crèmes or suppositories and can be inserted into the rectal area even when a person is in a midst of a grand convulsion. However, this method of administration also has drawbacks. It is considered more invasive, and (when conscious) individuals may not be comfortable having suppositories or creams inserted into this private area. In addition, since the substance is introduced into the large (rather then small) intestine, different absorption properties apply and the substance must be highly hydrophilic in order to be absorbed, and this presents its own challenges and drawbacks (as discussed in the next section). Generally, the vast majority of supplements are not delivered through rectal administration.

Parenteral

Parenteral administration delivers the compound into the body by means that bypass the GI tract. As outlined in Table 2.1, these methods include a variety of injections, as well as topical, transmucosal, and pulmonary routes. Delivering a substance by means that do not require absorption from the GI tract has many advantages. Usually, it is a faster method of delivery, since absorption from the GI tract is not needed. In some cases, the substance is delivered right into systemic circulation, bypassing the need for any absorption. However, some parenteral methods may be more invasive and unpleasant for most people, especially for children, and others may not be practical. For this reason, parenteral methods are generally reserved for those situations where oral administration of a compound is inappropriate.

Pulmonary administration takes place when the substance is inhaled – for example, when nicotine is delivered into the body while smoking a cigarette. Because the lungs are extensively perfused with blood vessels, absorption into general circulation is very rapid. In addition, since the wall between pulmonary cells and blood vessels is very thin, there is limited filtration that takes place, and virtually all chemical compounds that are inhaled end up in the blood stream.

Inhaling a substance has other drawbacks. In most cases, the bronchi and lungs become irritated when foreign substances (gasses or otherwise) are inhaled. This irritation is uncomfortable and often invokes the coughing reflex. Over time, coughing may diminish, but the irritation continues and may result in the destruction of pulmonary cells (as is seen in lung disease experienced by smokers). In the western world, few medicinal compounds are delivered by inhalation (except, for example, medications for asthma), and supplements are not generally administered in this manner, although smoking of a variety of substances (leaves, etc.) is common among native tribes and has been prescribed by shaman and tribal medics for thousands of years in order to deliver psychoactive substances into the body (for healing, precipitating a desired mind state during rituals, etc.).

Similar to smoking, transmucosal administration generally involves snorting a substance. A few centuries ago, this was a common method of delivering tobacco into the body, and continues to be used by some to take in various drugs of abuse (for example, heroin or cocaine). When a substance is snorted, it settles on moist cells that line the sinus passages, and since these cells are also extensively perfused with blood vessels, the substance will enter the blood stream and become distributed through the body (reaching the brain first). In addition, cells in nasal passages are involved in the sense of smell and reach deep into the brain. Substances that are snorted may not only activate these cells, but may also use this pathway to enter the brain, thus bypassing the circulatory system all together. Finally, a portion of the snorted substance ends up in the lungs and is absorbed from there. Thus, a substance that is snorted may simultaneously use three means to reach its target.

With intranasal delivery, absorption is not quite as rapid as it is when a substance is smoked, but it is still much faster than oral ingestion. However, there are risks associated with this method of delivery. The nasal passages may get irritated when a substance is introduced in this manner, and with repeated administration, the sense of smell may adversely be affected. In addition, since snorting substances may dry out nasal passages, sinus cells may become damaged and nasal bleeding is common. Generally, very few medications are given in this manner (except for nasal decongestants, and DDAVP, a hormone used with children to reduce bed wetting), and in the western world, nutritional and herbal supplements usually are not introduced into the body through this route of administration.

Surface absorption involves placing the substance in contact with a portion of the body and allowing it to become absorbed on site. Transdermal administration is the most common method, and a variety of topical medications are given by applying skin creams or patches. The substance must be able to traverse various layers of skin tissue, but if it becomes absorbed into the skin, it comes in contact with blood vessels that perfuse the skin, and enters general circulation. Some delay is evident, but the onset is at least as fast as that for compounds taken orally, and often it is faster. On the other hand, creams can easily be wiped off the skin, especially by an active child who plays and moves around quite a bit, and patches tend to irritate the skin of many patients and, again, may easily come off during activities that involve water, or when the person begins perspiring. Transdermal administration is generally reserved for creams that act on site (for example, delivering an antiseptic or antibiotic to the wound), although some medications meant for general circulation are administered through patches (for example, Daytrana, a stimulant medication used to treat symptoms of ADHD). Generally, nutritional and herbal supplements are not administered in this manner.

Another form of surface absorption involves placing the compound under the tongue, thus allowing absorption through the cells that line the mouth and the tongue. Because these cells are moist and extensively perfused with surrounding blood vessels, absorption is more rapid than it is with transdermal application. In addition, since a portion of the substance will be swallowed with saliva, some enteral administration takes place as well, although it is generally a minor portion of the compound. However, since swallowing some of the substance is unavoidable, the compound must be one that will not hurt or irritate the mouth, tongue, or esophagus. Although in the western world most herbal and nutritional supplements are not administered in this manner, it is common for some people in South America, Asia, Africa, and Australia to chew on leaves or plants, thus delivering the desired compound into the body.

A variety of injections can also be used to introduce a substance. Of these, intravenous (IV) injections provide the fastest possible route of administration. Since the injection is given right into the blood vessel, the substance immediately enters systemic circulation and no delay associated with any form of absorption takes place. This is the method used when a medication must begin to work immediately, and the patient is able to remain relatively still, allowing the injection to be administered. Most medications administered in this manner are given in emergency situations, or in inpatient settings when the patient remains in bed much of the time. Some drugs of abuse are also taken in this way (for example, heroin and cocaine), since the onset of the 'high' is immediate and very pronounced. However, IV injections are risky. Over time, blood vessels become irritated and may collapse, thus making this form of delivery impractical in the long run. In addition, any substance injected IV must be meant for this route of administration, and some substances are lethal when injected IV (although are able to safely be administered in other ways).

There are other forms of injections that are also utilized. Intramuscular injections (IM) are commonly used when a substance is introduced into the body and will be stored in a muscle for a long period of time, allowing gradual release into the system. This method is used with some long-acting psychotropic medications – for example, injectable forms of antipsychotics. Subcutaneous injections involve the delivery of the compound into the body by injecting it right under skin. Similar to IM injections, this method allows for local storage of the substance and gradual release into circulation. These injections tend to be very painful and are rarely used, although some drugs of abuse are delivered in this way (for example, 'skin popping,' a common method of injecting 'speedballs' – a mixture of heroin and cocaine).

There are other forms of injections that are meant for local delivery of a compound into specialized tissue. Intrathecal and intracerebroventricular injections are sometimes used to deliver pain blockers into the spinal cord. Intraperitoneal injection may be utilized to deliver medication into the body cavity, and is sometimes used when treating some forms of cancer. Generally, injections of any sort are very rarely used to deliver any nutritional or herbal supplements.

Methods of Absorption

Since the vast majority of supplements are administered orally, the compound must pass through the digestive tract (see Figure 2.1) and be

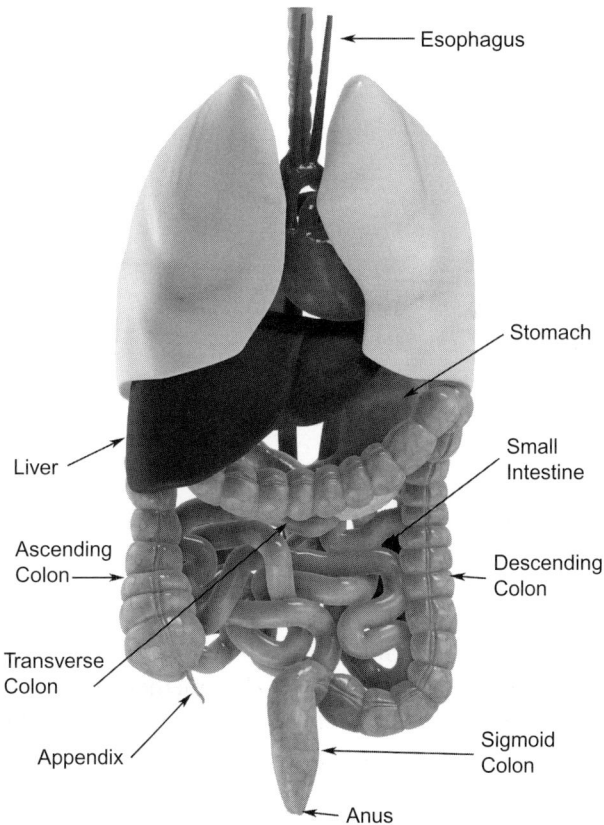

FIGURE 2.1 The digestive tract.

TABLE 2.2   Membrane transfer processes

Passive

   Diffusion

   Osmosis

    Filtration

Active

    Channels and Pumps (sodium, potassium, etc.)

   Binding

absorbed into the blood stream in order to become able to reach the target site (the brain).

Absorption involves travel of the substance across the walls of the small intestine. The inside wall of the small intestine is filled with villi – folds and protrusions that increase the surface contact and allow greater proportion of the foodstuff to come in contact with the intestinal wall. Propelled by smooth muscle contractions, the contents of the small intestine slowly move along and gradually become absorbed across the intestinal wall. Within it, the absorbed molecules encounter blood vessels and glands, and enter systemic circulation. Various factors must be considered that aid or hinder this process. These are summarized in Table 2.2.

Passive Transfer

Passive transfer takes place when a compound is able to pass across the wall of the small intestine into the blood vessel without requiring any assistance. The simplest of these is the process of diffusion, when a compound is simply able to dissolve into the surroundings. For example, water is able to freely pass across the intestine wall and enter the blood vessels.

Most compounds, however, are not able to diffuse as freely as water, and are subject to a more complex form of membrane transfer involving the process of osmosis. When osmosis takes place, there is a gradient that determines the degree to which a compound will traverse the membrane, and various factors affect the ease with which any compound will find its way across, including the molecular size, atomic structure, and electrical charge. The wall of the small intestine is made up of layers of cells, each of which has its own membrane. In order to get across the wall, compound molecules must either be small enough to pass through tiny openings between these cells, or must be able to pass through the membranes of these cells.

When compound molecules attempt to pass through membranes, they encounter those that are preprogrammed to keep them out, and others that may invite them in. To a large extent, this depends on whether the compound is endogenous (usually present in the body in its current form) or exogenous (essentially, foreign to the body). Although there are exceptions, generally speaking, the closer the compound molecule is to an endogenous compound the more likely it will be allowed to pass through. This means that those nutritional supplements that contain endogenous elements are more likely to be absorbed, although they are also more likely to be metabolized, as described in the next section.

Active Transfer

Those substances that are not able to freely traverse the membrane through osmosis may have another mechanism through which they may become absorbed. In order to maintain a normal life cycle, a constant exchange of chemicals between the inside and the outside of a cell must take place. Cells have various mechanisms that facilitate such transfer, one of which is a system of channels embedded in the cell membrane that selectively allows certain molecules to pass in or out of the cell. Some of these channels may also attract these molecules, and therefore they may be referred to as pumps. It is common for cells to have channels and pumps for sodium, potassium, and chloride. If a nutritional compound includes molecules of these chemicals, or ones that closely resemble them, they will be able to pass through the membrane more easily.

If the supplement does not contain molecules that closely resemble these endogenous ions, a substance may still be able to utilize these channels for active transfer. If the supplement molecules can easily bind to sodium, potassium, or other substances that have their own transport channels, the supplement may be able to get across these channels while bound to these endogenous molecules. Of course, this depends on how many endogenous molecules are available. This is one reason why supplements are sometimes recommended for concurrent administration with other nutrients that may increase the rate of absorption of the supplement.

DISTRIBUTION

Once the substance is absorbed, it becomes available for distribution through the body in systemic blood circulation. To a lesser extent, the substances may also enter the lymphatic system. As molecules circulate through the body, additional processes take place, especially involving metabolism and excretion (discussed in the next two sections). However, the degree to which supplement molecules will be metabolized and excreted depends on what happens to them while in circulation.

Supplement molecules may remain on their own without significantly dissolving in water or lipids. If that is the case, the degree to which the substance will be allowed to remain in circulation will depend on the extent to which the liver will metabolize it (described in the next section) and the kidneys will excrete it (described in the following section). However, most substances dissolve, and the degree and type of solubility significantly impact the time the molecules are allowed to remain in systemic circulation. The most important aspects of solubility are summarized in Table 2.3.

Water Solubility

The degree to which a substance dissolves in water determines how quickly the substance will be excreted. The kidneys are programmed to filter blood plasma and eliminate exogenous molecules from the body. Endogenous molecules may also be eliminated, but that depends on the feedback that the kidneys receive about whether there is sufficient or excessive presence of a nutrient. For example, when sodium levels in the body are low, kidneys will leave most of it in the plasma. However, when sodium levels are high, kidneys will eliminate excess sodium from the body by removing it into the urine.

When a compound easily dissolves in water (hydrophyllic), it will readily be taken up by the kidneys each time it passes through them.

TABLE 2.3 Solubility
Water solubility
Hydrophyllic vs. hydrophobic
Lipid solubility
Lipophillic vs. lipophobic
Lipid storage
Competition
Displacement

This means that a substance that is highly hydrophyllic may quickly be removed from the blood stream by the kidneys and become excreted. Because compounds that enter systemic circulation from the GI tract do so 'up-stream' from the kidneys, the filtration in the kidneys will occur before the compound has a chance to circulate to the brain. Thus, a highly hydrophyllic substance is likely to be eliminated without any psychoactive effect.

A hydrophobic substance, on the other hand, will resist elimination and is more likely to remain in systemic circulation. Such a substance will resist filtration by the kidneys and is more likely to reach the brain. However, a hydrophobic substance will not necessarily remain in circulation, since it may be metabolized the first time it passes through the liver (as discussed in the next section). In other words, water solubility and the degree to which a substance is metabolized are often inversely related.

Lipid Solubility

Even if a substance is relatively hydrophobic, and does not quickly become metabolized, it will not remain in circulation for very long, because gradually the kidneys will remove it. Thus, another property determines whether a substance will remain in circulation for a long time. Molecules exhibit both water solubility and lipid solubility, and both properties are independent. When a substance is lipophobic, it will not easily bind with fat cells (in the blood and elsewhere) and therefore will remain in systemic circulation for the time period it takes the body to metabolize and excrete it. Thus, a substance that is simultaneously hydrophyllic and lipophobic would be eliminated the fastest, usually before it has a chance to travel to its target site of action (the brain).

On the other hand, substances that are lipophyllic bind with fat molecules and become stored. This storage may occur wherever the substance encounters fat cells on its way through absorption and distribution. Lipid storage allows the substance to remain bound to the fat cells and release gradually into circulation. Thus, a substance that is highly lipophyllic, even if it is also hydrophyllic, is likely to remain in the system much longer – although some of it will be excreted quickly, the portion that binds to fat cells will remain in the system much longer. A substance that is both lipophyllic and hydrophobic may be expected to remain the longest.

Although both water and lipid solubility are independent of metabolism, lipid solubility does affect the metabolic rate of a substance. The portion of a compound that has bound to fat cells will generally pass through the liver unmetabolized. Thus, the degree to which a substance is lipophyllic plays an important part in the length of time the substance will remain in circulation.

Lipid solubility is very important to consider not only to understand how long a substance will remain in circulation, but also to predict whether gradual release from lipid storage will continue. We ingest a large number of nutrients, and these have various degrees of lipid solubility. When several compounds are present simultaneously, they will compete for lipid solubility, and that which is the most lipophyllic will 'win' and bind the most. Because lipid storage is finite and fat cells can become saturated, thus not allowing additional storage, other nutrients, even though also at least somewhat lipophyllic, may no longer find remaining storage space and may readily be metabolized and/or excreted. Thus, it is important to keep in mind not only the lipid solubility of any given compound, but also the relative lipid solubility of compounds and nutrients that are administered (or eaten) at the same time.

Lipid solubility becomes especially important when nutritional supplements are administered with medications (or when multiple compounds are used). Danger may particularly be likely when a person who has been taking a given dose of medications or supplements for some time is now given a new medication or supplement. It is likely that the compounds given thus far entered lipid storage at least to some degree. If a new compound is now administered that has a higher lipid solubility, this new compound will be more readily absorbed by the fat cells. If other compounds were already stored within them, they will be displaced by this new compound, and will rapidly enter systemic circulation, possibly at high levels. This may pose significant risk of side effects and toxicity, and in some cases may be life threatening. Thus, if multiple supplements are used, or if supplements are used in conjunction with medications, careful monitoring is needed. It is best to make sure that qualified prescribers (physicians, prescribing psychologists, nurse practitioners, etc.) monitor such cases.

Systemic Circulation

Because compounds in systemic circulation are delivered throughout the body, they are delivered to every body compartment and organ, not just to the desired target site. This is important to remember, since the same compound may exert different effects in various parts of the body. For example, even though a supplement is taken to change an aspect of brain function, that same supplement may exert undesirable effects in the GI tract (by changing gastric motility and causing diarrhea), in the heart (by affecting the heart rhythm), and in muscles that control movement (by causing tremors). Often the desired effects (change in brain function) may take some time, while other effects in the body may be more immediate. The balance between the two must always be carefully monitored.

When a substance begins to be absorbed, it starts to enter systemic circulation. The rate of absorption can be measured, and is often indicated in reference literature. The time it takes for half of the compound generally available for distribution to reach systemic circulation is referred to as distribution half-life, and it reflects the rate and extent of absorption (this is different than the elimination half-life discussed later in the chapter). Sometimes referred to as terminal half-life, this is especially relevant in multiple dosing regimens, because it determines the concentration, fluctuation, and the time required to reach equilibrium (also discussed later in the chapter).

As the compound enters systemic circulation, and assuming it is able to cross the blood–brain barrier (as reviewed below), the supplement may begin to exert the therapeutic effect. The more compound enters the blood stream the more clinical effect may be evident. However, as the compound enters systemic circulation, it also begins to be metabolized and excreted. Thus, what remains in circulation at any point in time is the result of the additive processes of absorption, and the subtractive processes of metabolism and excretion. The onset and strength of the therapeutic effect are determined by these pharmacokinetics, and generally speaking the onset of the effects (desired and adverse) will occur during the specified distribution half-life of the substance. Once this period elapses, unless additional doses are administered, additional effects are not likely.

When a substance is administered, we are not only interested in the time it takes to produce the onset of any effect, but also in the time it takes for a compound to exhibit efficacy. Efficacy is usually defined as a clinical effect that sufficiently lowers target symptoms. The degree of this effect is not well established, and varies depending on the definition that particular researchers choose to impose. Often, a substance is considered to have sufficient efficacy when it is able to produce a statistically significant drop in symptoms. This may only reduce symptoms by 50 percent, and often less. Clearly, the reader can note that all symptoms will not be eliminated, and another 50 percent (or more) of the symptoms remain. For this reason, a therapeutic response, as defined by research studies, may be very different than a therapeutic response that is sought during treatment.

The onset of therapeutic effect, and efficacy, need to be differentiated from the maximum effect that can be sought with the use of the compound. The maximum effect is generally defined as the maximum reduction in symptoms that can be attained with the use of the substance. Usually the maximum effect is established as the maximum dose above which further improvement in symptoms is not likely or may produce side effects that make further use impractical. Medications often have maximum dose limits established from prior research, and such limits for some supplements have also been established, although the majority of nutritional and herbal compounds have not undergone such careful research, so the maximum dose may need to be determined on a case-by-case basis by monitoring response and adverse effects. Generally, the dose above which improvement in symptoms is not evident and/or the side effects become difficult to manage needs to be regarded as the maximum therapeutic dose for the patient in question.

Potency is the strength of the compound in exerting its effect. Although the 'effect' usually refers to the desired changes in target symptoms, adverse effects are also related, since many substances exhibit dose-related increases in both, desired and adverse effects. Potent supplements require low doses to produce an effect, and compounds with low potency require much higher doses. However, potency in and of itself usually has little effect on efficacy. Even though less potent compounds require much higher doses, this does not necessarily mean that higher doses will also result in more adverse effects. Usually, the potency of a substance is only important in determining the strength of the dose that must be administered. Varying potency is the factor that determines that one substance may be effective at 10 mg, while another may require 100 or 1000 mg before efficacy is evident.

Toxicity is the level at which a substance becomes dangerous to the system. It is sometimes related to potency, in that substances that exhibit stronger binding affinities may also be more likely to cause toxic effects. However, in some cases less potent supplements are more likely to become toxic, since more of the compound needs to be taken to exert clinical effect, and dose-response curves may be different for desired effects and side effects (meaning that side effects become evident before clinical effects begin). Although doses or plasma levels that are likely to result in toxicity are sometimes established, adverse effects always must be carefully monitored in order to watch for signs of toxicity. As an example, St. John's Wort is a compound with low potency that must be taken at high doses (usually, above 1000 mg/day) in order to be effective. However, toxicity becomes more likely with high doses, and may be signaled by tremors, agitation, and other symptoms of so-called 'serotonin syndrome.' When a patient takes this compound it is necessary to carefully monitor both desired and adverse effects to maximize therapeutic gains, and a dose must be sought that simultaneously maximizes clinical effects while avoiding serious side effects and toxicity.

In some cases, toxicity may become life threatening. Although not all compounds exert such a threat, some do, and those must carefully be monitored. Those supplements that pose a significant danger may have a lethal dose established from prior research and experience. Often expressed as LD_{50}, the lethal dose is one that is presumed to cause significant risk of death in 50 percent of patients to whom it is given. By contrast, the effective dose, often expressed as ED_{50}, is the dose that is likely to be effective for 50 percent of the patients taking it. Both numbers are then used to determine the therapeutic index of a compound, which is derived by calculating the ratio of LD_{50}/ED_{50}. The higher the ratio, the safer the compound. For example, lithium is a mood stabilizer that is lethal for many people at the plasma level of about 2.5 mEq/L. By comparison, the effective dose required for acute stabilization is about 1.2–1.5 mEq/L. Thus, it can be said that the therapeutic ratio for lithium is less than 2, meaning that the lethal dose is less than twice the effective dose. By contrast, fluoxetine (brand name Prozac) is an antidepressant with a therapeutic range of about 20–60 mg, and has been known to be lethal at a dose of about 1000 mg (Eli Lilly, 2000). (However, in another case a patient took about 3000 mg and survived with no long-term damage (Eli Lilly, 2000).) Consequently, it is clear that the therapeutic ratio for fluoxetine is at least several hundred times higher than lithium. Similar statistics are sometimes established for supplements, but usually are not widely publicized. For example, lethal doses for caffeine and some stimulants have been established (as discussed later in the book). Individuals who intend to administer (or take) nutritional and herbal supplements should always remember that safety, above all, is paramount.

Blood–Brain Barrier

Even when a portion of a compound is able to survive metabolism and excretion and reaches the brain, there is no guarantee that the substance will be allowed to enter the brain. Blood vessels in the brain are surrounded by an extra coating of lipid cells that provide additional protection and filtration of what is allowed to enter brain tissues. The blood–brain barrier is made up of various cells, especially including glial cells that surround the capillaries in the majority of the brain. These cells form a tight membrane that does not allow the passage of many molecules.

Several factors determine whether a substance will be able to cross the blood–brain barrier, including the size of the molecule, its ionization, and its lipid solubility. Generally, those molecules that are small and highly lipophyllic pass through, while those that are highly ionized, large, and lipophobic are filtered out (Julien, 2008). It is important to know the particular substance's molecular size, ionization, and lipid solubility in order to determine how likely it is to pass the blood–brain barrier. Since herbal and nutritional supplements are essentially unregulated in the US, manufacturers often make claims that are not supported by actual data. However, most pharmacologic references (for example, Medical Economics, 2008b), including those that focus on nutritional and herbal supplements (Medical Economics, 2007, 2008a) provide in-depth information about the chemical properties of the compounds. Consequently, those who desire to use supplements in the treatment of psychological disorders should carefully review the information provided in those volumes and make an informed decision about whether any substance in question is likely to enter the brain to exert any therapeutic effect.

METABOLISM

Metabolism refers to the chemical transformation of a substance that usually reduces its effect and increases excretion. In many cases, metabolism is the chemical breakdown of a substance. Usually, administered compounds are complex chemicals that can be metabolized by splitting them into more basic components that are further metabolized or excreted by the body. When a compound is transformed, the product of this metabolism is usually referred to as a metabolite. A substance may be transformed into one or more metabolites, and consequently these metabolites may undergo further changes. It is not unusual for complex substances to undergo many stages of metabolism, and in some cases, metabolites go through a process of retroconversion, where one metabolite is converted to another, but then may partially be reconverted back. For example, Omega-3 oils undergo multistage transformations, and retroconversion between various components is common. When this is evident, metabolic processes become complex and are sometimes hard to anticipate. This is one reason why the clinical response to many supplements is somewhat unpredictable.

Some metabolites are inactive and essentially await excretion by the kidneys (or the bowels). However, in some cases the metabolites are clinically active and exert an effect that may be similar to that of the parent compound. In that case, there will be a period of time when the parent compound and the active metabolite will be in circulation at the same time, and may add to each other's clinical effects. In some cases, the active metabolites are more potent than the parent compounds, and may have a much longer systemic life. These active metabolites may also exert varying clinical effects that are not always additive. Consequently, understanding the behavior of those metabolites is crucial. In rare instances, the parent compound may be inactive and does not exert any clinical effect until it is metabolized into an active metabolite. In pharmacology, this is referred to as a prodrug, and there are few nutritional and herbal supplements where such a pattern is evident.

Understanding metabolism is particularly important when considering nutritional and herbal supplements. While medications are complex substances, they usually only contain one active ingredient, and because extensive pharmacological studies (which usually begin well before the release of the drug) are performed to understand how the substance behaves in the body, metabolic processes, including the rate and the behavior of metabolites, are relatively well established. On the other hand, nutritional and herbal supplements usually are not purified and contain many active ingredients (sometimes, dozens of them). To release them to market, pharmacological studies are not required. The ingredients may all exert varying clinical (and adverse) effects, and because their rate of metabolism may vary, different ingredients may become predominantly active as the substance goes through metabolism and some components are metabolized before others. This is another reason why it is often hard to predict the onset of effect and duration needed before improvement of symptoms can be expected.

Small Intestine

The small intestine serves very important gastric functions, including the metabolism and absorption of nutrients. Most of the chemical digestion takes place in the small intestine. As the contents slowly move through it, various enzymes are released and mix in the foodstuff to break down complex ingredients into more basic components that are then absorbed and become available to fuel cell function. In the small intestine, peptides are deconstructed into individual amino acids. Lipids (fats) become decomposed into various fatty acids and glycerol. Triglycerides are broken down into fatty acids and monoglycerides. Carbohydrates are degraded into glucose and other simple sugars. All of these basic nutrients are then absorbed through the blood vessels in the intestinal wall and enter systemic circulation. The peristalsis is slow enough to allow the foodstuff to remain in various portions of the small intestine for sufficient amount of time for these chemical processes to take place.

The ingredients in many nutritional and herbal supplements include basic nutrients typically consumed on a regular diet, although in larger amounts. Since the small intestine is programmed to break down a lot of these nutrients into subcomponents, many of them may not become available for absorption in the form in which they were ingested, and may undergo metabolism before absorption can begin. When supplements become transformed in the small intestine, the resulting substances may not have psychopharmacological relevance. For example, dopamine and serotonin, neurotransmitters involved in the pathophysiology of many psychological disorders, are available in pill form for oral supplementation. However, these substances undergo extensive metabolism before absorption, and the metabolites are not psychoactive. Thus, taking these supplements has no therapeutic value.

The small intestine is divided into several sections. The duodenum is the upper portion into which contents of the stomach gradually empty. Here, absorption begins, particularly including the absorption of iron and other metals. Thus, of all nutrients, metals are the first to become bioavailable, although this does not necessarily mean that those compounds have the fastest onset of effect. Clinical response is determined by a wide variety of pharmacologic properties, not only including the specific pharmacokinetic properties of the substance, but also the relevant pharmacodynamics (discussed in the next chapter).

Jejenum is the next portion of the small intestine, and the majority of nutrients are absorbed here. This includes lipids, electrolytes, and sugars. The ilium constitutes about the last half of the small intestine, and vitamins (for example, B_{12}) and salts are primarily absorbed there. The ilium empties into the first section of the large intestine. The large intestine includes various sections of the colon (ascending, transverse, descending, and sigmoid), and the rectum. As the foodstuff travels through the colon, nutrients have already been absorbed and no further absorption takes place, with the exception of water, which continues to be absorbed through the entire length of the colon. The anus defecates the remains of the undigested and unabsorbed foodstuff as feces.

Liver

Although some biotransformation takes place in the small intestine, the majority of metabolism takes place in the liver. It is further important to note that our circulatory system is designed to direct all nutrients into the liver before they are able to circulate through the rest of the body. When absorption takes place in the small intestine, the capillaries embedded in the intestinal wall lead to a system of blood vessels that empty into the hepatic portal vein. Thus, everything absorbed from the gastrointestinal tract enters the liver to undergo further metabolism before passing into systemic circulation.

When compounds initially pass through the liver, it is likely that only some of the absorbed contents may be metabolized. Various aspects determine what portion becomes broken down during the first pass through the liver, but it is likely that the majority of the compound will not be metabolized. Thus, a significant portion may exit the liver and become available to enter systemic circulation. The portion that does become metabolized in the liver the first time it passes through is said to become subject to the first pass effect. What remains after the first pass effect becomes available to circulate through the body (after it passes the kidneys, as discussed later in the chapter) and may find its way to the brain. However, since only a portion is likely to get through the blood–brain barrier, the remainder will remain in the blood and will enter the venous system that travels back into the liver. Once again, the liver will metabolize another portion, and the remainder will travel back to the brain (providing it is not excreted), and a smaller portion will again return to the liver to undergo another round of metabolism. Thus, when it comes to the metabolism of substances, it is common to identify the first pass effect, second pass effect, third pass effect, etc. Each time, another portion gets metabolized, and an ever decreasing portion remains in the blood stream. Eventually, all of the compound becomes metabolized (and/or excreted), but the clinical effect may still remain, based on the duration of time during which the portion that entered the brain may continue to be pharmacodynamically active.

As outlined in Table 2.4, liver metabolism (during each pass) takes place in two distinct phases, and each phase contains several types of reactions. Although these usually occur in sequence, sometimes they take place concurrently.

Phase I Reactions

Phase I has particularly been found to be relevant to the metabolism of psychoactive substances. Oxidation involves the addition of oxygen molecules or the removal of hydrogen. This is usually done by oxidase enzymes. Reduction is the reverse of oxidation. Hydrolysis involves the splitting of water molecules into hydrogen and hydroxide ions, which may then become candidates for further reactions. Cyclization and

TABLE 2.4 Phases of liver metabolism

Phase I
Oxidation
Reduction
Hydrolysis
Cyclization
Decyclization
Phase II
Methylation
Sulphation
Acetylation
Conjugation

decyclization are processes in which open-chain molecules are transformed into closed rings, or vice versa. As with the other reactions, these molecules are then available for further reactions.

CP450 System

Phase I reactions of particular interest are oxidative reactions that involve a group of liver enzymes known as the cytochrome P450 system (CP450). These enzymes reside within the endoplasmic reticulum of hepatic cells. The vast majority of medications undergo metabolism through this system. Twelve gene families of CP450 enzymes have been identified, and these are summarized in Table 2.5. By convention, each enzyme is labeled by a number that identifies the main family (the first numeral, one or two digits), a letter that identifies the subfamily (an alphabetic letter), and the specific gene within the subfamily (the second numeral, one or two digits). Although many specific enzymes have been identified, the vast majority of psychoactive drugs are metabolized by the CYP1, CYP2, and CYP3 families.

When molecules absorbed from the small intestine pass through the liver, they become substrates upon which these enzymes act in order to transform them. Although some substrates are transformed by only one specific CYP450 enzyme, others may be metabolized by several enzymes. The levels of liver enzymes may be affected by many factors,

TABLE 2.5 Cytochrome P450 families of enzymes

1A1	2A6	3A3 (30%)**	4A9	11A1	17	19	21	27
1A2 (13%)	2A7	3A4	4B1	11B1				
	2B6	3A5	4F2	11B2				
	2C8 (20%)* 3A7		4F3					
	2C9							
	2C18							
	2C19							
	2D6 (2%)							
	2E1 (7%)							
	2F1							

Note: Listed percentages are portions of all liver enzymes attributed to a given enzyme, as per Battista & Schatzberg (2006). Enzymes with no percentages constitute, as a group, approximately 28% of all CYP enzymes.
* Percentage listed is for all 2C enzymes combined,
** Percentage listed is for all 3A enzymes combined.

including age, genetics, disease, and presence of other substances and molecules. Younger individuals, especially children, exhibit higher levels of most liver enzymes, and therefore the rate of metabolism is much higher. For this reason, when medications or supplements are administered, children usually require higher plasma levels than those sought with adults, since greater proportions of the substrate is likely to be metabolized. Conversely, older individuals, whose liver function slowed with age, usually require lower plasma levels and dosage adjustments must be made, or toxicity may develop. In addition, those who have liver (or other metabolic) diseases must also take lower doses since their ability to metabolize substrates is compromised.

It is also important to note that genetics often influence the levels of CP450 enzymes. For example, some estimated 20–30 million Americans have low CYP2D6 levels (some have none), and another 15–20 million have significant CYP2D6 duplications, resulting in much higher levels of the enzyme (Julien, 2008). Thus, individuals with little or no CYP2D6 will be at risk for toxic levels of substances that are substrates for that enzyme, while those with increased levels will metabolize those same substrates so rapidly that clinical effect may not be evident. Generally, research on ethnopsychopharmacology has revealed that certain ethnic groups are more likely to exhibit CYP450 deviations. For example, one-third of Asian Americans and one-third of African Americans have a genetic alteration that decreases the levels of CYP2D6 (Risby, 1996). In cases where genetic differences of liver enzymes are suspected, genetic testing is available (through a simple blood test) to identify whether alterations in CYP450 genes are evident.

In addition to factors associated with age, disease, and genetics, the presence of various molecules, together with a substrate of interest, may affect levels of the enzymes that metabolize that substrate. Generally, some substances may act as inducers, increasing the levels of the enzymes, while others may act as inhibitors, decreasing the levels of the enzymes. Both are important to consider.

Inducers

Those substances that induce greater production of liver enzymes have an important effect on the rate of metabolism of the substrates. Usually, this means that levels of the substrate decrease and clinical effect is diminished. In some cases, the increased metabolism may result in a complete breakdown of the substance, leaving none to reach the brain. Thus, the presence of an enzyme inducer is an important pathway through which pharmacologic interaction effects take place.

When it comes to medications, the research that was done on each compound before it reaches the market identifies the pathways responsible for its breakdown, and the CYP450 enzymes involved in metabolism are clearly identified. In addition, pharmacologic studies not only identify the enzymes for which the medication is a substrate, but also whether or not that medication exerts its own effect on any liver enzyme. Because a medication may be a substrate for one enzyme and may alter levels of another (for example, by inducing it), both properties are then entered into a database, and pharmacists and medical prescribers have a wide variety of electronic and printed reference sources available to cross-reference whether two medications used concurrently will affect the liver in such a way as to interfere with each other's metabolism.

In addition to drug–drug interactions, some foods have also been identified that may induce some liver enzymes. For example, alcohol has been found to have inducing effects on many liver enzymes, and many medications carry warnings that they should not be consumed with alcohol (although these warnings may be even more likely because of risk of pharmacodynamic interactions, described in the next chapter). Generally speaking, however, ingestion of nutrients in the diet has not been shown to result in major induction of specific liver enzymes, although more general inducing effects are common. For example, after a meal, the levels of all liver enzymes generally increase.

Although medications are carefully researched with regard to liver metabolism, most nutrients are not. Consequently, when nutritional or herbal supplements are ingested, the specific effects on liver function are often unknown. This becomes especially important to consider when multiple supplements are used at once. Because they may affect the liver in all different ways, and all of these may impact how the supplements are metabolized, the effects of supplements are often unpredictable. Some of the supplements that are widely used have been researched with regard to their effects on the liver. For example, St. John's Wort has been shown to be a potent inducer on the CYP3A subfamily. Because these enzymes are responsible for the breakdown of many drugs (for example, theophylline and birth control pills), those who take this supplement need to be carefully monitored, especially when St. John's Wort is used in combination with other medications. Generally, supplements should only be used with individuals who are not taking any medications, and if concomitant use with any medications is planned, careful monitoring by a medical prescriber is necessary.

Inhibitors

It is not only important to monitor substances that may induce liver enzymes, it is even more important to monitor substances that may inhibit them. When a liver enzyme is inhibited, the metabolism of the substrates for this enzyme is significantly reduced. As a result, blood levels of the substrates are likely to rise unpredictably, since the pathway responsible for breaking them down is being slowed or inactivated. When the substrate is a psychoactive substance, the inhibition of the metabolism may result in dangerously high levels, toxicity, and death.

This is especially crucial when a substance is metabolized by only one enzyme, as is often the case with medications. When that enzyme is inhibited, the only way to break down the medication is reduced or eliminated, and consequently the medication will remain in the system, at levels much higher than desired, until it is gradually excreted. When a substance is a substrate for more than one enzyme, this is less of a risk, because inhibition of one enzyme does not affect the levels of the other enzymes also involved in its breakdown. As mentioned before, it is important to identify the relationship between any given substance and the relevant liver enzymes – which enzymes break it down, and whether the substance induces or inhibits any liver enzymes – in order to understand the factors that must be monitored when the compound is

administered. Data about these pharmacokinetics are available in medical reference publications (for example, Medical Economics, 2008b),
although most sources do not include much information about the pharmacokinetics of supplements. Some sources about naturopathic substances are available (for example, Medical Economics, 2007, 2008a),
but the pharmacokinetics of the vast majority of supplements are not
widely researched. When data about relevant liver enzymes (or other
pathways of metabolism) is not available, clinicians must follow the old
dictum recognized by most medical prescribers – 'start low and go slow.'

Although dietary considerations do not seem to play a major role
in enzyme induction, the same is not true for enzyme inhibition. Some
foods have been shown to have a significant effect on reducing the
enzymes that metabolize some supplements and medications. For example, grapefruit juice has been shown to have a significant inhibitory
effect on the CYP3A4 isoenzyme. Consequently, individuals who take
medications that are substrates for this enzyme will exhibit higher levels of these medications, possibly resulting in toxicity. For this reason,
some medications carry warnings that they should not be taken with
grapefruit juice, or close to the time when grapefruit juice is consumed.

Phase II Reactions

Phase II reactions are not as commonly associated with the metabolism of medications. However, supplements that contain nutrients may
be metabolized by those processes. For example, methylation involves
changes in the methyl group portion of various substrates. This process
is especially relevant to the metabolism of heavy metals and some proteins. Thus, methylation is involved in the metabolism of some supplements, including those that contain iron.

Sulphation involves the transformation of a molecule by attaching
a sulphonate, thus transforming a substance into one that is more easily recognized by the body. This process is very relevant to metabolism
of herbal supplements, since many of them are xenobiotic (foreign to
the body) and become transformed during the process of metabolism.
Usually, this renders the substance inactive, but in some cases this may
activate the compound. For example, sulphation may strengthen some
protein–protein interactions, and is involved in producing some important amino acids, like tyrosine, that may have psychoactive properties.

Acetylation describes a reaction where an acetyl group is introduced
into an organic compound. This may involve the substitution of an
acetyl group for an active hydrogen atom, resulting in the formation of
acetates, compounds that become involved in the metabolism of further
substances. The majority of proteins are modified in this manner.

Conjugation is the process by which genetic material is passed between substance molecules. In the process, the substrate becomes transformed and may be activated or deactivated. Many nutrients are transformed in this manner, and conjugation may be bidirectional. For example, Omega-3 fatty acids are often converted, and retroconverted, through conjugation.

Nutritional and herbal supplements, more so than medications, may become metabolized by any of the wide variety of metabolic processes associated with Phase I and II reactions, and consequently the effects of liver metabolism on naturopathic supplements are more unpredictable. In addition, because so many supplements contain a wide variety of active compounds, each of which may be metabolized through a different sub-set of liver reactions, it is difficult to accurately predict (or research) the exact effects of any given compound. For this reason, even though reference volumes (such as this one) attempt to summarize what is known about the action of these supplements, much remains unknown, and clinicians are again reminded that they must proceed cautiously and carefully monitor both desired and adverse effects ('start low and go slow').

Metabolites

When compounds become transformed, the result of the process is called a metabolite. A substance may be transformed into many metabolites. Technically, the transformation of any substance during metabolism results in the creation of metabolites. However, this term is usually reserved for those molecules that, after metabolism, still remain xenobiotic, meaning that the product of metabolism remains a substance that is exogenous to the body. Conversely, if substances become transformed into proteins, amino acids, and other substances naturally occurring within the body, the products of metabolism are not usually referred to as metabolites.

Metabolites may be active or inactive. An inactive metabolite is one that is not clinically relevant or psychoactive. Thus, when it remains in the blood stream, it essentially awaits excretion without exerting any effects. By comparison, active metabolites are those substances that are clinically relevant and produce some effects. There is no way to predict whether a substance will be transformed into active or inactive metabolites – evidence for one or the other must be obtained from research studies.

When a substance (like a medication or a supplement) is metabolized, it may result in a complete transformation into basic nutrients or other endogenous substances, or it may be transformed on to one or more metabolites. It is common for a substance to be transformed into many secondary compounds, some of which may be active and others that may be inactive.

Because metabolites will further contribute to clinical effects, it is important to identify those substances that are metabolized into active metabolites.

In some cases, the parent compound will remain in the system while the active metabolites are created and also enter general circulation. In such a scenario, the parent compound and the active metabolite will exert additive effects, thus magnifying the clinical reactions. When active metabolites are identified, and especially when it becomes evident that the metabolites become active while the parent compound is still in the system (and exerts effects of its own), dosage must appropriately be adjusted to allow for such additive effects.

Because nutritional and herbal supplements contain many active ingredients, these usually become transformed into a wide variety of molecules and metabolites. Some of these may be clinically active, and it is not unusual for the various active compounds to be transformed into metabolites that have clinical effects that are at least somewhat contradictory. For example, a supplement may be transformed into many metabolites, some of which have anxiolytic qualities while others activate the fight–flight mechanism. For this reason, once again, it is necessary to proceed very cautiously and methodically monitor all effects.

EXCRETION

Remnants of ingested compounds are excreted from the body by two separate systems. Substances administered orally pass through the GI tract in order to be absorbed and enter circulation. In most cases, ingested substances do not become absorbed in their entirety, and a portion remains unabsorbed as the substance concludes its travel through the small intestine. Since only water continues to be absorbed in the large intestine, any remaining solids become congealed into a mass that forms the feces. These solids not only include undigested food remains, they also contain any remnants of the ingested compound.

Since medications undergo a significant amount of research to identify the pharmacokinetic properties, the proportion of the substance that is usually excreted in feces is established, and the dosage is appropriately adjusted so that the portion that becomes absorbed is sufficient to produce clinical effects. Supplements, however, do not generally undergo such detailed research, and it may not be known what portion remains excreted in the feces. While it is more likely that nutritional supplements may become absorbed more completely, herbal supplements, which generally contain xenobiotic substances, may only be absorbed partially, and a significant portion of the ingested dose may be excreted unabsorbed.

As discussed above, the proportion that was absorbed enters circulation, and proceeds on to the liver. After passing the liver, the remaining portion remains in the blood stream. The human circulatory system is designed to pass all contents of the blood through another set of organs before the blood is allowed to circulate through the rest of the body. These organs are the kidneys, and the blood travels there right after it passes through the liver.

Kidneys

The kidneys have numerous biological roles, including maintenance of the balance of bodily fluids by filtering metabolites and minerals from the blood. The kidneys sense plasma concentrations of sodium, potassium, hydrogen, oxygen, and other compounds (such as amino acids and glucose), and are important regulators of glucose metabolism and other bodily functions (for example, blood pressure).

The kidneys clear waste products from the blood by removing them and concentrating them in a liquid that travels down urinary tracts, gets collected in the bladder, and becomes eliminated from the body as urine. As the blood passes through the kidneys, nephron cells filter out the contents of the blood and selectively reabsorb into the blood those molecules that should remain, while the remainder is sent down the urinary tracts. Thus, each time the blood passes through the kidneys, many contents are removed and not allowed to remain in systemic circulation. As discussed above, the circulatory system is designed so that this process occurs before the blood is allowed to circulate back into the heart, the lungs, and the rest of the body (in arterial vessels).

Many aspects determine what will be filtered out by the kidneys, but two are the most crucial. The most important factor is the water solubility of the substance. Those that are highly hydrophyllic are easily removed by the kidneys and are not likely to be reabsorbed. These substances become cleared very quickly, and are eliminated in the urine. Since the contents of urine are not reabsorbed, anything that enters urine has effectively left the circulatory system and will not be available to travel to the target sites of effect. By contrast, those substances that are highly lipophyllic are dissolved into lipids and become reabsorbed by the kidneys, thus resisting elimination. Those substances remain in the blood stream and travel through the remainder of the body.

While each substance has its own inherent water solubility, metabolism can alter this property. Some aspects of liver metabolism change the water solubility of the substance, potentially making it more water soluble. In such a scenario, the substance that passes through the liver becomes more hydrophyllic, and is mostly excreted by the kidneys. Such a substance is not able to travel to the targets sites of effect (like the brain). Thus, not only the baseline water solubility of the substance, but also the type of liver metabolism the substance undergoes determines whether the substance will be able to pass through the kidneys.

Another aspect has a significant impact on the filtering performed by the kidneys. The kidneys regulate the level of acidity (pH level) of the blood. As the pH level of the blood drops (the blood becomes more acidic), the kidneys work harder to remove acidic contents to restore the proper pH balance of 7.35–7.45. Consequently, those supplements that lower the blood's pH balance are likely to increase the kidney's efforts to remove acidic content from the blood. This may have an impact on blood levels of those supplements that have pH levels below 7.4.

Half-Life

An important aspect of all drugs and supplements is the elimination half-life of the compound, usually symbolized by $T_{1/2}$. An elimination half-life is the time that it takes for 50 percent of the drug to be eliminated from the body. While in the strictest use this term refers to the elimination of a substance, usually the half-life refers to the time period during which one-half of the absorbed amount becomes inactive, through the combination of metabolic deactivation (liver effects) and excretion (kidney effects).

The half-life is an important pharmacodynamic property. Generally, blood plasma concentrations at levels less than 50 percent of the absorbed dose do not produce full clinical effects, and therefore the elimination half-life usually refers to the length of time that the substance will exert the desired clinical effects within the body.

The half-life is important to establish, and research studies usually aim to discover the half-life of a given substance. The length of the half-life usually determines the frequency of the dosing. Thus, a substance with a half-life of 24 hours is usually taken once per day, while another with a half-life of 12 hours will usually require twice per day (BID) dosing. Substances with half-lives fewer than 12 hours need multiple daily dosing, and therefore are often inconvenient. Since much of the time it is desirable to attain a clinical effect that remains constant through the entire day, the dosing must be established in accordance with the half-life. Usually, repeated doses are taken at times when the half-life of the previous doses elapses. Thus, substances that last the whole day are taken once per day, substances that last half of a 24 hour day are taken twice per day, etc.

When doses are taken consistently at time intervals equal to the substance's half-life, a steady state is gradually reached where the blood levels of the substance remain consistent with each additional dose, and

TABLE 2.6 Half-life elimination

Number of half lives	Percent of substance eliminated	Percent of substance remaining
0	0	100
1	50	50
2	75	25
3	87.5	12.5
4	93.75	6.25
5	96.87	3.13
6	98.44	1.56
7	99.22	0.78

each subsequent dose is counteracted by ongoing elimination, resulting in constant blood levels of the substance. Generally, five to seven doses are required to reach this steady state.

Conversely, when it is necessary to discontinue a substance, it is important to calculate how much of the substance may remain in the blood stream at any given point after the last dose. This is done by dividing in half the amount in the blood stream that remains after each half-life period has elapsed (as evident in Table 2.6). Thus, after five half-lives elapse, almost 97 percent of the substance has been cleared, essentially resulting in complete elimination. In some cases, when complete elimination is sought, it is desirable to wait seven half-lives (at which time more than 99 percent of the substance has been cleared). Such a period is sometimes referred to as a washout, and it is desired when the patient is switched from taking one substance into another that has a potential for dangerous interactions with the first. A washout period assures that almost all of the initial substance is cleared before the second substance is started.

PEDIATRIC CONSIDERATIONS

Although the principles of pharmacokinetics apply to all individuals, regardless of age, some aspects of the pharmacokinetic phases are likely to differ between adults and children. Some specific considerations are outlined below.

As teenagers grow older, their rate of absorption, distribution, metabolism, and excretion begins to resemble those of young adults. Thus, the discussion below focuses specifically on children, and readers should consider that pharmacokinetic considerations with adolescents will fall somewhere between the characteristics described for children and those that are established for adults.

Absorption

Most supplements are administered through the enteral route, and become absorbed in the small intestine. However, routes of administration, and rate of absorption, may pose specific challenges when supplements are used with children.

Routes of Administration

Most herbal and nutritional supplements are available for oral administration, primarily in the forms of pills (tablets, capsules, etc.). However, as discussed earlier in the chapter, many children do not like to take pills. While some supplements may be able to be prepared as tinctures, most do not provide this method of administration. In addition, the majority of nutritional and herbal supplements cannot be crushed, or opened and 'sprinkled,' since such use may result in premature metabolism of the substance, essentially rendering it useless as a psychopharmacological compound. For this reason, children who are able (and willing) to take oral supplements in available forms are best candidates for this form of treatment.

Absorption Considerations

As discussed earlier in the chapter, many aspects affect absorption. Because children's diets may not resemble the diets of adults on whom the supplements may have been researched, rates of absorption may differ significantly between children and adolescents. Generally, children absorb substances faster than adults, but this is affected by the types of foods that are consumed, as well as the fluid intake. Some children eat a lot of sugary foods, and therefore substances that are highly reactive to glucose intake may be absorbed at different rates (faster or slower, depending on a substance). Similarly, some children do not drink many fluids, and substances that require water for absorption may be absorbed more slowly and/or eliminated more completely without being absorbed. Generally, when supplements are administered, parents should also regulate the children's diets to make sure that a normal intake of fluids and nutrients is evident.

Distribution

Children's circulatory rates are much higher than those of adults. For this reason, children tend to exhibit faster rates of distribution of absorbed compounds through the circulatory system. This tends to be especially evident among children who are very active. Because pulse depends (at least in part) on motor activity, those children who are physically active have much higher rates of blood circulation. This means that children are likely to exhibit a faster rate of distribution of compounds than teenagers or adults.

In addition, volume of distribution must be considered. Since children are much smaller than adults, doses must appropriately be adjusted for their size. Some supplements are dosed at an established ratio of milligrams of substance per each kilogram of body weight. When such guidelines are established, it is easy to convert an adult dose into one that is appropriate for the child's size. However, doses for many supplements are not established by body weight. Instead, the starting doses and the usual effective doses are identified, and these are generally established for adults. In those situations, appropriate calculations must be performed to determine the right starting dose for the child.

It is prudent to start any child on the lowest dose available, and slowly titrate upward at sufficient time intervals (at least 1–2 weeks between dose increases) while carefully monitoring clinical and adverse effects. With older children and adolescents, it may be useful to calculate the starting dose by adjusting the adult dose downward based on body size. According to the National Center for Health Statistics (2002), the weight of an average adult male in the US is about 190 pounds (about 86 kg), while the average weight of a woman is 162.9 pounds (about 74 kg). This information allows the calculation of the usual mg/kg ratio that has been used with adult men and women. The obtained ratio can then be multiplied by the weight of the teenager to determine the appropriate dose.

For example, the usual effective doses of SAM-e with adult males has been established to fall between 1600 and 2400 mg per day. Thus, the dose-to-weight ratio for adults is about 18–28 mg/kg per day. If a teenager weighs about 100 pounds (about 45 kg), his effective dose may fall somewhere between 816 and 1269 mg per day. Obviously, it is necessary to start at the lowest dose, but providing adverse effects are minimal, the dose can gradually be increased until the teen is given a dose that falls somewhere within that range, and if clinical effects are not adequate, rather than raising the dose above that range, another supplement should be tried.

Metabolism

As with rates of distribution, children exhibit much higher rates of metabolism. The liver of a child works much faster at metabolizing the nutrients, and the levels of liver enzymes are much higher (when considering the weight ratio). For this reason, children tend to metabolize medications and nutrients much faster than adults and teenagers.

When mg/kg ratios are established for a medication or a supplement, the ratios for a child must generally be higher than those for adults. In other words, mg/kg levels that may be effective for adults may be too low to be effective for children. In the example above, the dose-to-weight ratio for using SAM-e with adults has been estimated to be about 10–28 mg/kg per day. However, given the faster metabolism of children, the same ratio may be too low. Thus, adult mg/kg ratios can not easily be adopted for children, and a higher dose-to-weight may need to be used. Unfortunately, such ratios are rarely established in research literature, and therefore much trial and error is needed in order to arrive at an effective dose. As recommended several times in this chapter, clinicians and parents must 'start low and go slow,' and carefully monitor any and all effects that result from the use of the supplement. However, as long as children do not exhibit adverse effects, clinicians and parents should not be surprised if children will require higher mg/kg ratios than adults before significant clinical effects are observed.

Higher metabolic rates not only determine the effective dose, but also change many other aspects of pharmacokinetics. For example, the onset of effect may be faster (providing a sufficient dose is used), and the duration of effect may be shorter (because of faster metabolism). It is not uncommon for children to require twice per day doses of supplements that may only be administered once per day with adults.

Excretion

Since distribution and metabolism are faster, so is the rate of excretion. Children's kidneys work faster, thus increasing the rate at which urinary excretion takes place. This means that the blood gets filtered more quickly, and often more vigorously, eliminating from the blood stream greater proportions of supplements than are usually seen with adult kidneys. Once again, this may affect significant pharmacokinetic properties, including the plasma levels, rates of onset of effect, and frequency of dosing.

As with metabolism, rates of elimination are affected by many factors, including nutrition (which may affect the pH levels of the blood) and fluid intake. Children who take in large amounts of fluids (perhaps because participating in sports makes them sweat and increases their thirst) are likely to exhibit higher rates of clearance of many supplements, and doses may need to be adjusted to allow for these lifestyle factors.

Chapter 3

Pharmacodynamics

Since psychopharmacology is the study of the mechanisms, effects, and use of substances that act on the brain, it is necessary to be familiar with the structure of the brain, as well as principles of brain function, in order to understand the action of psychoactive compounds. As our knowledge of the brain increases, we are becoming more aware of the complex nature of brain changes that underlie many psychological disorders. In some cases (for example, depression), the structure of the brain may change, and some parts of the brain may be larger or smaller. In other cases (for example, attention deficit hyperactivity disorder (ADHD)), structural changes may not be dramatic, but significant functional changes may clearly be apparent and parts of the brain may be underactive. In some disorders (for example, schizophrenia), both functional and structural changes may underlie the psychopathology.

Two related disciplines examine the brain structure and function. Neuroanatomy is the study of the structure of the nervous system, including the brain. When brain structure is examined, it is necessary to understand not only what parts may exhibit deviations from normal size, but also what cognitions, emotions, and behaviors are associated with these structures. Conversely, neurophysiology is the study of the function of the nervous system. When brain function is examined, the amount of activity in specific areas is measured, and deviations from expected levels of activity are correlated with the functional aspects associated with those areas. In addition, understanding neurophysiology requires the knowledge of neurons and important aspects of neurotransmission (for example, the action of neurotransmitters). Accordingly, this chapter will review neuroanatomy and neurophysiology in order to help readers understand the relationship between the brain changes associated with various psychological disorders (as discussed in later chapters of this book) and the specific changes in mood, cognition, and behaviors that may be expected when psychoactive compounds act on the brain and alter brain function.

Nutritional and Herbal Therapies for Children and Adolescents
47

NEUROANATOMY

The human nervous system is divided into many branches, reminiscent of a tree structure. The most basic division is between the central nervous system (CNS, including the brain and the spinal cord) and the peripheral nervous system (PNS, including all nerves outside the CNS). Although the vast majority of our discussion will primarily relate to CNS (especially the brain), various aspects of PNS should also be reviewed, because they have some involvement in several psychological symptoms (for example, anxiety).

Peripheral Nervous System

The PNS is further divided into sub-branches. The somatic nervous system sends information pertaining to sensory and motor functions, while the autonomic nervous system regulates the function of bodily organs and smooth muscles.

Somatic Nervous System

The somatic nervous system (SNS) includes all nerves that run to and from the spinal cord and send information to and from the muscles and senses. Generally, efferent pathways send information from the spinal cord to the muscles, and regulate motor functions involved in the movement of the body and limbs. By contrast, afferent pathways run toward the spinal cord and carry information from sensory organs. Although peripheral injury or severe electrolyte (and neurotransmitter) depletion can affect the functions of these pathways, most psychoactive substances do not act peripherally and effects evident in sensory and motor areas are primarily the result of CNS (not SNS) changes.

Autonomic Nervous System

The autonomous nervous system (ANS) includes all nerves that run between the spinal cord and bodily organs (and smooth muscles involved in the function of internal body organs). The ANS has two divisions of particular interest in psychopharmacology, the sympathetic nervous system, and the parasympathetic nervous system.

The sympathetic nervous system is involved in the activation of the fight–flight mechanism. When an anxiety reaction is provoked, the pituitary releases a number of hormones, some of which trigger portions of the sympathetic nervous system directly, and others communicate with remaining portions of the glandular system (for example, the thyroid and the adrenal cortex) to release additional activating hormones. When large amounts of these hormones are present, changes typically associated with panic reactions are evident.

The activation of sympathetic nervous system affects many bodily organs, and portions of the sensory and motor systems. Pupils dilate, salivation decreases, respiration becomes faster and shallower, pulse and blood pressure increase, gastric motility slows down, the urge to eliminate increases, and muscles in the motor system become more tense and rigid. This activation is intended to handle physical stressors, and the body readies for a physical 'fight' of the threat or a 'flight' away from it. Because our system has no ability to discern physical from emotional/psychological stress, the same sympathetic activation occurs with all types of stressors. Symptoms of anxiety disorders (for example, panic disorder) involve regular episodes of significant sympathetic nervous system activation. When the body prepares for this fight or flight, it enters a state of significant autonomic arousal. Regular and significant activation of these mechanisms is likely to result in gradual systemic damage that is evident with many disorders commonly considered to be stress related.

After the sympathetic system activates the stress reaction, a system is necessary to restore the body to a level of arousal that is typical of normal functioning. This is regulated by the parasympathetic nervous system, which counteracts sympathetic activation. The levels of stress hormones decrease and the body organs and muscles return to normal function. Pupils constrict to a normal level, salivation increases and digestive processes restart, respiration slows and becomes deeper, pulse and blood pressure return to normal, and muscles in the motor system relax.

When individuals experience stress reactions, common with many anxiety disorders, sympathetic nervous system chronically becomes activated, and compounds with anxiolytic action have to calm this stress reaction. Usually, this is attained by targeting the function of brain structures responsible for the triggering of anxiety reactions (for example, the locus coeruleus and the hypothalamus). However, some of these substances also act peripherally to reduce sympathetic activation and return the respiration, circulation, and other systemic function to normal levels.

Central Nervous System

The central nervous system (CNS) includes the brain and the spinal cord. While the brain will obviously be the major target of this discussion, a few words about the spinal cord may also be helpful.

The spinal cord contains thick nerve bundles that are arranged in afferent and efferent pathways. The afferent pathways carry information from sensory organs as well as sensory receptors on the muscles and in the organs. These inform the brain about the world outside and within the body. Conversely, efferent pathways carry nerve impulses to muscles responsible for bodily and motor functions. Generally, the function of the nerves within the spinal cord is to carry information as quickly and efficiently as possible, and provide an interface with the vast network of nerves within the somatic and autonomic systems. Most psychoactive drugs have little effect on neuronal transmission within the spinal cord, although those substances that affect neuronal transmission globally (for example, by increasing amounts of GABA or glutamate) exert their effect within the entire nervous system, and those substances that affect a specific type of neurotransmission (for example, analgesics), may interfere with neuronal transmission of that signal along the whole length of those nerve pathways.

Most psychoactive substances, however, target the brain to exert their action. The brain is divided into several regions, each of which has many subcomponents. While the discussion of all of those is beyond the scope of this book, those brain regions that have specific relevance to psychological function are reviewed below. Most basically, the brain can be divided into the cerebral cortex and those areas located under it. Each of those general regions has different functions and makes different contributions to psychological and emotional functioning. Sometimes brain structures are divided in accordance with evolutional progression. The brain stem and the cerebellum are referred to as hindbrain, and are responsible for the most basic life and motor functions. The midbrain encompasses areas that sit on top of the brain stem but still under the cortex, and is surrounded by the cortex on all sides. The forebrain, the cortex, is the most evolved and is responsible for the 'highest' forms of mental functioning, including planning and thought.

The cortex also surrounds two ventricles, openings filled with cerebrospinal fluid, located bilaterally. The third ventricle is located in the area of midbrain, and the fourth ventricle is located close to the brain stem as part of the central canal that runs down the length of the spinal cord. The ventricles allow the cerebrospinal fluid to circulate and cushion the brain, and serve as additional supply of protein and glucose. The cerebrospinal fluid also allows brain cells to deposit waste products into it, which get transported into venous blood circulation.

Cerebral Cortex

The cerebral cortex is the largest area of the human brain. Like all parts of the brain, it contains neuronal cells that have cell bodies and appendages (called axons and dendrites, discussed later in the chapter). The cortex is generally organized with cell bodies located on the outside, and connections between the neurons running toward the inside. These connections combine to form thick bundles running cross-laterally, known as the corpus callosum. Because cell bodies are darker than some of the connections (the axons, which are covered by myelin sheath), they are sometimes referred to as 'gray matter,' and the connections are referred to as 'white matter.'

As visible in Figure 3.1, the cortex is organized along a major division that splits it in half, laterally, and the corpus callosum connects the two hemispheres. In accordance with cross-lateral organization, the left side communicates with the right side of the body, and vice versa, although this is only true of sensory and motor functions. Portions of the cortex that process content not relevant to sensory or motor function is still divided across the two hemispheres, and generally the left side is considered to process content related to sequential and verbal processing, while the right side is more involved in holistic thinking and simultaneous processing. However, significant sex-based differences exist, and brains of men and women show differences in how the cognitive

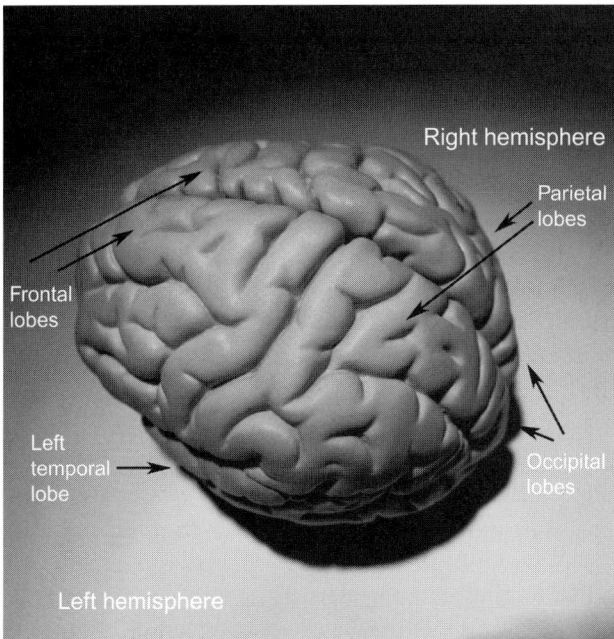

FIGURE 3.1 Major division of the cerebral cortex.

functions are split between the two hemispheres. In addition, significant interpersonal differences within the sexes are also apparent.

Each hemisphere is divided into four lobes (see Figure 3.1). The frontal lobes, together with the pre-frontal areas located right above the eyes, are involved in the processing of many important psychological functions. The upper regions, closer to the top of the head, control movement. Together with some subcortical areas (like the basal ganglia and cerebellum, discussed below), they are involved in the planning and coordination of motor behavior. The frontal lobes also process important executive functions. These include planning, recall of information, decision making, impulse control, and working memory (to assist with planning and decision making). When frontal lobes are underactive, individuals may exhibit problems with motor coordination and/or control of motor output, as well as difficulties with executive functions – problems with planning, exercising good judgment, controlling impulses and emotional urges, and using working memory. Several psychological disorders, including ADHD, are associated with changes in frontal lobe function (especially, underactivity of those areas).

Temporal lobes occupy the areas of the cortex surrounding the ears on both sides of the head. Temporal lobes are involved in processing of auditory information, but also make significant contributions to other aspects of emotional functioning. Temporal lobes are also involved in the regulation of memory functions, especially those memories that involve some emotional content. Temporal lobes are also involved in mood and anxiety disorders, and changes in the structure and function of the temporal lobes has been implicated in many psychological disorders, including symptoms of depression and mania.

Occipital lobes occupy the rear-most portion of the cortex, extending sideways toward the ears, where the occipital lobes meet the temporal lobes. The primary function of occipital lobes is to process visual information. Although most psychological disorders do not seem to involve impairment evident in occipital lobes, some psychological functions are very complex and involve the majority of the cortex. For example, the ability to pay attention is so complex that it involves areas in all of the cortical lobes, including areas of the occipital lobe (Mirsky, 1987).

Parietal lobes occupy the top portion of the brain and extend sideways about mid-way toward the ears (where they meet the temporal lobes). The anterior (toward the front) areas of the parietal lobes process information received from tactile senses (for example, touch). The remainder of the parietal lobes serves integrative functions. Parietal lobes are centrally situated and junction with the three other cortical lobes.

Consequently, they process information that combines visual, auditory, tactile, and motor functions. Disturbances in parietal lobes are commonly associated with low cognitive functioning and problems with attention.

Subcortical Areas

Those parts of the brain that lie directly under the cortex, and extend between the cortex and the top of the spinal cord, are collectively referred to as subcortical. As a group, these parts of the brain are involved in regulating basic life functions, as well as emotional processing. Many subdivisions are recognized, and those with the greatest relevance to psychological and emotional symptoms are illustrated in Figure 3.2 and discussed below. As with cortical lobes, the subcortical structures are symmetrically located bilaterally.

The thalamus is the largest portion of the diencephalon region of the brain. The thalamus serves as a major relay station between the cortex and the remaining parts of the nervous system. The thalamus processes

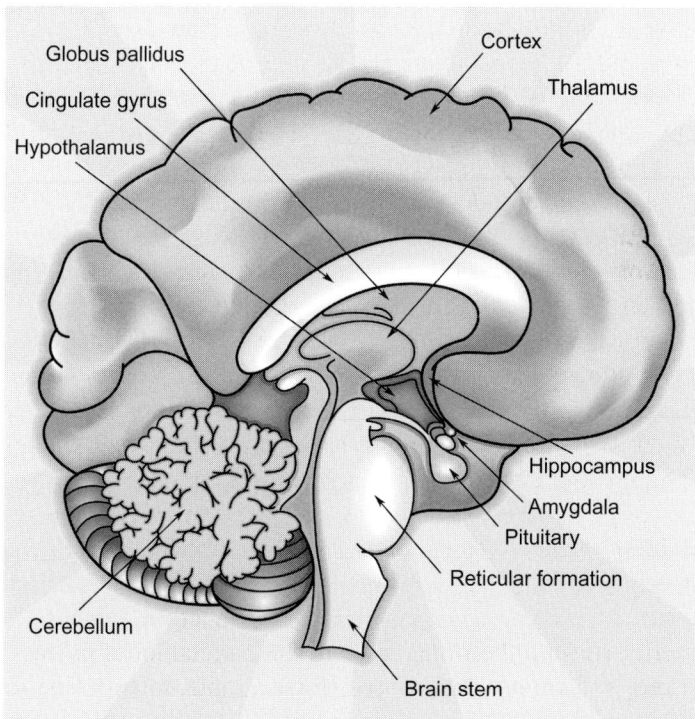

FIGURE 3.2   Major subcortical regions.

sensory and motor information and relays it to the appropriate portions of the cortex. This involves the auditory, visual, gustatory (but not olfactory), and somatosensory functions, especially including the perception of pain. The thalamus may also play a role in regulating sleep and consciousness (including cortical arousal and awareness). Symptoms of sleep disorders and ADHD may involve some thalamic functions.

The hypothalamus lies under the thalamus and is much smaller. However, it serves crucial psychological functions. The hypothalamus regulates crucial life functions, including hunger, reproduction, and the perception of danger. When a stressor is perceived, the hypothalamus invokes the activation of the sympathetic nervous system and many subsequent physiological and psychological changes associated with the fight–flight reaction. Thus, hypothalamus is involved in many psychological symptoms, especially anxiety. In addition, hypothalamus may also be involved in the regulation of sleep, and sleep disturbance commonly seen in depression may partially be due to hypothalamic dysregulation.

The hypothalamus lies very close to the pituitary. Included as part of the glandular system, the pituitary is a small (pea-size) part of the brain that regulates hormones involved in maintaining homeostasis. The pituitary releases many hormones, including those that activate the remainder of the glandular system, especially the thyroid and the adrenal cortex. Under stress, or at other times when the anxiety reaction is provoked (for example, during a panic attack), the pituitary stimulates the endocrine system to release additional hormones that activate the sympathetic nervous system. Physiological changes associated with the fight–flight reaction – for example, rapid heart beat and respiration – are precipitated by the presence of those hormones within the blood stream, acting as long-distance messengers to provoke these reactions in various muscles and organs.

The hippocampus is an oblong structure that extends around the diencephalon, encircling it on both sides. Its primary role is in the encoding of memory. Damage to the hippocampus results in severe impairment in the ability to store new memories, although the recall of stored memories usually remains relatively intact. Damage to cholinergic cells associated with Alzheimer's dementia usually begins in and around hippocampus, and gradually spreads outward as functional deficits become more broad and severe. Memory enhancers typically target this part of the brain, although some exert their action by increasing vigilance and attention to task (mediated by other brain structures). More recently, hippocampus has been implicated in symptoms of severe anxiety disorders, especially post-traumatic stress disorder (PTSD). When severe trauma takes place, the hippocampus can become overactivated – probably by the amygdala, as discussed below – and trauma-related memories are written so strongly into long-term storage that they do not become subject to the gradual extinction that naturally occurs with the vast majority of memories. Consequently, preventing hippocampal overactivation after trauma has been associated with better adjustment and less risk of PTSD (Stahl, 2008).

The amygdala, a peanut-shaped structure, lies adjacent to the hippocampus at its anterior end points. The amygdala is involved in mediating the sense of smell, as well as the activation of memory systems (through its connection with the hippocampus). The amygdala also takes part in regulating strong emotional reactions, especially anxiety and anger, and may be involved in mood disorders. Patients with depression have been shown to have exaggerated amygdala activity (especially on the left side), while patients with bipolar disorder have been shown to exhibit smaller amygdala volumes (Blumberg *et al.*, 2003).

The amygdala, hippocampus, hypothalamus, pituitary, and the thalamus are sometimes referred to collectively as the limbic system. Other brain structures commonly are also included, including the cingulate gyrus (involved in the mediation of cognitive and attentional processes) and the fornix (another part that contributes to memory processing). As a group, the limbic system regulates the majority of human emotions. It is highly connected with the brain's pleasure center (especially the nucleus accumbens) and may play a role in addictions, as well sexual behavior. By communicating with the endocrine system, the limbic system is an important component of the stress reaction and is involved in producing symptoms of anxiety. Overactivation of the limbic system is implicated in those psychological disorders that include features of anxiety, while the underactivation of this system may be related to disorders where hypoemotionality and/or lack of empathy is the prominent feature (for example, psychopathy).

The striatum is located under the cerebral cortex and communicates extensively with all cortical lobes. It is divided into the putamen (which regulates movement and learning) and caudate nucleus (which is involved in learning and memory). A related brain structure, the globus pallidus, mediates attentional and cognitive processes. Positioned nearby, the substantia nigra plays an important role in the regulation of movement, pleasure, and reward. It is involved in motor planning as well as addictive behaviors. The subthalamic nucleus is adjacent, and contributes to motor planning (especially action selection) and impulse control.

The striatum, globus pallidus, subthalamic nucleus, and substantia nigra are collectively referred to as basal ganglia. As a group, these structures are involved in motor coordination and planning, as well as self-control. Impairment in the function of basal ganglia seems to be an important contributory factor in disorders that include problem behaviors, for example ADHD (especially, the hyperactive-impulsive type), tic disorders, and obsessive compulsive disorder (OCD). The basal ganglia's contribution to self-control may be broad, and most disorders in which poor self-control is evident are thought to involve underactivity of the basal ganglia at least to some extent.

The reticular formation is an oblong structure, located vertically along the top of the spinal cord, in the brain stem. The reticular formation regulates the onset (and maintenance) of sleep/wake cycles and contributes to the filtering of incoming stimuli required for attentional processes. The pons relays information between the cerebellum and the rest of the brain, and contributes to the regulation of arousal and respiration. The medulla oblongata, located adjacent to the pons and the cerebellum, regulates life-sustaining autonomic functions, including respiration, pulse, and blood pressure.

The reticular formation, pons, and medulla oblongata are sometimes referred to as the reticular activating system (RAS). The RAS is extensively connected with the rest of the brain and regulates the basic level of arousal in the brain and in the body. Underactivation of the RAS is a contributory factor in disorders caused, at least in part, by insufficient neuronal activity. Symptoms of ADHD, sleep disorders, and autism, and damage to the RAS may result in permanent coma. Conversely, overactivation of RAS may be involved in producing symptoms of hypervigilance, for example those seen in patients with PTSD.

Finally, the cerebellum, located at the base of the brain, posterior to (in back of) the brain stem and inferior to (below) the cortex, is the largest of all subcortical areas, and plays important roles in the regulation of sensory and motor functions. The cerebellum stores functional motor units – precise sequence of specific movements that make all motor tasks, including walking, writing, grasping an object, etc. Disorders in which problems with motor control are apparent (such as ADHD) have been shown to be associated with smaller volumes of the cerebellum.

NEUROPHYSIOLOGY

Although structural changes in brain function have been identified in many psychological disorders, merely identifying those changes usually is not clinically helpful. For example, while it is important to understand how the size of frontal lobes determines (at least in part) the degree to which one can perform planning and utilize impulse control, this knowledge usually does not meaningfully guide effective clinical interventions. After all, we have not identified ways in which the size of any portion of the brain can be altered.

However, the function of various parts of the brain can be influenced. To do so, it is important to understand the function of neuronal cells, and how that function can be targeted by psychoactive substances. Thus, in order to learn about the function of the brain, it is important to understand the principles of neurophysiology.

The Neuron

The neuron (see Figure 3.3) is the basic building block of the brain. When brain parts 'communicate' with each other, neurons send and receive information. To understand the principles of this process it is necessary to understand the parts of the neuron and what each component is designed to do. Essentially, the neuron is like any other cell in the body, except that it has appendages designed to allow the cell to communicate with other neurons.

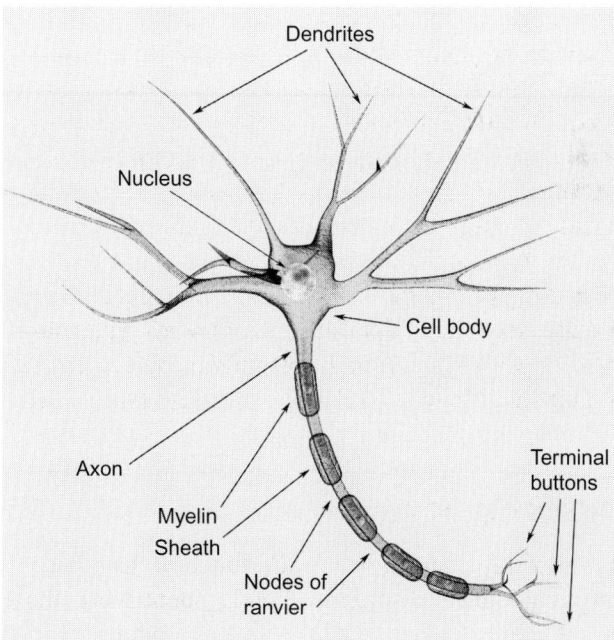

FIGURE 3.3 Major parts of the neuron.

The Cell Body

Like all cells, the neuron has a cell body. A number of organelles are located within it. These serve a wide variety of functions related to metabolism, cell life, production of neurotransmitters, etc.

At the heart of the cell is the nucleus. Contained within it are tiny nucleoli that contain deoxyribonucleic acid (DNA), a macromolecule that contains the genetic instructions used in the development and functioning of all cells. In order to influence the cells, information from the DNA must become available to be distributed through the cell. To do so, transcription of the genetic material must take place. This occurs within the nucleus. Enzymes transcribe portions of DNA into molecules of ribonucleic acid (RNA). RNA molecules then travel out of the nucleus and become available to come in contact with a variety of enzymes, electrolytes, proteins, lipids, and other molecules, many of which are ingested into the body during meals. A variety of molecules and proteins make up a 'molecular machine' that decodes RNA molecules and uses the contents to form proteins, amino acids, and other vital molecules. As these continue to undergo a multitude of complex conversion processes, some of those eventually become neurotransmitters.

The endoplasmic reticulum is an extensive network of cisternae (sacs and passages) that is usually (but not always) attached to the cell membranes (for example, the membrane around the nucleus). These sacs and passages allow proteins to collect and become available to be enacted upon by various enzymes, allowing transformation to occur. Ribosomes, made up of fragments of RNA and proteins, often become embedded, changing the appearance of the organelle's texture (thus becoming a rough endoplasmic reticulum). These ribosomes await contact with transported proteins and enzymes to take part in metabolic processes. The smooth endoplasmic reticulum does not contain ribosomes, but is also involved in many metabolic processes, including gluconeogenesis (the production of glucose). Smooth endoplasmic reticulum consists of a network of tubules and vesicles that create an increased surface area for the action or storage of enzymes and the products of these enzymes. The sarcoplasmic reticulum is found in smooth muscles and it is involved in the storing and pumping of calcium ions. It contains large deposits of calcium that are released when the muscle is stimulated. The calcium, in turn, plays a major role in stimulating the neuron to fire.

Neurons contain many other organelles. The mitochondria are involved in the production of adenosine triphosphate (ATP), the main source of the cell's chemical energy. In this way, mitochondria regulate cellular metabolism. In addition, mitochondria are involved in signaling, cellular differentiation, and the control of the cell's life cycle (including cell growth and cell death). The mitochondrion has also been shown to have its own genome. When the function of mitochondria is disturbed, the consequences can be very severe. For example, many forms of cardiac dysfunction, diabetes, and neuropathies have been shown to be related to mitochondrial dysregulation. Although research findings have not specifically implicated mitochondrial dysfunctions in psychological disorders, it is possible that those disorders characterized by underactive brain pathways may be related to metabolic abnormalities, and these in turn may partially be caused by mitochondrial dysregulation. For these reasons, introducing supplements that increase levels of ATP have been tried, although these generally have not met with much success. However, supplementation with other nutrients may affect mitochondrial function, although this effect has not specifically been identified in research studies.

The golgi apparatus is similar to the endoplasmic reticulum, and contains a complex of cisternae. In fact, contents of the endoplasmic reticulum and the golgi apparatus are often exchanged between the two. However, the function of the golgi apparatus is to package molecules for transport. There, molecules are concentrated and formed into vesicles. These vesicles are then prepared for transport outside of the cell. Some of these are bound for channels in the cell membrane that will allow the vesicles to leave the cell. However, vesicles of most relevance to the topic of this book are those that contain neurotransmitters. Those vesicles gradually travel to the terminal button (discussed below) and become released into the synapse.

The Cell Membrane

The membrane of the neuron is composed of two layers of lipids. These provide an effective barrier keeping intracellular fluid and the contents of the cell body inside of the cell, while keeping outside molecules from entering the cell. However, the membrane has many channels. These are programmed to allow certain molecules in or out of the cell. Some channels remain open, at least to some degree, most of the time. These transport crucial electrolytes in and out of the cell, including sodium and potassium. In fact, a particular type of a channel, called a sodium/potassium pump, is programmed to pump two molecules of potassium into the cell for every three molecules of sodium out of the cell. This precise proportion is designed to maintain a fragile balance of electrolytes inside the cell.

Other channels embedded in the membrane usually remain closed, but may open when a receptor attached to these channels becomes activated. Examples of these include channels that allow chloride and calcium into the cell. Because these electrolytes can significantly change the electrical charge across the membrane of the cell, they have a major impact on whether or not the cell will fire. More details about such channels are discussed in the next section, and in the next chapter.

The Dendrites

Dendrites are appendages that are designed to receive communications from other cells. They resemble a tree-like structure, forming projections that become stimulated by other neurons and conduct the electrochemical charge to the cell body (or, more rarely, directly to the axons). The surface of the dendrites is filled with receptors that become enacted upon by neurotransmitters that traversed the synapse after the presynaptic neuron fired and released neurotransmitters into the synapse. Dendrites integrate this stimulation (from a multitude of receptors) and play a crucial role in determining the extent to which the received stimulation will result in an action potential. Although dendrites have traditionally been regarded as receivers of the neurotransmission, recent research has found that dendrites can also release neurotransmitters into the synapse (Stuart *et al.*, 2008). This new data adds to our understanding of the incredible complexity of neuronal transmission.

The Axons

Axons, sometimes referred to as nerve fibers, are long appendages (in some cases, several feet in length) that transmit the action potential down its length during cell firing. When the cell becomes stimulated and firing begins, the electrochemical changes travel down the length of the axon. The axon terminates in a network of small appendages each of which contains terminal buttons. These buttons release the neurotransmitter into the synapse when the neuron fires.

The speed of the neural transmission depends on various properties of the axon, especially the nature of its membrane. Some axons are only encased in the same membrane that surrounds the rest of the cell body. However, others are additionally surrounded by sections of fatty tissue formed by glial cells. This insulation is called a myelin sheath, and it is produced in sections, separated by short gaps called nodes of Ranvier. The presence of myelin sheath greatly increases the speed with which an axon will transmit the action potential down its length. Indeed, most neurons are myelinated, and demyelination is a pathological process that is a common feature of disorders such as multiple sclerosis.

The Synapse

Synapses are microscopic gaps that separate the terminal buttons of one neuron from receptors (usually, located on the dendrites) of another neuron. When neurons communicate, they release chemicals that must travel across this gap to stimulate the post-synaptic receptors. The human brain contains trillions of neurons, although it contains about 100 billion neurons (see Figure 3.4). Thus, on average, each neuron communicates through tens of synapses, although in reality the range is very wide – some neurons terminate in few synapses, while others may be involved in communicating through thousands of synapses. Neurons also communicate with other cells. For example, neurons that control the motor system communicate with muscle cells and synapse with them.

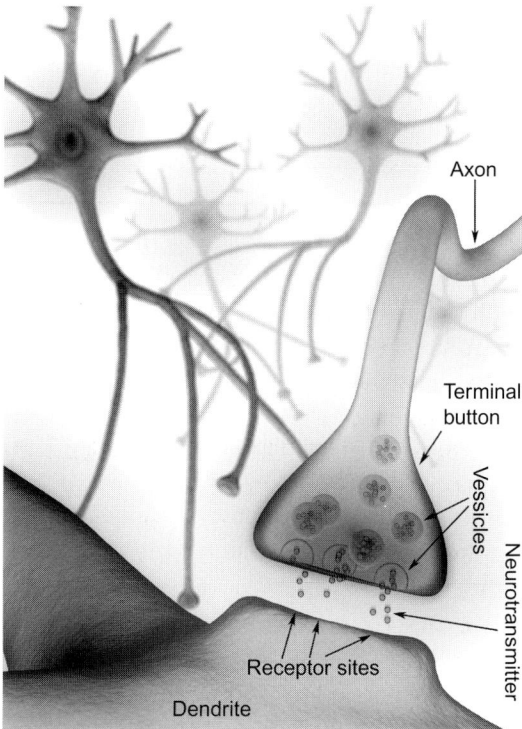

FIGURE 3.4 The synapse.

Although the typical structure of a synapse involves a gap that separates axonic terminal buttons of the pre-synaptic neurons with dendritic receptors of the post-synaptic cells, other types of synapses also exist. For example, some synapses separate axonic terminal buttons from receptors on cell bodies of the post-synaptic neurons, and other synapses separate pre-synaptic buttons from receptors on axons of the post-synaptic cells. Thus, although axodendritic synapses are the most common, axosomatic and axoaxonic synapses also exist.

Neuronal Communication

Neurons communicate with each other by transmitting messages across synapses. Communications usually flow one way, with pre-synaptic axons firing on post-synaptic receptors. However, some variation exists, and some neurons have several axons, some of which fire back upon the sending cell. This is evident in some cells that are responsible for the stimulation of the brain. For example, some neurons in areas of the brain stem that stimulate the stress response (like the locus coeruleus) are equipped with a feedback system where neurons simultaneously fire on post-synaptic cells and also on their own autoreceptors, turning off further firing. This feedback loop is designed to prevent overfiring, and defects in these autoreceptors may be responsible for symptoms of some anxiety disorders (like panic attacks).

At rest, the neuron is in a slightly polarized state. This means that the electrical charge across the membrane is about $-70\,mV$. When this occurs, the neuron is said to be in a state of a resting membrane potential. If changes within the neuron increase this negative charge, the neuron is said to be in a hyperpolarized state, and getting the neuron to fire is more difficult. Conversely, when changes within the cell cause the charge across the membrane to drop in the direction of a positive charge, the neuron becomes hypopolarized and firing becomes more likely. Hyperpolarization and hypopolarization is determined by many factors, one of which is the flow of ions in and out of the cell. Some molecules, for example chloride, carry a negative charge, so when membrane channels are open that allow chloride to flow into the cell, the neuron will become hyperpolarized and much more stimulation will be necessary to get it to fire. Conversely, calcium molecules carry a positive charge. When membrane channels open that allow calcium to flow into the cell, the neuron quickly becomes hypopolarized, and firing becomes much more likely.

When the neuron fires, the membrane becomes permeable to a number of exchanges between the inside and outside of the cell. This phenomenon 'travels' down the length of the axon, in a manner analogous to the way that electricity travels across a wire. However, because this is an electrochemical process, the charge must constantly be 'refueled' along the axon, and the exchange of electrolytes between the inside and outside of the cell maintains that charge. When the axon is unmyelinated, constant refueling of this impulse across the cell membrane takes place, and the impulse travels down the axon more slowly. By contrast, myelinated axons fire more quickly because sections of myelin sheath prevent the exchange of molecules across cell membrane and the electrical impulse inside the neuron 'jumps' from one node of Ranvier to another, where it undergoes chemical refueling. Thus, the majority of neurons are myelinated.

As discussed above, neurotransmitters are generally synthesized in the cell body and packaged into vesicles. These vesicles travel down the length of the axon and become grouped in terminal buttons. With axonal firing, the vesicles flow into the membrane of the terminal buttons and the vesicle membrane fuses with the terminal button membrane, spilling the contents into the synapse. The neurotransmitters then 'swim' across the synapse and become available to junction with post-synaptic receptors, exerting some effect on the post-synaptic cell.

Post-Synaptic Effects

As discussed in the next chapter, there is a large variety of neurotransmitter substances. In the most general terms, neurotransmitters act as agonists or antagonists on post-synaptic cells. Agonists increase the likelihood that the post-synaptic cell will fire. Usually, this is accomplished by affecting the polarization of the post-synaptic cell, but more subtle effects also take place. For example, one type of receptor (discussed below) does not result in immediate changes in polarization, but affects intracellular changes that may result in an increase of the cell's action potential, an increase in the production of a neurotransmitter, or other similar changes. Thus, although the effects may not be as immediate, the activity of the post-synaptic cell will nevertheless be increased in some way.

Antagonists exert the opposite effects. They decrease the likelihood that the post-synaptic cell will fire. This may be accomplished by activating receptors that allow negatively charged ions to flow into the cell to hyperpolarize it, or by exerting intracellular changes that decrease the metabolism of the neurotransmitter or otherwise decrease the action of the post-synaptic cell. Agonist effects are commonly exerted by both of these mechanisms, while antagonist effects are primarily the result of the activation of channels that hyperpolarize the post-synaptic cell.

Types of Receptors

As may be evident from the discussion above, two types of receptor cells are primarily present in the brain. Some receptors are attached to ion channels and are referred to as ionotropic. When these receptors are activated, the adjacent channels change in size. Usually, a receptor causes a channel that is completely or mostly closed to open more widely. As a result, molecules for which the channel is programmed flow into the cell, and the cell may become hyperpolarized or hypopolarized. Agonist effects are evident when a neurotransmitter binds to an ionotropic receptor and causes a channel to open that allows positively charged molecules (for example, calcium) to flow into the cell. Antagonist effects are evident when a neurotransmitter binds to an ionotropic receptor and causes a channel to open that allows negatively charged molecules (for example, chloride) to flow into the cell.

Ionotropic receptors may also change the size of channels that are usually open. For example, sodium channels must remain open in order to allow sodium to be exchanged between the inside and the outside of a cell. When neurotransmitters bind to receptors that change the size of these channels, the cell may become dysregulated. These effects are evident when some substances interfere with cardiac function. In addition, this is the mechanism of action of some poisons. Some plant extracts contain molecules that interfere with the action of sodium channels, and these compounds should generally be avoided.

Some molecules act as allosteric modulators. This means that the chemical exerts little effect of its own on an ionotropic channel, but has an effect on the degree to which another neurotransmitter can exert its effect on the post-synaptic cell. For example, alcohol is a substance that directly binds to post-synaptic receptors connected to chloride channels. When present together with gamma aminobutyric acid (GABA), a neurotransmitter that causes chloride channels to open, those channels open much wider. Thus, alcohol is considered to be an agonistic allosteric modulator of GABA.

Allosteric modulator effects may also be antagonistic. For example, phencyclidine (PCP) is a psychoactive compound that binds to receptors on calcium channels. When present with glutamate, a neurotransmitter that causes these channels to open, PCP seems to decrease the size of these channels. Thus, PCP is an antagonistic allosteric modulator of glutamate.

Another type of post-synaptic receptor is the metabotropic receptor. Rather than being attached to channels programmed to allow specific ions to pass through the membrane, metabotropic receptors are embedded in the cell wall and have extracellular and intracellular portions. The extracellular part is a sensor programmed to be activated by a specific molecule (the neurotransmitter). The intracellular part is a storage mechanism to which various g-proteins are attached. When the extracellular portion is activated, the intracellular part releases the g-proteins and allows them to swim into the cell body. These g-proteins then become involved in a variety of intracellular metabolic processes. They may bind to a variety of proteins and amino acids and may affect various cell functions. For example, they may contribute to the hyperpolarization or hypopolarization of the cell, thus affecting the cell's likelihood of firing. These g-proteins may also become building blocks for the conversion of neurotransmitters, and may increase the amount of neurotransmitter that the cell produces. Consequently, when the cell fires, more neurotransmitter may become released into the synapse, making it more likely that post-synaptic effects will increase.

Psychoactive effects are usually exerted by a combination of ionotropic and metabotropic effects. Since ionotropic receptors affect ion channels, their action is usually more rapid and the effects of substances that rely on this mechanism of action will generally be seen more quickly. However, long-term changes in the sensitivity of these receptors are less likely, and therefore the brain is more likely to return to baseline when the use of the substance is discontinued. By contrast, metabotropic effects take longer but may have more lasting effects, since they cause changes in the metabolic functions of the cell. Of course, this discussion is greatly simplified, and many substances exert clinical effects by both of these (as well as other, more complex) mechanisms.

Synapse Regulation

When a neurotransmitter is released into the synapse, various mechanisms are involved in controlling the amount of effect that it will be able to exert on the post-synaptic cell. The first of these is the process of reuptake. Autoreceptors on terminal buttons are programmed to react to the presence of the neurotransmitter in the synapse, and open channels that allow the neurotransmitter to flow right back into the releasing cell. In this way, the amount of the neurotransmitter that will remain in the synapse to become available to active post-synaptic receptors is carefully controlled. Back in the terminal button, golgi apparatuses may be present that will repackage the neurotransmitter into another vesicle, which may then be available for release with the next cycle of cell firing.

Chemical processes are also used to regulate the amount of neurotransmitter that is available to exert its action. In the synapse, and inside the terminal buttons, enzymes are present that are programmed to attach to the neurotransmitter and break it down into more basic (and inactive) components. When the neurotransmitter is packaged in the vesicle, the vesicle membrane protects it from degradation. However, when contents of the vesicle are released into the synapse, some neurotransmitter molecules then come in contact with the enzymes and are degraded. Similarly, after reuptake, neurotransmitter molecules are not immediately repackaged by the golgi apparatuses, and may come in contact with the enzymes. Thus, enzymatic degradation is another mechanism of regulating the amount of neurotransmitter that will be available to activate the post-synaptic cell.

Some pre-synaptic neurons also have metabotropic autoreceptors. When activated, these autoreceptors exert intracellular changes that affect a number of cell functions. Some of these may hyperpolarize the cell, thus making further firing less likely. Others may interfere with neurotransmitter production, thus decreasing the amount of neurotransmitter available when further firing takes place. This is yet another mechanism that regulates the levels of neurotransmitters in the cell and in the synapse.

Synapse regulation also takes place as a result of competition between a variety of substances for the same target receptors. Neurotransmitters generally activate receptors that are programmed to respond when neurotransmitter molecules come in contact with them. However, neurotransmitter molecules are complex chains, and molecules may also be around that resemble the neurotransmitter very closely, but not entirely. Such 'imposter' molecules may still bind to the receptors, since the chemical match is pretty close, but may not activate them. These substances are called receptor blockers. When a blocker occupies a receptor, it does not allow the neurotransmitter to bind to it, and therefore the action of that neurotransmitter will be affected. When the neurotransmitter and the blocker are both present in the synapse, the one that is present in greater amounts is likely to 'win' the contest and exert its action (either activation or blocking).

Receptor blockers may exert either agonist or antagonist action, depending on the nature of the neurotransmitter that they resemble. For example, substances that occupy GABA receptors without activating them will act as antagonists for GABA, and will at the same time be agonists for general brain activation, since GABA is an inhibitory neurotransmitter and decreases brain action. The reverse is true when an excitatory neurotransmitter is blocked. This competition provides yet another mechanism by which post-synaptic excitation is regulated.

Mechanisms of Psychoactive Effects

As mentioned before, an agonist effect exists when the likelihood of action is increased, while an antagonist effect exists when the likelihood of action is decreased. However, because neurotransmitters themselves can be excitatory or inhibitory (as discussed in the next chapter), agonist and antagonist effects may sometimes seem contradictory. For example, a substance can have an antagonist effect on a neurotransmitter, but if that neurotransmitter is inhibitory, antagonizing it will actually agonize brain function. Conversely, if a neurotransmitter is excitatory, antagonizing it will also antagonize brain function. Consequently, it is necessary to be clear what is being referred to when agonist or antagonist effects are described. In the discussion below, antagonist effects will be those that decrease the effects associated with the neurotransmitter being affected, and agonist effects will be those that increase those effects.

Agonist Effects

Agonist effects increase the action associated with the neurotransmitter being affected. When a neurotransmitter is released, its targets are the post-synaptic receptors. Thus, a substance can exert an agonist effect by causing more neurotransmitter to be released into the cell. This can occur by making the cell membrane more 'leaky,' thus increasing the possibility that vesicles will fuse with the terminal button membrane and release their contents into the synapse. A number of psychoactive substances utilize this mechanism of action, especially those classified as psychostimulants.

After the neurotransmitter is released, reuptake removes it from the synapse. Thus, agonist effects will also be evident when the reuptake mechanism is blocked or significantly slowed. When this occurs, more neurotransmitter will remain in the synapse, and for a longer period of time, increasing the chance of stimulating post-synaptic receptors. Many medications and several herbal compounds affect neurotransmitters by interfering with reuptake mechanisms.

Most neurotransmitters are broken down by enzymes that degrade the molecules into more basic compounds. These enzymes are usually present in the synapse and in the releasing cell. Blocking these enzymes or degrading them will prevent the enzymes from deactivating the neurotransmitter. When enzymes are degraded, more neurotransmitter will remain in the synapse, and for a longer period of time, thus increasing the likelihood of post-synaptic stimulation. In addition, reuptake takes the neurotransmitter molecules back into the cell, and if degrading enzymes are deactivated, the neurotransmitter will more likely find its way to the golgi apparatus and become repackaged into another vesicle, thus increasing the amount of the neurotransmitter available for release with further neuronal firing. Many classes of medications, and some herbal compounds (for example, St. John's Wort), exert their effects at least in part by utilizing this mechanism.

When it is desirable to increase the amount of action associated with a neurotransmitter, it may be helpful to increase its production within the cell. When this takes place, more neurotransmitter becomes available to be released with each neuronal firing. Since neurotransmitters are primarily synthesized from precursors ingested in food, increases in the intake of these compounds (for example, by taking dietary supplements) are sometimes presumed to be effective. Generally, results of research studies reveal that this method of increasing the production of the neurotransmitter is not effective. However, there are other methods of increasing production of the neurotransmitter. The most effective involves the activation of metabotropic receptors that allow g-proteins to be released into the cell, thus increasing the production of many molecules, including the neurotransmitter. Indeed, this mechanism is exploited by many antidepressant and anxiolytic compounds.

Since allosteric modulator substances modify the magnitude of the effect of neurotransmitters, the presence of such molecules may enhance post-synaptic stimulation of ionotropic receptors. Thus, even if the amount of neurotransmitter available to exert stimulation is relatively low, the presence of an agonist allosteric modulator will increase the degree of the post-synaptic effect. Many plant extracts produce psychoactive effects by magnifying the action of endogenous neurotransmitters.

Substances can also exert synergistic effects by additive properties. Many neurons have receptors for several neurotransmitters. In addition, neurotransmitters within the same chemical families closely resemble each other's molecular structure. Consequently, cross-binding may be evident where neurotransmitters not only bind to its own receptors, but also bind to receptors programmed for neurotransmitters that bear a close resemblance. When it is desirable to increase the effects of one neurotransmitter, increasing the level of its sister compound may have broad effects that include the desired action. This method of effect is often evident with the use of medications and supplements that exert antidepressant and psychostimulant effects.

Antagonist Effects

Antagonist effects decrease the action associated with the neurotransmitter being affected. Since a neurotransmitter must 'swim' across the synapse, and avoid reuptake and enzymatic degradation in the process, decreasing the amount of the neurotransmitter being released will decrease the chances of post-synaptic stimulation. This can occur by making the cell membrane more impervious, thus decreasing the possibility that vesicles will fuse with the terminal button membrane and release their contents into the synapse. Some psychoactive compounds that exert antipsychotic action partially utilize this mechanism of action.

Since reuptake removes the neurotransmitter from the synapse, increasing the rate of reuptake will remove more neurotransmitter, thus decreasing the likelihood of post-synaptic stimulation. The neurotransmitter can then be more likely to be deactivated by degrading enzymes and may not become repackaged. Although most compounds do not rely on this mechanism to exert its primary action, this may be a secondary method in which some anxiolytics reduce anxiety.

Enzymes that degrade neurotransmitter molecules are often present in the synapse and in the releasing cell. Increasing the production of these enzymes will increase the rates of degradation of the neurotransmitter. As a result, less neurotransmitter will remain in the synapse and the likelihood of post-synaptic stimulation will be decreased. In addition, since reuptake takes in the neurotransmitter molecules back into the cell, increased presence of degrading enzymes will decrease the chance of the neurotransmitter becoming repackaged into another vesicle, thus decreasing the amount of the neurotransmitter available for release with further neuronal firing. Once again, this is not the primary action of most psychoactive compounds, but some anxiolytics and mood stabilizers may partially work through these mechanisms of action.

When it is desirable to decrease the amount of action associated with a neurotransmitter, it may be helpful to decrease its production within the cell. When this takes place, less neurotransmitter will be available to be released with each subsequent firing. Metabotropic autoreceptors generally trigger this mechanism in order to avoid excessive excitation of neurons. Compounds that activate these autoreceptors use this mechanism to produce their inhibitory effects, and anxiolytics, mood stabilizers, and antipsychotics often exert their effect at least in part by this action.

Allosteric modulator substances modify the magnitude of the effect of neurotransmitters, and the presence of such molecules may decrease post-synaptic stimulation of ionotropic receptors. Thus, even if the amount of neurotransmitter available to exert stimulation remains constant, the presence of an antagonist allosteric modulator will decrease the degree of the post-synaptic effect. Many plant extracts produce psychoactive effects by altering the action of endogenous neurotransmitters.

Substances can also exert effects by competitive properties. Some molecules may bind to receptors without activating them, and in the process make the receptors unavailable for binding with the neurotransmitter. Consequently, when receptor blockers are present, they will compete for receptor sites and decrease post-synaptic stimulation at least to some extent. Some psychoactive substances utilize these mechanisms, including those that are used to prevent brain overstimulation – for example, antipsychotics, tranquilizers, and compounds used to block the effects of heroin or other substances of abuse. Some naturopathic compounds for example, rauwolfia also work in this manner.

Chapter 4

Substances Involved in Neurotransmission

Neurons communicate with each other by way of releasing chemical transmitters that potentially affect the post-synaptic cells. Collectively, these substances are known as neurotransmitters. However, there are other substances that are actively involved in neurotransmission. Some chemical messengers only cross the synapse, while others travel long distances to affect target sites. All neurotransmitters are synthesized within the body, from precursors generally ingested during meals consumed as part of a normal diet. Thus, changes in levels of neurotransmitter precursors may, at least theoretically, change the amount of neurotransmitter substances synthesized by the cells. Even when sufficient amounts of precursors are present, a variety of other enzymes and related substances, collectively called second messengers, affects neurotransmitter synthesis. While some of these enzymes are also synthesized within the cells, others must cross the membrane in order to enter the cell, and molecules that regulate the permeability of cell membranes may affect the degree to which these substances can travel into the cell. Consequently, a comprehensive understanding of neuronal communication must include the knowledge of how all of these substances affect neurotransmission.

NEUROTRANSMITTERS AND HORMONES

Neurotransmitters are chemicals released from the neuron in order to exert potential effect on some receptors. Actually, neurons release chemicals that can act as neurotransmitters or hormones. Neurotransmitters communicate across the synapse and seek to exert some effect on the post-synaptic cell. By contrast, hormones are transmitters that are released into systemic circulation (for example, the blood stream) and travel longer distances to find their target sites. Thus, neurotransmitters are short-distance messengers, and hormones are long-distance communicators, and some chemical substances act as both. For example, epinephrine, a neurotransmitter within the central nervous system, also acts as a peripheral hormone.

Neurotransmitters and hormones can be grouped into various categories, based on their chemical structure, sites of effect, or type of influence on the receptors. Generally, neurotransmitter and hormones exert excitatory effects, stimulating relevant portions of the brain and body, but some are inhibitors, causing a decrease in activation of its targets. In addition, some of these chemicals are present in distinct pathways within the brain, while others are endogenous to the entire brain. The following discussion will point out these differences in order to help readers understand the complex nature of neuronal action and the homeostatic mechanisms employed by the brain.

Dopamine

Dopamine is a monoamine. Monoamines are neurotransmitters that belong to a chemical group that is composed of one amino group (organic compounds with a nitrogen atom and paired electrons of other molecules), an aromatic group (stable atomic molecules arranged into a circle), and a two-carbon chain. Monoamines comprise a large group of neurotransmitters, including catecholamines, indolamines, and histamine, and most are involved in many psychoactive effects.

Monoamines are synthesized through a process that initially involves the conversion of amino acid precursors, like tyrosine or tryptophan, into trace amines, like tyramine or tryptamine, which are then converted through enzymes into neurotransmitters. Thus, levels of monoamine neurotransmitters may be affected by the amount of available precursors, as well as the availability of enzymes necessary to complete the steps needed for neurotransmitter conversion.

Dopamine belongs to a subgroup of monoamines called catecholamines, since it also includes a molecule of catechol. The precursor of dopamine is tyrosine. Tyrosine is ingested from dietary protein, especially in foods that are aged, like most cheeses, types of meats (for example, salami), red wine, etc. Tyrosine is also converted in the body from another monoamine precursor, phenylalanine. This complex mechanism is needed in order to assure that regardless of dietary intake, sufficient amounts of tyrosine are available to produce this crucial neurotransmitter. Tyrosine is converted into levodopa (L-Dopa), which is then converted into dopamine. Since L-Dopa is also a naturally occurring amino acid found in food (for example, in some types of beans), dietary intake of L-Dopa may affect the amount of dopamine produced within the cell. In fact, L-Dopa is also a neurotransmitter involved in regulation of motor control, and supplementation with L-Dopa is a well-known treatment for some dementias (like Parkinson's). When L-Dopa is administered orally, its absorption is dependent on dietary considerations. For example, protein tends to interfere with the absorption of L-Dopa, and when L-Dopa supplements are administered, patients are advised to change their diet so that protein is not ingested when L-Dopa is administered (Kempster & Wahlqvist, 1994). However, this may only apply to L-Dopa supplements, and therefore intake of protein may have no effects on the degree to which endogenous L-Dopa is converted into dopamine.

Levels of dopamine are regulated by several mechanisms. Enzymes that break down this neurotransmitter are present in the synapse, as well as inside the neurons. These include Catechol-O-methyl transferase (COMT) and monoamine oxydase (MAO). These enzymes degrade dopamine and inactivate its neurotransmitting properties. In addition, dopamine is subject to reuptake by a pre-synaptic transporter that results in excess dopamine being taken up by the cell that just released it.

Dopamine stimulates five dopamine receptor types on post-synaptic cells, identified as D1 through D5, and the D2 receptors are also present pre-synaptically. All of these are metabotropic and are involved in the release of g-proteins into the post-synaptic cell, changing the intracellular concentration of the second messenger cyclic adenosine monophosphate (cAMP). Post-synaptically, activation of the receptors modulates the activity of various ion channels and increases the likelihood that the post-synaptic neuron will fire. Pre-synaptically, activation of the D2 autoreceptor decreases the amount of cAMP and decreases the pre-synaptic action potential. This system is in place to limit the extent to which a dopamine-releasing neuron will continue firing.

Dopamine is an excitatory neurotransmitter that stimulates neurons in four specific brain pathways. Dopaminergic projections start in the substantia nigra and ventral tegmentum areas of the brain stem and extend into various cortical and subcortical areas.

One pathway leads to the basal ganglia and regulates motor control. This is a crucial pathway for regulation of motor control as well as motor planning. Disturbances in dopaminergic control of this pathway results in a number of significant psychological symptoms. When basal ganglia are underactive, problems in motor control become apparent, such as those that are evident in Parkinson's dementia. However, underactivity of the basal ganglia also results in motor symptoms where the ability to control the movement, rather than produce it, is impaired. Tics evident in a variety of tic disorders (including Tourette's disorder), and compulsions evident in obsessive compulsive disorder (OCD) are the result of the underactivation of the basal ganglia. In addition motor hyperactivity evident in attention deficit hyperactivity disorder (ADHD) is also presumed to be caused, at least in part, by the underactivation of the D1 and D4 dopaminergic receptors in the basal ganglia.

Another dopaminergic pathway controls portions of the limbic system. This limbic pathway includes projections between the ventral tegmental area and the nucleus accumbens, and this short pathway is known as the reward center of the brain. Many drugs of abuse stimulate D1 and D2 receptors in this pathway, resulting in the 'high' that is associated with substance abuse. Overactivation of D2 receptors may also occur endogenously. For example, psychosis may be evident when D2 receptors in the limbic pathway are hyperstimulated. This has been shown to occur during active episodes of psychosis associated with schizophrenia and other psychotic disorders.

Dopaminergic projections also activate portions of the frontal cortex. The dorsolateral prefrontal cortex is involved in the control of cognitions – specifically, the ability to sustain attention and perform sequential problem solving. The ventromedial prefrontal cortex is similarly involved in cognitive and attentional processes. Both of these areas are stimulated by the mesocortical dopaminergic pathway. When these brain areas are underactive, symptoms of distractibility are apparent. Severe underactivation of these pathways, for example, when these areas become damaged as a result of the progressive brain degeneration evident in schizophrenia, so-called 'negative' symptoms of schizophrenia (severe cognitive deficits) become evident.

The fourth dopaminergic pathway runs from the hypothalamus to the pituitary, and stimulates the pituitary to release hormones. This is especially evident during stress reactions, but may also be involved in sleep regulation. Overactivation of this pathway causes difficulties with sleep and overproduction of stress hormones. Underactivation of this pathway may be evident in depression.

When dopaminergic pathways are underactive, several strategies can be employed to increase the levels of dopamine. First and foremost, taking dopamine as a supplement is ineffective. Dopamine easily becomes oxidized and supplemental dopamine does not make it into the brain, and therefore taking supplemental dopamine is useless. Consequently, other mechanisms must be utilized to increase cortical and subcortical levels of dopamine.

Some medications interfere with the enzymatic degradation of dopamine by decreasing the action of the MAO enzyme. Although these medications have been around for a long time, they pose life-threatening risks (for example, stroke) associated with non-reversible deactivation of this enzyme. Some herbal supplements (for example, St. John's Wort) may inhibit this enzyme to a more minor degree. Another strategy involves decreasing the reuptake and/or increasing the pre-synaptic release of dopamine. This mechanism is evident in the action of many drugs of abuse (like methamphetamine), as well as prescription stimulants (like methylphenidate). Some naturopathic compounds, like ephedrine, also work by utilizing this mechanism, but these supplements are often dangerous and generally are not recommended. Some compounds bypass pre-synaptic processes and stimulate post-synaptic receptors directly. Again, some drugs of abuse exert their effect in this manner, and most nutritional and herbal stimulants do not bind to post-synaptic receptors for dopamine. Finally, some naturopathic compounds (for example, phenylalanine) may increase the availability of the precursor for catecholamines (including dopamine), and this mechanism may have some efficacy in treatment of depression (as discussed in Chapter 6).

When dopaminergic pathways are overactive, mechanisms must be utilized to slow down the firing in dopaminergic pathways. Some nutritional and herbal supplements directly interfere with dopaminergic stimulation, although most compounds used to decrease dopaminergic activation (for example, to decrease psychosis) usually exert their action by effecting more global brain effects (discussed later in the chapter).

Norepinephrine

Like dopamine, norepinephrine is also a monoamine and a catecholamine. Also known as noradrenaline, norepinephrine is also converted from tyrosine. In fact, norepinephrine is produced from dopamine. Thus, tyrosine is gradually converted by various enzymes into L-Dopa, then dopamine, and then norepinephrine. Consequently, factors involved in regulation of the conversion of tyrosine will affect not only levels of dopamine, but also levels of norepinephrine.

As is the case with dopamine, levels of norepinephrine are regulated by several mechanisms. Enzymes that break down this neurotransmitter are present in the synapse, as well as inside the neurons, and include COMT and MAO. In addition, norepinephrine is also subject to reuptake by a pre-synaptic transporter that results in excess norepinephrine being taken up by the cell that just released it.

Norepinephrine stimulates two families of receptor types on post-synaptic cells, identified as alpha and beta, and alpha receptors are also present pre-synaptically. All of these are metabotropic and are involved in the release of g-proteins into the post-synaptic cell, changing the intracellular concentration of various second messengers, including cAMP. Post-synaptically, activation of the receptors modulates the activity of various ion channels (including calcium) and increases the likelihood that the post-synaptic neuron will fire. Pre-synaptically, activation of the alpha-2 autoreceptor decreases the amount of cAMP and calcium that flows into the cell, and consequently decreases the pre-synaptic action potential. This system is in place to limit the extent to which a norepinephrine-releasing neuron will continue to fire.

Norepinephrine is an excitatory neurotransmitter and hormone that stimulates receptors in several specific brain and peripheral pathways. Noradrenergic projections start in the locus coeruleus area of the brain stem and extend into various cortical and subcortical areas. In addition, noradrenaline activates autonomic projections, and is also released into the blood stream to exert its action as a hormone.

Two noradrenergic pathways stimulate the frontal lobes. The prefrontal pathway is involved in the regulation of mood and may have a role in symptoms of depression. The other frontal pathway contributes to the dopaminergic control of attentional and cognitive functions. Underactivation of these pathways may contribute to the symptoms of distractibility evident in ADHD, as well as symptoms of cognitive slowing associated with depression.

The limbic pathway is the most important projection that is involved in the activation of the fight–flight mechanism. When locus coeruleus activates the hypothalamus, the hypothalamus then activates the pituitary (through a dopaminergic pathway), and the pituitary releases hormones (including noradrenaline) that activate the sympathetic nervous system. Thus, overactivation of this limbic pathway plays a major role in producing symptoms of anxiety, especially panic attacks. This pathway is also associated with symptoms of psychomotor agitations commonly evident in some forms of mixed-manic and depressive episodes. Conversely, underactivation of this pathway has been associated with flatness of emotional tone and lack of the ability to experience empathy commonly associated with antisocial personality characteristics.

The cerebellar noradrenergic pathway activates the cerebellum and is involved in motor control. Together with dopaminergic projections that activate the frontal lobes and the basal ganglia, it is involved in the execution of motor behaviors, as well as motor control and planning.

Underactivation of this pathway may play a contributory role in symptoms of ADHD.

The remaining noradrenergic pathways are involved in the activation of smooth muscles and bodily organs. Norepinephrine plays a major role in the regulation of blood pressure, heart rate, and bladder control. This is important to consider, since changes in overall levels of norepinephrine are likely to affect many autonomic functions, including symptoms that may potentially be life threatening.

When noradrenergic pathways are underactive, similar strategies can be employed that are used to increase the levels of dopamine. Again, taking supplemental norepinephrine is useless, but some medications increase levels of norepinephrine by decreasing the action of the MAO enzyme, and some herbal supplements may increase levels of norepinephrine by inhibiting this enzyme to a minor degree. Substances may also decrease the reuptake and/or increase the pre-synaptic release of dopamine. This mechanism is evident in the secondary action of many drugs of abuse (like methamphetamine), as well as some prescription medications (like atomoxetine). Although some herbal preparations also work by utilizing this mechanism, some of these compounds are dangerous and their use must carefully be monitored. As with dopamine, some compounds may stimulate post-synaptic noradrenaline receptors directly, but most nutritional and herbal stimulants do not exert their action through such mechanisms. Finally, some naturopathic compounds (for example, phenylalanine) may increase the availability of the precursor for catecholamines (including norepinephrine), and this mechanism may have some efficacy in treatment of depression (as discussed in Chapter 6).

When noradrenergic pathways are overactive, some mechanisms may be utilized to slow down norepinephrine pathways. While some medications decrease norepinephrine activity directly (for example, alpha and beta-blockers, both of which are antihypertensives), most nutritional and herbal supplements do not directly interfere with noradrenaline stimulation, and those compounds used to decrease noradrenergic activation usually exert their action by effecting more global brain effects.

Epinephrine

Epinephrine (also known as adrenaline) is also a monoamine and catecholamine. It is produced in the final step of conversion of tyrosine. Thus, the complete cycle is evident when tyrosine is gradually converted by various enzymes into L-Dopa, then dopamine, then norepinephrine, and then epinephrine. Consequently, factors involved in regulation of the conversion of tyrosine will affect levels of epinephrine in the same ways previously discussed for dopamine and norepinephrine.

As with dopamine and norepinephrine, levels of epinephrine are regulated by several mechanisms. Enzymes that break down this neurotransmitter are present in the synapse, as well as inside the neurons, and include COMT and MAO. In addition, epinephrine is also subject to reuptake by a pre-synaptic transporter that results in excess epinephrine being taken up by the cell that just released it.

Epinephrine does not have its own receptors. Instead, since its chemical composition resembles norepinephrine very closely, epinephrine stimulates norepinephrine receptors both in the brain as well as peripherally. In fact, while norepinephrine is primarily a neurotransmitter, epinephrine is primarily a hormone. Consequently, the action of adrenaline is essentially that of noradrenaline, with more intense peripheral effects. Effects of epinephrine stimulation are especially evident during stress reactions, and epinephrine is one of the major hormones involved in the stimulation of the sympathetic nervous system. Stimulation of adrenergic receptors is likely to exert sympathetic effects, while blocking those receptors will result in parasympathetic reactions. Most nutritional and herbal compounds do not exert their effect by binding to adrenaline receptors, although some dangerous compounds, like ephedrine, exert their stimulatory effects by binding to a variety of catecholinergic receptors, including those usually stimulated by adrenaline.

Serotonin

Serotonin is a neurotransmitter that belongs to a subgroup of monoamines called indolamines, since it includes a molecule of indole (benzene and nitrogen). The precursor of serotonin is tryptophan. Tryptophan is an amino acid that is a routine constituent of most protein-based foods. Tryptophan is also one of the 20 amino acids present in standard genetic material. In several steps, tryptophan is converted into serotonin through various enzymes.

Levels of serotonin are regulated by several mechanisms. Because it is a monoamine, the MAO enzyme that breaks down catecholamines also breaks down serotonin. In addition, serotonin is subject to reuptake by a pre-synaptic transporter that results in excess serotonin being taken up by the cell that just released it.

Serotonin stimulates many subtypes of post-synaptic receptors, divided into four families (5HT1, 5HT2, 5HT3, and 5HT4), some of which have several subtypes (for example, 5HT1A and 5HT1C). Most of these are metabotropic and are involved in the release of g-proteins into the post-synaptic cell, changing the intracellular concentration of various second messengers, including cAMP. However, the 5HT3 receptor is ionotropic and regulates sodium and potassium channels. Post-synaptically, activation of the serotonin receptors modulates the activity of various ion channels and increases the likelihood that the post-synaptic neuron will fire. Pre-synaptically, activation of the 5HT1D autoreceptor decreases the amount of cAMP and decreases the pre-synaptic action potential. This system is in place to limit the extent to which a serotonin-releasing neuron will continue firing.

Serotonin is an excitatory neurotransmitter that stimulates neurons in four specific brain pathways. Serotonergic projections start in the raphe nucleus area of the brain stem and extend into various cortical and sub-cortical areas.

One pathway stimulates the frontal lobes. The pre-frontal pathway is involved in the regulation of cognitive functions. Underactivation of this pathway may contribute to the symptoms of cognitive deficits associated with depression. In addition, serotonin acts as a regulator of noradrenergic activity in the frontal pathway. Thus, cognitive deficits evident in depression may be the result of limited serotonin regulation of noradrenergic activity in this pathway.

Another serotonergic pathways leads to the basal ganglia and con-tributes to the regulation of motor control. Although dopamine is the major neurotransmitter in this pathway, serotonin tends to regulate its activity, and act as an inhibitor of dopaminergic activation. This regula-tory system is designed to control the amount of dopaminergic activa-tion in those areas of the brain. Thus, when dopaminergic stimulation in this pathway is insufficient, blockage of serotonin may restore appropri-ate level of activity within those areas. Such mechanisms are utilized by some medications (for example, atypical antipsychotics). Interestingly, however, although increasing dopaminergic activity within this pathway improves symptoms of ADHD, blockage of serotonin does not seem to produce similar benefits. Thus, the relationship between dopamine and serotonin in this pathway is more complex than we currently understand.

Another serotonergic pathway controls portions of the limbic system. Here, serotonin once again acts as an inhibitor that regulates the amount of noradrenergic stimulation of this pathway. Thus, when locus coeruleus stimulates the fight–flight response, serotonin acts to increase the amount of this stimulation and prevent the system from becoming dysregulated.

Similarly, serotonin also regulates the extent to which the hypoth-alamus activates the pituitary. By inhibiting dopaminergic activity, serotonin prevents overactivation of this pathway. As is the case in the limbic pathway, this system is probably designed to prevent overactivation of the fight–flight mechanism.

The remaining serotonergic pathways are involved in the regulation of the brain stem, smooth muscles, and bodily organs. Serotonin plays a major role in the regulation of gastrointestinal functions, including the vomiting reflex. It also plays a role in the regulation of sleep–wake cycles, although serotonin's function in sleep regulation may be related to the degree to which it is available as a precursor for melatonin (as discussed below).

When serotonergic pathways are underactive, similar strategies can be employed that are used to increase the levels of catecholamines. Compounds that decrease the action of the MAO enzyme will increase the availability of serotonin within the synapse, and some herbal supplements may inhibit this enzyme to a minor degree. Substances may also decrease the reuptake of serotonin, and this is a major action of many compounds with anxiolytic and antidepressant properties (for example, St. John's Wort). Although some compounds may also stimulate post-synaptic serotonin receptors directly, most nutritional and herbal stimulants do not exert their action through such mechanisms, although some drugs of abuse (for example, LSD) work in this manner. Finally, some naturopathic compounds (for example, tryptophan or 5-HTP) may increase the availability of the precursor for serotonin, and this mechanism may have some efficacy in treatment of depression, anxiety, and sleep disorders (as discussed in Chapters 6, 8, and 9).

Thus far, no disorders have been associated with endogenous overactivity of serotonergic pathways, although excessive supplementation with serotonin agonists has been known to produce symptoms of 'serotonin syndrome' that, in some cases, has been known to be fatal. Symptom onset is usually rapid, often occurring within minutes. Serotonin syndrome encompasses a wide range of clinical findings. Mild symptoms may consist of increased heart rate, temperature regulation problems (shivering or sweating), dilated pupils, muscle tremors or twitching, and hyperactive reflexes. Moderate toxicity includes additional symptoms of hyperactive bowels, high blood pressure, fever, and agitation. Severe toxicity includes heart dysrhythmia, hypertension, agitated delirium, muscular rigidity, seizures, and renal failure. Consequently, when administering supplements that may increase levels of serotonin, clinicians must use caution and carefully monitor the patient's response.

Melatonin

Melatonin is also a monoamine that belongs to a subgroup of indolamines. The precursor of melatonin is tryptophan. Thus, the conversion of tryptophan involves several steps, and serotonin and melatonin are produced in stages. Consequently, levels of serotonin affect levels of melatonin, and a serotonin deficiency may also result in decreased levels of melatonin.

Levels of melatonin are regulated by mechanisms similar to those that regulate serotonin. Because it is a monoamine, it is the MAO enzyme that breaks it down, and melatonin is subject to reuptake by a pre-synaptic transporter that results in excess serotonin being taken up by the cell that just released it. However, melatonin is primarily a hormone, released into the blood stream. Thus, levels of melatonin are primarily regulated by the retina and the pineal gland, which release most of the melatonin found in the central nervous system. Peripherally, melatonin is also released by the skin, and bone marrow. Although most of the melatonin is produced outside of the blood–brain barrier, it seems able to cross it and exert its effect both centrally and peripherally.

Melatonin binds to receptors on the brain and in various organs of the body. In the brain, melatonin contributes to other mechanisms that regulate circadian rhythms, and is involved in control of the sleep–wake cycle. Elsewhere, melatonin is thought to be an antioxidant and may interact with the immune system, although the specific mechanisms and effects of this relationship have not yet been identified. Consequently, melatonin is being researched as a potential treatment for cancer, immune disorders, and cardiovascular disease.

A deficit in melatonin has been implicated as one mechanism responsible for sleep disorders, especially insomnia. Those types of sleep difficulties where patients find it very hard to fall asleep after going to bed may be regulated by melatonin. In addition, melatonin supplementation has been shown to increase dreaming and has been used to address REM sleep deficits seen in patients with sleep disorders (including narcolepsy). Thus far, no disorders have been associated with excess levels of melatonin, and melatonin supplements are commonly used to treat sleep disorders (as discussed in Chapter 9), and may have some benefit in treating symptoms of mania (as discussed in Chapter 7).

Histamine

Histamine is a monoamine that does not belongs to either catecholamine or indolamine subgroups. It is metabolized from the precursor histidine. It is released into some synapses, and also into the blood stream where it acts as a hormone. It is also broken down by an enzyme, and may be removed from the synapse through reuptake.

Histamine stimulates four subtypes of post-synaptic receptors. These are concentrated in the brain as well as in smooth muscles, gastric cells, and in bone marrow. Histamine is also known as a neuromodulator, since it regulates the release of other neurotransmitters, like acetylcholine, norepinephrine, and serotonin. It also has pre-synaptic receptors that control the amount of histamine that is released. This system is in place to limit the extent to which a histamine-releasing neuron will continue firing.

Histamine is primarily associated with the functioning of the immune system. During an immune reaction, histamine is released and contributes to physical changes necessary for the immune system to fight a pathogen, including the increase in blood pressure, temperature, swelling, and bronchial constriction.

The psychoactive properties of histamine are not yet well understood. Histamine is known to contribute to the regulation of sleep and wakefulness. Histamine cells fire rapidly during states of wakefulness, fire slowly during states of rest, and do not fire during REM sleep. Blocking histamine is a well-known pharmacological approach used to induce sleep.

In addition, histamine also plays a role in sexual dysfunction, and supplementation with folic acid and niacin (used together), as well as L-histidine (an enzyme that metabolizes histamine from histidine) has been shown to be effective in addressing histamine deficiencies. Low levels of histamine have also been shown to correlate with schizophrenia.

Although some supplements are sometimes used to address deficits in histamine, it is more common for psychoactive compounds to exert antagonist effects on histamine receptors. Antihistamine side effects include drowsiness and fatigue, and these reactions are sometimes seen with a variety of psychoactive supplements and medications.

Acetylcholine

Acetylcholine is a non-monoamine neurotransmitter that is prevalent in the central and peripheral nervous systems. It is synthesized from choline and acetyl coenzyme A (AcCoA). Choline is a nutrient that is classified within the B-complex group of vitamins. Choline is present in many foods, including egg yolks, soy, and many types of meat. The human body synthesizes the other precursor, AcCoa from glucose in order to have needed sources of both precursors available for metabolism of acetylcholine. Some individuals who do not consume choline-rich foods in sufficient quantities may need to take choline as a supplement (usually, in the form of lecithin).

Levels of acetylcholine are regulated by several mechanisms. It is broken down by two types of cholinesterase enzymes, and it is also subject to reuptake by a pre-synaptic transporter that results in excess acetylcholine being taken up by the cell that just released it.

Acetylcholine stimulates two families of post-synaptic receptors, muscarinic and nicotinic. Muscarinic receptors are those that respond not only to acetylcholine but also to muscarine, a compound found in some mushrooms (including poisonous ones). Overstimulation of muscarinic receptors may result in death. These receptors are metabotropic and the associated g-proteins are involved in the gradual depolarization of acetylcholine transmission involved in slow peripheral nerve conduction. By contrast, nicotinic receptors are stimulated by acetylcholine and nicotine, and are ionotropic. Nicotinic receptors control ion channels for sodium and potassium, and opening of these channels causes quick depolarization of the neuron resulting in rapid firing. This type of neurotransmission generally occurs in junctional folds at neuromuscular junctions, and is involved in motor control.

Acetylcholine pathways originate in two distinct parts of the brain. Projections that start from the lateral tegmental area of the brain stem extend to the striatal regions of the basal ganglia, and are primarily involved in motor control. Acetylcholine is also the primary neurotransmitter that controls the somatic branches of the peripheral nervous system, innervating pathways that are responsible for motor control. Changes in levels of acetylcholine in these central and peripheral pathways result in many motor side effects, including tremors and problems with coordination of movements.

Another set of brain pathways start from the nucleus basalis of Meynert (in the vicinity of the thalamus) and project to the hippocampus, amygdala, and portions of the frontal lobes. These pathways are responsible for regulation of memory encoding, fear reactions, and cognitive functions. Thus, acetylcholine may play a contributory role to cognitive deficits evident in depression as well as symptoms associated with anxiety reactions. In addition, some naturopathic compounds (for example, lecithin and choline) may increase the availability of the precursor for acetylcholine, and this mechanism may have some efficacy in treatment of symptoms of mania, ADHD, and tic disorders (as discussed in Chapters 5, 7, and 10).

When acetylcholine function is depressed, many side effects are evident. Since acetylcholine is the major neurotransmitter involved in memory encoding, underactivation of these pathways (as evident in Alzheimer's) results in significant difficulties with forming new memories. Decrease in acetylcholine function is also associated with cognitive blunting and problems with motor control. Some compounds block cholinergic receptors and produce significant adverse effects, including constipation, dry mouth, blurred vision, and drowsiness.

Overactivation of acetylcholine pathways similarly results in unpleasant and potentially dangerous side effects. Direct overactivation of muscarinic receptors, evident when large amounts of muscarine are ingested, results in increased salivation, perfuse sweating, lacrimation, severe nausea, and diarrhea. Death from cardiac or respiratory arrest may then follow. More minor increases in acetylcholine stimulation are not lethal, but are unpleasant. In the motor system, in pathways where both dopamine and acetylcholine are present (for example, in the basal ganglia), dopamine acts as a regulator for acetylcholine release. When dopamine is suppressed, as is the case with some antipsychotic compounds, acetylcholine levels rise dramatically and motor rigidity, spasms, restlessness, drooling, tremor, and shuffling become evident. These are commonly called extra-pyramidal side effects (EPS). Persistent EPS is not only unpleasant, it may become permanent when tardive dyskinesia (TD) becomes evident. This disorder is caused by a permanent upregulation of receptors and the symptoms are permanent and untreatable. Obviously, clinicians must be very careful administering any compounds that may result in low levels of acetylcholine and/or choline depletion.

Glutamate

Glutamate, also known as glutamic acid, is an amino acid neurotransmitter that is very prevalent in the central nervous systems. It is synthesized from glutamine, a nutrient present in many meats, eggs, dairy products, wheat, and various vegetables (for example, cabbage, beets, beans, spinach, and parsley). It is also available as a flavor enhancer in many forms, including monosodium glutamate (MSG), a flavoring agent derived from sugar beets and commonly used in oriental cuisine.

Levels of glutamate are regulated by a mechanism that recycles glutamate into glutamine. Glutamate is taken up by glial cells that neighbor the releasing neurons. There, it is desynthesized into glutamine, passed back into the releasing neuron, resynthesized into glutamate, and packaged into vesicles to be released again into the synapse.

Rather than stimulating specific pathways, glutamate is present in the entire brain. It is the most abundant excitatory neurotransmitter and contributes to the stimulation of nearly every synapse. Four types of post-synaptic glutamate receptors have been identified, three of which are ionotropic. Glutamate receptors control the opening of calcium channels in the cell membrane. Because calcium ions are positively charged, influx of calcium into the cell rapidly depolarizes it, and the neuron will be induced to fire. In fact, influx of calcium into the cell depolarizes the cell so effectively that rapid firing may occur. When this continues, the cell may become overstimulated and continue to fire without sufficient refractory periods between impulses. This can damage the cell and, over time, cell death may result from overstimulation of glutamatergic neurotransmission.

Overactivation of glutamate neurons is also associated with other risks. Glutamatergic activity, especially when not properly synchronized, has been implicated as a causal factor in seizures, where a paroxysmal depolarizing shift causes spontaneous firing of large groups of neurons, about 1 second apart. Glutamate dysregulations may also be involved in symptoms of bipolar disorder, especially those of mania. Consequently, some medications and naturopathic supplements are used to suppress glutamatergic activity in the brain.

However, when glutamate function is depressed, significant side effects may become evident, especially including lethargy, fatigue, and, in extreme cases, respiratory arrest and death. Thus, excessive antagonism of glutamatergic neurotransmission can be dangerous. Interestingly, glutamate is also involved in memory mechanisms responsible for extinction (forgetting). When glutamate activity is too low within the memory circuits (for example, at the hippocampus), memories may become encoded too vividly, and the usual process of fading does not take place. This has been proposed as a mechanism responsible for recurring post-traumatic flashbacks experienced by individuals with post-traumatic stress disorder (PTSD).

No naturopathic compounds appear to exert their effects primarily by altering levels of glutamatergic activation, although some anxiolytics work by changing the relative balance of glutamate–GABA activation (as described below).

GABA

Gamma aminobutyric acid, commonly referred to as GABA, is an amino acid neurotransmitter that is also prevalent in the central nervous systems. It is synthesized from glutamate, the neurotransmitter described above. When glutamate is synthesized from glutamine, some of it is packaged into vesicles and released into the synapse, and some neurons further transform glutamate into GABA and then release it into the synapse.

Levels of GABA are regulated by two mechanisms. Through a process of reuptake excess GABA is taken up by the releasing neurons. GABA is also degraded by an enzyme that breaks it down into more basic constituents. These two mechanisms are utilized to prevent excessive GABAergic effects within the brain.

Like glutamate, GABA is present in the entire brain. It is the most abundant inhibitory neurotransmitter that balances glutamate's stimulation of synapses. Four types of post-synaptic GABA receptors have been identified, three of which are ionotropic. GABA receptors control the opening of chloride channels in the cell membrane. Because chloride ions are negatively charged, influx of chloride into the cell rapidly hyperpolarizes it, and causing the neuron to fire will require much more stimulation. In fact, influx of chloride into the cell depolarizes the cell so effectively that rapid inhibition of synapses in the entire brain may occur, possibly leading to cardiac and respiratory arrest, coma, and death. Thus, supplementation with drugs and supplements that agonize GABA activity must be done with caution.

In lesser amounts, increase in GABA function may result in lethargy, fatigue, muscle relaxation, and difficulties remaining awake. Because the action of GABA opposes glutamatergic stimulation of neuronal firing, increase in GABA activity is a strategy utilized by most anticonvulsant medications. Because the pathophysiology of seizures and bipolar (especially, manic) is somewhat similar, increasing GABA is also a mechanism of action utilized by many mood stabilizers.

Underactivation of GABA pathways is also associated with risks that are similar to glutamate overactivation. Because GABA balances glutamate's effects, a decrease in GABA activity will result in an increase of glutamatergic excitation of neurons. Consequently, symptoms of mood dysregulation, extreme hyperactivity and impulsivity, and possibly seizures and death may occur. Because the appropriate balance of GABA and glutamate is so crucial to maintain, clinicians must proceed with much caution when disturbing the endogenous balance of these crucial neurotransmitters.

Increasing GABA neurotransmission and/or decreasing glutamate activation has been shown to be effective in treating various psychological disorders (including mania, anxiety, and sleep problems), and substances that act in this manner are discussed in Chapters 7, 8 and 9. In addition, naturopaths sometimes recommend supplementation with GABA, and various forms of GABA tablets and capsules are available on the market. Unfortunately, these are of very limited value. GABA does not easily cross the blood–brain barrier, and the majority of GABA becomes metabolized and/or excreted before it can enter the brain. In addition, at high doses, supplemental GABA appears to cause a mix of sedation and increased anxiety (as discussed in Chapters 8 and 10). Thus, GABA supplements appear to show no benefits and their use is discouraged.

Glycine

Glycine is an amino acid commonly found in proteins. It is synthesized in the body from serine, another proteinogenic amino acid naturally synthesized within cells. As one of the 20 most common amino acids found in proteins, it serves multiple metabolic functions, but some of it is also released into synapses as a neurotransmitter.

Levels of glycine are primarily regulated by enzymatic degradation. Various enzymes are responsible for the breakdown of glycine. Some of these processes reverse the metabolism of glycine and convert the amino acid back to serine. Other enzymatic processes transform glycine into other molecules, including gloxylic acid.

Like glutamate and GABA, glycine is present in the nervous system and is an important building block for many chemical processes. As a neurotransmitter, it binds to several families of ionotropic and metabotropic receptors, but its primary inhibitory action seems to be the result of regulating chloride channels in a manner similar to the action of GABA. These effects are primarily seen in the spinal cord. In the brain, the effects of glycine are less predictable. For example, it seems to be involved in regulating glutamatergic neurotransmission at the NMDA glutamate ionotropic receptors that are involved in opening calcium channels and causing rapid depolarization of the post-synaptic cell. Thus, glycine may be an alosteric modulator for glutamate.

Increase in glycine function may result in effects similar to the increase of GABAergic neurotransmission (fatigue, drowsiness, etc.). However, since glycine seems to have varying effects in different parts of the brain, supplementation with glycine may also result in excitatory effects. For example, in overdose, glycine causes death by hyperexcitability of the brain. Supplementation with glycine seems to offer limited benefits, although some preliminary evidence exists that it may be helpful in treating the symptoms of psychosis (as discussed in Chapter 11).

Inhibition of glycine action is also associated with serious risks. Strichnine is a potent glycine antagonist, and causes muscular convulsions and death by asphyxia. In smaller doses, it was once used as a stimulant. Interestingly, bicuculine is a weaker antagonist that seems to exert its effect by antagonizing glycine and GABA. Thus, the effects of the inhibition of glycine may be similar to those seen when GABA transmissions are antagonized.

Adenosine

Adenosine is a glycosamine found in almost all cells. It is synthesized from uridine, and through other chemical processes in complex steps that involve transcription of RNA information. Uridine is a nutrient found in tomatoes, yeast, organ meats (such as liver), and broccoli, but adenosine is so crucial to cellular function that ample amounts become synthesized even in absence of sufficient dietary intake of uridine.

Levels of adenosine are regulated by several mechanisms. When released into synapses, it is rapidly reabsorbed through reuptake. In addition, adenosine is rapidly transformed through a variety of complex processes. Various forms of adenosine are present in cells, including cyclic adenosine monophosphate (cAMP), adenosine diphosphate (ADP), and adenosine triphosphate (ATP). All of these are crucial second messengers that are transformed into a variety of molecules, and their action is discussed in more detail later in the chapter. In addition, when adenosine enters systemic circulation, it is broken down by enzymes present in red blood cells.

Because adenosine has several crucial roles in the life function of almost all cells, it is abundant in all neurons and only some of it is released into the synapse and into the blood stream. It binds to several families of metabotropic receptors, and some of its effects mediate the action of calcium channels. Thus, the overall effect of adenosine release, especially as a neurotransmitter, is inhibitory. As a hormone, it may have anti-inflammatory effects and it also acts as a vasodilator. Adenosine is sometimes used intravenously to diagnose heart dysrhythmias and arterial blockages.

Increase in adenosine results in inhibitory effects both centrally and peripherally. Fatigue and drowsiness are expected, although central agonism of adenosine is rare. Instead, when used intravenously to diagnose cardiovascular problems, injection of adenosine causes a brief heart block. Adenosine is also released by the brain during epileptic attacks, perhaps in an attempt to protect the cells from damage.

Inhibition of adenosine action is the best adenosine-related effect. Since adenosine is an inhibitory neurotransmitter, inhibiting its action exerts a stimulating effect, and this mechanism of action is responsible for caffeine's stimulating effects that may be beneficial in treating symptoms of ADHD (as discussed in Chapter 5). In higher doses, anxiety, irritability, muscle twitching, insomnia, and respiratory cardiac problems become evident. Although very rare, death after overdose of caffeine has been reported.

PRECURSORS

Changes in brain function may be accomplished through a variety of mechanisms. Usually, it is desirable to alter the rate at which neurons fire in various areas of the brain. Increasing or decreasing the amount of neurotransmitter will usually change the amount of activity evident in the corresponding neurons. Although in some cases changing the amount of neurotransmitter available at the synapse may be accomplished through other means (for example, by inhibiting reuptake), the most straightforward way, at least theoretically, is to alter the amount of neurotransmitter that is being produced by the releasing cell. Consequently, availability of the relevant precursors may impact the degree of neurotransmitter synthesis.

While in some cases it may be desirable to decrease neurotransmission, in most cases, an increase in the availability of a neurotransmitter is sought. Thus, when a deficiency in a neurotransmitter is apparent, it may be desirable to consider whether neuronal cells have enough precursors available to synthesize the neurotransmitter. Sometimes, it may be desirable to introduce additional amounts of precursors, in the hope that additional amounts of neurotransmitters will be produced. However, this strategy is subject to many regulatory mechanisms that often impose a small window within which neurotransmitter synthesis will fall. Since most precursors are ingested during meals, insufficient amounts of precursors may be consumed. However, in such a situation, the cell usually utilizes other means to metabolize the precursor. Conversely, when excess precursor is available, the cell excretes it or utilizes it during other metabolic transformations. Thus, changing the amount of precursor may or may not have a potential impact on the amount of neurotransmitter that will be produced.

Many precursors are amino acids. Our genetic code is programmed to covert 20 amino acids regarded as 'standard,' 'normal,' or 'primary.' These are listed in Table 4.1. Some of these are essential, meaning that they are required by the body but are not produced endogenously, and

TABLE 4.1   Standard amino acids

Alanine	Leucine
Arginine	Lysine
Asparagine	Methionine
Aspartic Acid	Phenylalanine
Cysteine	Proline
Glutamic Acid	Serine
Glutamine	Threonine
Glycine	Tryptophan
Histidine	Tyrosine
Isoleucine	Valine

therefore must be ingested from diet. Non-essential amino acids are produced by the body, but may also be ingested in food. Because the standard amino acids are required by the body to perform many metabolic functions, the World Health Organization lists recommended daily intake values for these important nutrients (WHO, 2007).

Because the regulatory mechanisms are different for each precursor, it is beneficial to specifically discuss the precursors for those neurotransmitters with significant psychoactive effects, and identify the mechanisms that regulate the amount of precursor that the cells use to synthesize neurotransmitters.

Tyrosine

Tyrosine is one of the 20 standard amino acids present in the body and used by cells to synthesize proteins. This is a non-essential amino acid, meaning that when it is not only ingested from diet, it is also synthesized by the body. Tyrosine is found in casein, a protein in milk and other milk-based products (like cheese). Tyrosine is also present in non-dairy foods that are aged, including some types of meats and red wine.

Since tyrosine is a non-essential amino acid, it is produced by the body when insufficient amounts are ingested. However, tyrosine pairs with phenylalanine to form an amino acid pair, and phenylalanine is an essential amino acid, meaning that it must be ingested in food. Thus, the WHO has set typical recommended daily intakes for these molecules, and the recommended daily amount for the pair of phenylalanine and tyrosine is set at 25 mg/kg of body weight (WHO, 2007). Since one mechanism of producing tyrosine is by converting phenylalanine into tyrosine, the recommended daily intake of the phenylalanine/tyrosine pair should be weighed more heavily toward phenylalanine.

When food is ingested that contains tyrosine, the molecule is extracted during metabolic processes that take place in the small intestine, and absorbed into circulation. There, it travels through the body, crosses the blood–brain barrier, and enters neurons, where it gets metabolized into catecholamine neurotransmitters. The body employs a complex mechanism to regulate the amount of tyrosine in cells. If too little is ingested, tyrosine is produced through various metabolic processes. When too much tyrosine is ingested, tyrosine is broken down through phosphorylation, sulfation, oxidation, and other metabolic processes.

Because these regulatory processes enforce a narrow range of tyrosine presence within cells, supplementation with tyrosine has not been found to be effective. Even though tyrosine is the precursor of a family of neurotransmitters extensively involved in the regulation of mood, administering tyrosine in supplements has been found to result in no improvements in mood states (Lieberman *et al.*, 1985). In fact, some research has shown that supplementation with tyrosine may actually reduce levels of dopamine within the brain (Chinevere *et al.*, 2002). Similarly, supplementation with tyrosine has no effect on symptoms of anxiety, but may be beneficial in reducing the harmful physical effects of stress hormones (Reinstein *et al.*, 1985).

Clinicians are generally advised against using tyrosine supplements. The WHO recommendations about dietary intake should be observed and in cases where it is apparent that the dietary intake falls significantly below recommended levels, supplementation may be attempted. However, clinicians should make sure that combined dietary intake and supplementation produces a combined intake close to WHO recommendations and does not significantly exceed those levels. On the other hand, supplementation with tyrosine precursors (for example, phenylalanine or phenylethylamine) may have some efficacy in treatment of depression (as discussed in Chapter 6).

Tryptophan

Tryptophan is also one of the 20 standard amino acids present in the body and used by cells to synthesize proteins. This is an essential amino acid, meaning that it is only ingested from diet. Tryptophan is found in a wide variety of protein-containing foods, including eggs, cheese, meat (especially turkey), fish, wheat, rice, potatoes, and bananas. Since tryptophan must be ingested in food, the WHO has set a typical recommended daily intake for tryptophan at 4 mg/kg of body weight (WHO, 2007).

When food is ingested that contains tryptophan, the molecule is extracted during metabolic processes that take place in the small intestine, and absorbed into circulation. There, it travels through the body, crosses the blood–brain barrier, and enters neurons, where it gets metabolized into indolamine neurotransmitters, as well as niacin. Because the body does not produce tryptophan, it has limited abilities to regulate the amount of tryptophan in cells. When too much tryptophan is ingested, it is broken down through various metabolic processes, and can sometimes be retroconverted if needed. However, when limited amounts are ingested, tryptophan deficiency may be apparent, resulting in suppressed amounts of serotonin, melatonin, niacin, and other important molecules. Depression and sleep disorders may partially be caused by limited amounts of tryptophan in the body.

For this reason, supplementation with tryptophan has been attempted, and was popular until the late 1980s, when over 30 deaths were caused by contaminated batches of tryptophan. The supplement was then banned in the United States (and many other countries), but, more recently, it was revealed that problems in manufacture were responsible for these deaths and the supplement is potentially safe. Consequently, sales of tryptophan as a supplement were allowed to resume in 2001, and the FDA ban on tryptophan supplement importation was lifted in 2005.

Clinicians are advised to carefully consider whether supplementation with tryptophan is indicated. First, the WHO recommendations about dietary intake should be observed. In cases where it is apparent that the dietary intake falls significantly below recommended levels, supplementation may be attempted. Otherwise, supplementation with tryptophan may be helpful in addressing sleep problems (as discussed in Chapter 9), and supplementation with 5-HTP, a transformed form of tryptophan, may be effective in treating symptoms of depression (discussed in Chapter 6) and anxiety (covered in Chapter 8).

Glutamine

Glutamine is another standard amino acid. It is non-essential and supplied from food or synthesized by the body. Glutamine is found in meat, fish, eggs, dairy products, wheat, beans, and some vegetables. Small amounts may also be present in fermented foods, such as miso.

Since glutamine is a non-essential amino acid, it is produced by the body when insufficient amounts are ingested. It is metabolized from glutamic acid, another non-essential amino acid. However, under certain conditions it becomes partially essential, since the body may not always be able to produce sufficient amounts. This may be the case during illness or after severe injuries.

When food is ingested that contains glutamine, the molecule is extracted in the small intestine and absorbed into circulation. Although most is metabolized during first pass effect, the remainder travels through the body, readily crosses the blood–brain barrier, and enters neurons, where it gets metabolized into glutamate. The amount of glutamine in cells is regulated through a variety of metabolic processes. If too little is ingested, more glutamine is converted from glutamic acid. When too much glutamine is ingested, only a portion is converted to glutamate, and the remainder is metabolized into many protein chains involved in various cellular processes.

As with all precursors, a narrow range of glutamine is permitted within cells, and supplementation may be of limited value, at least when it comes to treating symptoms of psychological disorders. Although glutamine is considered a nutraceutical, its benefits seem to be most significant when it is used as a supplement to treat injuries, burns, and other forms of physical trauma (Morlion *et al.*, 1998). It is also used by bodybuilders and may show benefits in improving muscle growth (Ivy & Portman, 2004). When used as a psychoactive compound, its effects seem inconsistent. Non-peer reviewed sources sometimes list it as effective in treatment of depression, ADHD, and schizophrenia. However, there seems to be a dearth of empirical research to support these claims. Although supplementation with glutamate is not associated with significant adverse effects, limited benefit is likely, and therefore clinicians are advised to avoid using glutamine supplements, or use them as a last resort with careful monitoring and oversight.

Serine

Serine is another standard amino acid. It is non-essential and supplied from food or synthesized by the body from a number of metabolites, including glycine. Serine is found in soybeans, nuts (especially peanuts, almonds, and walnuts), eggs, chickpeas, lentils, meat, and fish (especially shellfish). Serine is produced by the body when insufficient amounts are ingested. It is metabolized from ketones and glycine, and retroconversion with glycine also occurs.

As with most amino acids, when food is ingested that contains serine, the molecule is extracted in the small intestine and absorbed into circulation. There, it travels through the body, crosses the blood–brain barrier, and enters neurons, where it gets metabolized into glycine and many other molecules. Thus, the amount of serine in cells is regulated through these metabolic processes. If too little is ingested, more serine is converted from various sources. When too much is ingested, only a portion is converted to glycine, and the remainder is metabolized into folate and many other proteins.

As with all precursors, only a limited amount of serine will be converted to glycine, and supplementation may be of limited value. Although non-peer reviewed sources list it as effective in treatment of a variety of symptoms of psychological disorders (especially depression and anxiety), there is no empirical research to support these claims. Thus, although supplementation with serine is not associated with significant adverse effects, benefits are unlikely, and therefore clinicians are advised to avoid using serine supplements.

Uridine

Rather than an amino acid, uridine is a nucleoside, a molecule that consists of a nucleobase (a molecule formed when transcribing the DNA) and a ribose (a naturally occurring molecule). It is non-essential and supplied from food or synthesized by the body from uracil. Uridine is primarily found in sugar beets, sugarcane, tomatoes, yeast (especially the types used to make beer), organ meats, and broccoli. Uridine is produced by the body when insufficient amounts are ingested.

When food is ingested that contains uridine, the molecule is extracted during digestive processes and enters systemic circulation. There, it travels through the body, crosses the blood–brain barrier, and enters neurons, where it gets metabolized into adenosine and other molecules. Thus, the amount of uridine in cells is regulated through metabolic processes. If too little is ingested, more serine is converted from uracil. When too much is ingested, only a portion is converted to adenosine, and the remainder in metabolized into other molecules.

Only a limited amount of uridine will be converted to adenosine, but supplementation with uridine has nevertheless been attempted. Because adenosine is an inhibitory neurotransmitter, supplementation with uridine to treat symptoms of anxiety has been investigated, with mixed results. The chapter in this handbook that discusses the treatment of symptoms of anxiety disorders includes discussion of this nutraceutical. In addition, some researchers have used uridine supplements, in conjunction with Omega-3 acids, to treat symptoms of depression, and it is hypothesized that uridine may act as a co-factor in magnifying the effects of these fatty acids. However, uridine supplements are not yet available and, thus far, only animal studies report potential benefits. Thus, at this time, use of uridine supplements is not recommended.

Glucose

Glucose is a monosaccharide, a simple sugar used by all cells as a source of energy. It contains carbon atoms and hydroxyl groups, and therefore it is called a carbohydrate. It is non-essential and supplied from food or synthesized by liver and kidneys in a process called gluconeogenesis (from lactate, glycerol, and other molecules). Glucose is found in a wide number of sweet-tasting foods, including most fruit, some vegetables, and refined sugar. Glucose is produced by the body when insufficient amounts are ingested.

When food is ingested that contains glucose, the molecule is extracted and broken down during digestive processes in the duodenum, where insulin, a hormone produced by the pancreas, is deposited. As a hormone, insulin is also present in systemic circulation where it aids the body (especially, the muscles) absorb and metabolize glucose into energy. Glucose readily crosses the blood–brain barrier, and enters neurons, where it undergoes extensive metabolism and, among others, may be involved in the synthesis of acetylcholine. Thus, the amount of glucose in cells is regulated through complex processes, including levels of insulin and the type of enzymes available to perform glucose metabolism. If too little glucose is ingested, more is produced by the body. When too much is ingested, lipid storage increases, and high sugar intake is often associated with significant weight problems.

Since the body is able to produce ample amounts of glucose, supplementation with glucose is not needed. On the other hand, excess of glucose intake has been implicated in a wide variety of psychological disorders, especially ADHD. Sugar is believed by many to cause hyperactivity, and a wide variety of elimination diets have been developed that limit the intake of glucose. Unfortunately, unequivocal evidence exists that sugar does not cause hyperactivity, and elimination of sugar from the diet does not improve symptoms of ADHD or any other behavioral disturbances (Wolraich et al., 1995). Clinicians are advised to steer parents away from these time-wasting approaches. While limiting sugar intake is a prudent nutritional strategy that is likely to contribute to the prevention of obesity, it has no effect on any symptoms of any psychological disorders.

SECOND MESSENGERS

When a change in brain function is sought, the most straightforward way to accomplish it is to agonize or antagonize the effects of the neurotransmitters associated with these brain functions. Increasing the release of the neurotransmitter, blocking its reuptake or enzymatic degradation, or (in some cases) increasing the amount of the precursor may accomplish this goal. However, there are many methods utilized by cells to regulate the extent to which these changes increase or decrease the available neurotransmitter, and, in some cases, the mechanisms described above exert limited effects. In those instances, it may be necessary to attempt to change internal aspects of cell function to change the rate of neurotransmitter synthesis or the degree of cell membrane permeability.

As discussed in the previous chapter, post-synaptic receptors can be ionotropic or metabotropic. While ionotropic receptors regulate the extent to which a channel coded for specific molecules opens or closes, metabotropic receptors produce effects by changing the inner workings of the cell.

Metabotropic receptors are coupled with g-proteins that are released when the receptor is stimulated. These proteins may produce a wide variety of changes, and many molecules can serve as g-proteins. In fact, g-protein is a generic term that refers to a large number of molecules that serve as molecular switches to activate (or inactivate) various intracellular functions. For example, g-proteins may stimulate or inhibit the production of cAMP, regulate cell migration, and change membrane fluidity.

Although g-proteins are generally synthesized within the cell, in some cases they can be synthesized outside of the cell and enter the cell by crossing the membrane. This section will describe some of the better known molecules that are involved in various intracellular functions.

Cyclic Adenosine Monophosphate

Cyclic adenosine monophosphate (cAMP) is a second messenger used for intracellular signal induction. It is synthesized from adenosine triphosphate (ATP) by enzymes (g-proteins) that are attached to metabotropic receptors and become released when the receptor is activated. Cyclic AMP is involved in the regulation of glycogen, sugar, and lipid metabolism.

Cyclic AMP may affect brain function in many ways. In some cases, increase in levels of cAMP may result in an increase in the production of a neurotransmitter, contributing to an agonist effect. This action has been presumed to be responsible for some of the beneficial effects of psychotropic medications, like selective serotonin reuptake inhibitors (SSRIs), a category of antidepressants that includes the medication Prozac. However, cAMP may also regulate cyclic nucleotide-gated ion channels, resulting in membrane hyperpolarization and resultant antagonist effects. Thus, the overall effect of changing the activity of cAMP is poorly understood and may be may be unpredictable.

Similarly, supplementation with cAMP or ATP has not proven effective. Some on-line pharmacies promote the sale of ATP, claiming that the human body may not produce sufficient amounts of cAMP. In fact, one such facility claims that an adult human at rest requires 40 kg of ATP per day, and during strenuous activity, the demand may increase to 500 g per minute (Mason, n.d.). However, these claims are not supported by any empirical evidence, and, even if true, there is no data that supports the notion that the body is not able to produce sufficient amounts of cAMP. Consequently, clinicians are advised against recommending supplementation with cAMP, ATP, or any similar compound.

Choline

Choline is a partly essential nutrient that is usually grouped within the Vitamin B complex. Although not a standard amino acid, it is a natural amine found in the lipids that make up cell membranes. As described above, it is a co-factor required for the synthesis of acetylcholine. Although small amounts are produced by the body, most choline must be ingested in food. Choline-rich foods include egg yolks, soy, and organ meats (especially liver), and many vegetables contain choline in smaller amounts. Adequate daily intakes of this micronutrient have been established by the Food and Nutrition Board of the Institute of Medicine of the National Academy of Sciences and are reported to be between 425 and 550 mg/day for adults (Veenema et al., 2008), or between 5 and 6.4 mg/kg/day. Although no guidelines have been established for adequate intake for children, the mg/kg ratio can be used to calculate the range appropriate to the size of the child or adolescent.

When food is ingested that contains choline, the molecule is absorbed into circulation and travels through the body. It crosses the blood–brain barrier, and enters neurons. Choline is involved in the metabolism of acetylcholine, as well as maintaining structural integrity and signaling roles for cell membranes, and donating methyl molecules during various metabolic processes. Thus, the amount of choline in cells is regulated through a variety of metabolic processes. When too much choline is available, only a portion is converted to acetylcholine, and the remainder is metabolized through other means. If too little is ingested, choline deficits may become evident.

Choline deficits may result in a variety of medical problems, including heart disease and liver damage. Those who do not consume choline-rich diets may need to take a choline supplement and various health benefits have been associated with choline supplements. Similarly, choline has been implicated in a variety of psychological functions. Since it may regulate membrane permeability, it may have an effect on neurotransmission and may be beneficial in potentiating the action of many neurotransmitters. However, this hypothesis has not borne out in research, although lecithin (a precursor for choline) is showing promise as a mood stabilizer and is discussed in Chapter 7. At this time, the only well-documented psychotropic benefit of choline seems to be the possible improvement of memory in those who may begin to exhibit early signs of dementia, although evidence is beginning to emerge of some potential benefits in treating symptoms of ADHD (as discussed in Chapter 5) and tics (as discussed in Chapter 10). In addition, those who take inositol (to treat symptoms of depression, anxiety, or ADHD) may also benefit from augmentation with choline.

Taurine

Taurine is an organic acid that is sometimes grouped with standard amino acids, although in the strictest sense it does not belong in that group and is a product of metabolism of cysteine, a standard amino acid. It is a non-essential nutrient and is synthesized by the liver. However, some children lack the enzymes necessary to metabolize taurine, and taurine has been added to baby food since the 1980s. In addition, taurine is a nutrient present in shellfish, most meats, and (in smaller amounts) in milk. It is sometimes added to energy drinks, but its energy-promoting effects have not been proven.

Taurine is absorbed into circulation and travels through the body. It crosses the blood–brain barrier, and enters neurons. Taurine has been hypothesized to play a role in membrane stabilization, calcium homeostasis, glutamate regulation, and inhibitory neurotransmission. In the cell, taurine may keep potassium and magnesium inside the cell while keeping sodium out. Thus, it may affect neuronal firing. Remaining taurine is conjugated to form the bile salts and is excreted into bile, where it is transported to the duodenum to take part in the metabolism of various lipids.

Taurine deficits may result in a variety of medical problems, including heart disease and liver damage. Taurine supplementation has been shown to produce some benefits in reducing cardiovascular problems and obesity (Tsuboyama-Kasaoka et al., 2006), and may reduce blood levels of cholesterol (Zhang et al., 2004). When given to patients with congestive heart failure, taurine may also increase the force and effectiveness of heart-muscle contractions (Azuma et al., 1983). Taurine supplementation has been investigated as an anxiolytic, and some studies have reported promising results. This aspect of taurine supplementation is discussed in the chapter that reviews treatment of anxiety (Chapter 8). Taurine is also expected by some to have mood stabilizing effects, and is briefly discussed in Chapter 7. Because it binds to glycine receptors, some have also hypothesized possible antipsychotic benefits (see Chapter 11).

Essential Fatty Acids

Essential fatty acids are lipids that are not metabolized by the body and therefore must be obtained from the diet. These fatty acids are involved in various biological processes, and produce many compounds when they are metabolized. There are two primary families of essential fatty acids, Omega-3 and Omega-6, with constituent lipids within each group. Fatty acids within each of these families may be converted from each other, but not across families, and therefore both families must be consumed in food. Western diet typically includes Omega-6 fatty acids in large amounts, and foods like grains, plant-based oils, poultry, and eggs are rich in Omega-6 lipids. However, Omega-3 fatty acids, primarily present in cold-water fish, are not as commonly consumed, and consequently supplementation with Omega-3 has been recommended.

Along with other lipids, essential fatty acids are extracted in the small intestine, absorbed into circulation, and travel through the body. Once transported into cells, essential fatty acids serve numerous functions. They influence membrane fluidity and may be involved in the regulation of neuronal firing. They are also transformed into many other molecules, including ecosanoids and lipoxins that are involved in anti-inflammatory effects. Thus, levels of essential fatty acids within the cells are regulated by complex metabolic processes.

Essential fatty acid deficits may result in a variety of medical problems. Cardiovascular disease is often the result of a variety of pathological processes, including chronic inflammation, and use of essential fatty acid supplements has been associated with cardioprotective benefits. In addition, those cultures where high consumption of foods rich in Omega-3 is evident have lower incidence of dementia, and therefore essential fatty acid supplements may have protective effects against future dementia (although have not been shown to arrest or reverse current symptoms of dementia).

More recently, psychotropic benefits of Omega-3 have been investigated. Thus far, research studies have shown that supplementation with these fatty acids may offer benefits in treating symptoms of bipolar disorder, depression, ADHD, and psychosis. In this handbook, chapters that review the treatment of these disorders include sections that discuss Omega-3's potential utility.

Chapter 5

ADHD

In 1885, a German physician named Heinrich Hoffman wrote about some interesting patients that he saw in his practice, including a case of 'Fidgety Phil' that he found particularly intriguing (Stewart, 1970). This description is commonly regarded as the first important reference to a boy with hyperactivity. Still (1902) described some three dozen children who had significant difficulties with maintaining focus and also exhibited symptoms of notable overactivity. These two dimensions of symptoms were accompanied by problems with aggression, defiance, and emotional overreactivity. Thus, for over 100 years we have recognized that children who exhibit problems with overactivity and difficulties sustaining attention present with significant emotional and behavioral difficulties. Today, this syndrome is known as attention deficit hyperactivity disorder (ADHD).

To diagnose ADHD, the current version of the *Diagnostic and Statistical Manual of Mental Disorders* (DSM-IV, American Psychiatric Association, 2000) requires clinicians to assess two dimensions of symptoms, hyperactivity/impulsivity, and inattention. Depending on the specific variant evident in a given person, ADHD can be diagnosed as 'Predominantly Hyperactive–Impulsive Type,' 'Predominantly Inattentive Type,' or 'Combined Type.' Individuals who present with enough symptoms from either (or both) clusters to negatively affect their adaptive functioning, but not enough symptoms to meet all diagnostic criteria in either cluster, can be diagnosed with ADHD 'Not Otherwise Specified.'

SYMPTOMS OF ADHD

Children and teens with ADHD commonly exhibit a variety of problems across different settings. In accordance with the DSM-IV-TR diagnostic guidelines, these symptoms fall along the dimensions of hyperactivity/impulsivity and inattentiveness, and they are often referred to as the 'primary' or 'core' symptoms, since they are presumed to be directly caused by the underlying etiology. However, a child with ADHD is a member of his family, his class, and his peer group, and his interactions with his parents, siblings, teachers, and peers are negatively affected by the core symptoms. Consequently, children and teens with ADHD commonly develop secondary symptoms that stem out of the primary difficulties and further exacerbate their difficulties with adaptive behaviors.

Core Symptoms

Behavioral dimensions of hyperactivity/impulsivity, and distractibility are presumed to be separate clusters, and impairment in at least one of these is required for diagnosis, but patients sometimes exhibit symptoms that overlap and may fall into either cluster. In addition, symptoms in each cluster may present differently in diverse settings and situations.

Impulsivity/Hyperactivity

Impulsivity and hyperactivity are especially common in males with ADHD. These children and teens often act with little forethought and exhibit a knee-jerk reactivity to environmental events. When they feel urges to do and say things, they utilize minimal cognitive processing and convert these impulses into behaviors. Some symptoms of impulsivity are relatively obvious to recognize. For example, a young child may run out into the street chasing a ball, forgetting to look whether or not a car may be coming his way. However, by the time children reach school age, they are expected to utilize sufficient self-control to be able to suppress such impulses. Children with ADHD find this difficult, and so they may place themselves in danger because they seemingly act without thinking. This tendency is also evident in many decisions they make – for example, problems suppressing the impulse to continue playing when it is time to start doing homework, or difficulties accepting that it is time to stop watching television because it is time to start getting ready for bed.

Many patients who are impulsive are also hyperactive and exhibit a 'driven by a motor' quality, a restlessness, and a need to constantly move about. These children exhibit additional management difficulties. They have problems sitting still at meals. They tend to utilize high levels of physical activity during play and can be very noisy. They are likely to roughhouse with siblings, which often results in conflicts. In restaurants and stores, they find it difficult to remain still and often wander away and require parents to chase after them. In school, they are often disruptive and may not be able to remain at their desk during class. They may call out answers without waiting to be called upon. When playing with other children, they are often bossy and argumentative, since they find it hard to accept it when things do not go their way. All in all, parents, teachers, and peers often find these behaviors frustrating, and children with ADHD frequently get reprimanded, scolded, and punished.

When children become teens, hyperactivity usually becomes less apparent, but impulsivity may persist. Teenagers primarily display the symptoms of impulsivity in their decision making and are more likely to exhibit poor judgment, spontaneously break rules (for example, go out of the home to see friends at inappropriate times, such as close to bedtime), and frequently change their mind about activities and interests. While all teenagers may exhibit some of these problems, teens with ADHD display these behaviors so frequently that their day-to-day existence is adversely affected to a significant degree.

Distractibility/Disorganization

Individuals with ADHD exhibit problems with distractibility because it is hard for them to filter out distractions in the environment that interfere with sustaining attention on the primary task. Often, distractibility is most apparent in school, and children and teens with ADHD often daydream during class and exhibit difficulties completing their work. Students who do not pay attention gradually exhibit difficulties with academic performance, gaps in academic skills, and a significant drop in grades. As children become teens, their workload increases and they are expected to be able to independently perform more complex academic tasks. Teens who are distractible often find it difficult to sustain attention during homework assignments, and often hand in work that is incomplete.

Children and teens who are distractible usually are also disorganized. As a result, they have difficulties keeping track of their things and they frequently lose toys, homework assignments, books, etc. The disorganization they exhibit is often frustrating to their teachers. The book bags, desks, and lockers of children with ADHD are often very messy and unkempt. It is common for them to lose track of what they have in their book bag or desk, and retain items in there long after they are no longer necessary, further frustrating their parents and teachers. Distractibility and disorganization are conceptually related. Mental effort is required to be able to sustain attention and filter out distractions. It takes similar mental effort to remember to do something or memorize where an item was placed. Those individuals who have difficulties with these mental activities frequently have problems with both distractibility and disorganization.

Secondary Symptoms

When children and teens with ADHD to go through life with symptoms of this disorder their existence is filled with frequent stress and conflict. Some symptoms (especially those in the impulsive cluster) predispose them to interpersonal conflicts and related difficulties, and all symptoms of ADHD are likely to affect self-esteem and motivation.

Children and teens who are impulsive often exhibit limited ability to deal with frustration. When a person, any person, faces a situation that did not come out as planned, or one where preferred action is not possible, that person experiences an internal feeling of frustration, an urge that may be accompanied by a thought, 'I don't like this.' Day-to-day life frequently places one in such situations – a sibling is playing with a toy or a game that you would like to play with, a parent is not allowing you to continue playing and tells you to start doing something else, or a video game activity does not come out as you expected and you did not achieve the score you hoped for. Children who are not particularly impulsive gradually learn to accept such situations as part of normal life. However, those who exhibit symptoms of ADHD have difficulties dealing with this frustration, and usually display it more strongly and openly, by defying the parent or exhibiting an emotional outburst (like throwing the game controllers across the room).

When a child is playing with a video game and a parent says, 'Stop playing because it's time to do your homework,' the initial reaction will likely be to resist the change and continue with the activity that he is enjoying at the moment. A child who has good impulse control will experience that internal urge to resist, but before he chooses a response, he will process the situation and recognize that resisting will only result in a negative outcome (for example, getting yelled at). Instead, an impulsive child has difficulties delaying the reaction to perform such processing, and in likely to express the negative urge through protests, arguments, and downright defiance. Indeed, children and teens with ADHD who are impulsive are usually also described as defiant.

When children and teens with ADHD face a situation where an emotional reaction was invoked, their limited self-control makes it hard for them to suppress that reaction. This is especially evident where negative feelings were awakened, like when they became frustrated or saddened. Consequently, they are 'reactive,' in that they have difficulties suppressing the initial urge to react, and externalize whatever they feel inside. However, because they tend to overreact when things do not go their way, they are more likely to get scolded and punished, and over time they may internalize a sense of frustration, low self-esteem, and anger.

Children and teens with ADHD are more likely to incur academic failure and adverse consequences, like detentions, suspensions, and expulsion from school. These experiences affect their self-concept and self-esteem, and children with ADHD often feel 'dumber' than their peers. As they internalize these feelings, their sense of self-efficacy becomes compromised. Children with ADHD often conclude that they cannot succeed academically, and their motivation to try hard to do their homework and study becomes increasingly limited.

RULE-OUTS AND COMORBID DISORDERS

It is recognized by most researchers and mental health professionals that symptoms of ADHD are commonly accompanied by other difficulties. In fact, some estimate that about half of children with ADHD present with symptoms of at least one other disorder (Barkley, 2006), and that the rate of co morbidities increases with age (Ramsay & Rostain, 2008). In order to appropriately target all symptoms that may be contributing to overall impairment, clinicians need to be vigilant to recognize all symptoms and develop a comprehensive treatment plan. This will require mental health professionals to consider whether symptoms of ADHD account for all difficulties, or symptoms of additional disorders need to be recognized and treated.

Disruptive Disorders

Children and teens with ADHD often present difficulties with aggression, oppositional behaviors, and conduct problems. By some accounts, up to 84 percent of children and adolescents with ADHD also exhibit symptoms of oppositional or conduct disorder (Barkley, 2006). Some have suggested that problems with self-control underlie all of these disorders, thus explaining the comorbidity (Lynam, 1998).

Individuals who present with symptoms of ADHD, especially variants that include the hyperactive–impulsive cluster of symptoms, commonly exhibit comorbid defiance and argumentativeness. The overlap between the two is well documented, and it is likely that problems with impulsivity underlie difficulties with judgment as well as problems controlling one's reaction to frustration (Burns & Walsh, 2002). Thus, poor self-control commonly results in combined symptoms of ADHD and oppositional defiant disorder (ODD), especially in males. On the other hand, if problems with self-control are only evident in situations where the client has difficulties controlling his feelings of frustration, the clinician must determine whether other symptoms exist to justify the diagnosis of

ADHD. If symptoms of impulsivity or agitation do not appear present outside of frustrating situations, it is likely that a diagnosis of ODD (without ADHD) is appropriate. In such a situation, behavioral approaches, rather than medications or supplements, are usually most effective.

When severe aggression, destruction of property, serious violations of rules, and violation of laws (through theft, truancy, etc.) is apparent, symptoms of conduct disorder (CD) may be evident. When these problems are present, they cannot be accounted for by symptoms of ADHD, since the vast majority of individuals with ADHD do not perform these behaviors, and only 1–3 percent of children with ADHD are also diagnosed with CD (Pfiffner *et al.*, 1999). CD, however, is more likely to occur in the context of a history of comorbid ADHD and ODD. When ADHD (Hyperactive–Impulsive, or Combined Type) and ODD are present together, about half of those patients later go on to be diagnosed with CD in adolescence (Wilens *et al.*, 2002). When comorbid ADHD and CD are present, treatment planning must include interventions that focus on symptoms of ADHD (for example, nutritional and herbal supplements) and CD (such as contingency management).

Mood Disorders

Mood disorders commonly co-exist with ADHD. Up to 32 percent of children with ADHD present a comorbid depressive disorder, and up to 13 percent are diagnosed with some variant of bipolar disorder (Biederman *et al.*, 1991). In addition, mood disorders commonly mimic symptoms of ADHD – for example, depression is associated with distractibility and some variants of depressive symptoms include motor restlessness, and manic symptoms typically include impulsivity. Consequently, clinicians must be able to differentiate symptoms of ADHD from those that accompany mood disorders.

Symptoms of depression may include irritability, fatigue, and poor concentration. Clinicians need to determine whether motor restlessness and distractibility is the result of depression or ADHD. Generally, if these symptoms seem to accompany a chronic presentation of depression that also includes sadness, fatigue, and low self-esteem, a separate diagnosis of depression may be needed. Depending on length, severity, and course of symptoms, dysthymia or major depression may be diagnosed. When symptoms of ADHD and depression are present, a comprehensive treatment plan will have to address both sets of symptoms. Some supplements, discussed later in the chapter, may be able to simultaneously address symptoms of ADHD and milder forms of depression (such as dysthymia). In addition, milder forms of depression may be able to be addressed through psychotherapeutic interventions. However, if symptoms of major depression and ADHD are present, it is likely that both sets of symptoms will need to be addressed pharmacologically, and use of multiple supplements may be needed. Clinicians should address these situations with extreme caution, since the simultaneous use of multiple stimulants is rarely studied and the effects may be unpredictable.

At times, children or adolescents may exhibit symptoms of ADHD and mania or hypomania. It is relatively uncommon for children and adolescents to present with symptoms of 'classic' mania – excessive pursuit of pleasure, grandiosity, severe flight of ideas, decreased need for sleep, and rapid/pressured speech. Rather, hypomanic or mixed episodes are more likely, where patients present with significant agitation, restlessness, and difficulties with concentration. When such symptoms seem to wax and wane, while hyperactivity, impulsivity, or distractibility seems more consistently apparent, it is possible that symptoms of ADHD and bipolar disorder are present. In those cases, the use of multiple supplements is likely to be necessary.

Anxiety Disorders

Anxiety disorders are also common in individuals with ADHD, and studies report that 25–35 percent of individuals with ADHD also present symptoms of at least one anxiety disorder (Tannock, 2000). Symptoms of anxiety can usually be differentiated from symptoms of ADHD with little difficulty. However, when symptoms of both disorders co-occur, each may change the expression of the other (Barkley, 2006). For example, individuals with ADHD and anxiety tend to exhibit less impulsivity (Barkley), and comorbid ADHD and anxiety may result in more aggression (Tannock).

Children who exhibit chronic symptoms of anxiety may also be restless and distractible. When significant symptoms of anxiety are present, it is important to examine the behavioral expression of these symptoms. If restlessness and distractibility are primarily evident in situations when anxiety is apparent, symptoms of ADHD may not be present. However, if symptoms of ADHD occur at times when anxiety is not experienced, both disorders may need to be diagnosed. In those cases, use of supplements that simultaneously address both sets of symptoms may be beneficial, and if these are ineffective, use of multiple supplements may be needed.

In addition, clinicians must also remember that it is not uncommon for children with anxiety to present with comorbid symptoms of depression. In fact, Pfiffner et al. (1999) reported that about 23 percent of clinic-referred children had comorbid symptoms of anxiety and depression.

Thus, it possible that triple comorbidity may be apparent – depression, anxiety, and ADHD. In these complex situations mental health professionals must carefully assess the symptoms, timeline, and accompanying features to determine which symptoms may be associated with which disorders, and which symptoms should initially be targeted for treatment.

Medical Disorders

When considering disorders that result in ADHD-like impairment, medical factors should also be considered. While uncommon, some children with symptoms that resemble ADHD actually suffer from medical conditions. For decades, it has been known that children who experience lead poisoning exhibit symptoms of hyperactivity, poor self-control, and focusing difficulties. Consequently, a belief developed that deleading may be beneficial for those who exhibit these symptoms even if they are not known to suffer from lead poisoning. Unfortunately, results of research studies clearly point out that this approach is not effective. True, studies have shown that chelation decreases hyperactivity (David *et al.*, 1976), but subjects in the study were children who were shown to have abnormal lead levels in their blood. Although limits for acceptable lead levels in the blood have been steadily dropping, most children do not exhibit lead levels that are near the limit, even when conservative criteria are utilized, and deleading seems to provide no benefit for children who do not exhibit abnormal plasma levels of lead. However, those who grow up in impoverished backgrounds are at a higher risk, and so this possibility should be considered. A referral for appropriate work-up may be needed, and clinicians may try to locate a social service agency that may be performing screening for lead poisoning within the community.

Needless chelation is not only useless, it is also very dangerous. Deleading is associated with dangers of kidney failure, bone marrow depression, shock, hypotension, convulsions, cardiac arrhythmias, and respiratory arrest. A number of deaths have been linked to chelation therapy. While much of the unnecessary chelation is done with autistic children, some is also done with children with symptoms of ADHD. Parents should be warned that chelation is potentially deadly and totally useless, unless it can be proven that the patient exhibits abnormally high levels of lead, in which case it must be done under very intensive medical supervision.

Other medical problems may also contribute to formation of ADHD-like symptoms. Respiratory problems, especially severe allergies or uncontrolled asthma, commonly cause children to exhibit motor restlessness and inattentiveness. Similarly, endocrine problems have a significant influence. For example, an overactive thyroid commonly causes motor overactivity, and an underactive thyroid affects the ability to concentrate. These disorders are important to rule out, especially when there is evidence of family history of these problems in close biological relations (such as siblings or parents). A careful and thorough medical examination should always accompany the initiation of any mental health treatment. If present, these disorders should be addressed medically, not with the use of nutritional or herbal supplements.

Finally, when problems with distractibility are apparent (especially in school), dietary considerations should be reviewed. Children who do not consume an appropriate breakfast are known to be distractible (Arnold, 2002). When children are hungry or malnourished, their brains are not able to generate sufficient activity to sustain attention. Thus, eating a good breakfast is a prerequisite to being able to focus. The caloric content varies by the age and size of the child, but a nutritious breakfast should include a mix of three primary nutrients that correlate with brain function, carbohydrates, proteins, and fibers. Of these, the carbohydrates should primarily include complex nutrients (for example, whole grain breads and cereals, oats, or bran), since these are broken down more slowly, gradually releasing energy. Foods with high sugar content should be avoided. Although much research has shown that sugar does not contribute to hyperactivity (Barkley, 2006; Conners, 2001), simple carbohydrates are broken down very quickly and provide a quick burst of energy for the brain, but the effects wane very quickly. The discussion that follows assumes that supplements are being used with children and adolescents who are not malnourished and consume a normal breakfast, and yet continue to exhibit symptoms of ADHD.

ETIOLOGY

Our understanding of the etiology of this disorder has evolved over the past several decades. Today, the vast majority of clinicians recognize that the symptoms of ADHD stem from neurophysiological differences evident in the brains of children with ADHD. Consequently, this chapter will review those factors to help the practitioners develop an appropriate framework to conceptualize the treatment strategies that are most likely to result in effective symptom reduction.

Hyperactivity and Impulsivity

Humans are impulsive by nature. This means that every moment our brain generates a large number of impulses. Some of these impulses are thoughts, and some others are urges to say things or perform some movement. As various portions of the brain generate those impulses, those urges are relayed into the anterior portion of the frontal lobes to perform decision making and determine whether or not the urge should be converted into action. Thus, when the frontal lobes are not fully activated, are smaller, or otherwise do not function to capacity, the urges that are sent to them are not processed sufficiently and too many of them become quickly converted into behaviors. In this context, it becomes clear that impulsivity and hyperactivity are closely interrelated – hyperactivity is merely the reduced ability to control motor impulses, so that too many of them become converted into overt behaviors. In other words, hyperactivity is really motor impulsivity.

Anterior frontal lobes not only process motor urges, but also play an important role in decision making. Usually, when we decide on a course of action, it is beneficial to review alternatives (based on prior learning and experiences), organize the decision-making process into discrete steps, and implement the solution. These are commonly known as executive functions, and, according to Barkley (1997) require the use of verbal and non-verbal working memory; self-regulation of affect, motivation, and arousal; and planning. Thus, interference with the normal function of the frontal lobes potentially results not only in hyperactivity but also in deficit in executive functions.

To understand why the complex brain system responsible for motor control and executive functions may malfunction, one more aspect must be considered. Brain function occurs by the coordinated action of brain cells, or neurons. Neurons work by 'firing,' or transmitting messages. Neurons are not actually connected to each other, but are separated by small spaces called synapses. In order for one neuron to communicate with another, a chemical messenger (a neurotransmitter) most be released into the synapse and affect the post-synaptic neuron. While there are some neurotransmitters that are found throughout the entire brain, others are more localized and are involved in the processing of discrete brain functions. The frontal lobes (especially the aspects of frontal lobe function discussed herein) are primarily controlled by the action of dopamine. Thus, levels of dopamine are likely to affect the extent to which motor control and executive functions are appropriately performed.

Inattentiveness and Disorganization

Inattentiveness and disorganization are brain functions that also involve the frontal lobes (Stahl, 2008). To filter out distractions, one must suppress the urge to attend to an event that comes into one's awareness, like a sound that is heard or an item that comes into view. This requires self-control. In addition, when one strives to organize one's things, keep track of possessions, and plan to complete assignments or perform assigned responsibilities, the use of executive functions is also necessary. However, the organization of thoughts and the ability to filter out distractions are more purely cognitive tasks that do not require the use of the motor system, and therefore do not require the activation of basal ganglia and the cerebellum. Indeed, it is apparent that different portions of frontal lobes are involved in attention and concentration, and those parts of the brain have been found to be primarily activated by both dopamine and norepinephrine. Consequently, changes in the levels of either of those neurotransmitters may have an effect on inattentiveness.

In addition, another subcortical part of the brain is crucial to consider. The reticular formation, also known as the reticular activating system (RAS), is an oblong bundle of nerve cells located within the brain stem. The RAS is extensively connected with various portions of the brain, including all cortical lobes. The RAS can conceptually be understood as the 'gas pedal for the brain,' since it plays a major role in activating the brain to sustain a baseline level of arousal. If the RAS does not activate sufficiently, the brain (including the frontal lobes) will not function at capacity and symptoms of distractibility will be much more likely.

There are various reasons why the RAS may have difficulties activating the brain. One of these may be related to the corpus callosum, a longitudinal fissure densely packed with connections between neurons. Much of brain action involves communication between various brain areas, and those messages must be transmitted through the corpus callosum. Thus, if the corpus callosum exhibits any difficulties in efficiency or capacity, deficits in brain functions are likely to be apparent.

As discussed above, regions of the frontal lobes that are involved in motor control and executive functions (like planning) appear to be regulated primarily by dopamine, while regions that are involved in arousal and the control of attention are regulated by both dopamine and norepinephrine. The RAS activates the brain by releasing dopamine in its substantia nigra and tegmentum regions, and dopaminergic projections activate regions of the frontal lobes, basal ganglia, cerebellum, and other brain areas not directly related to ADHD. RAS also releases norepinephrine in the locus coeruleus and projections activate portions of the frontal lobes responsible for attentional control, as well as other brain structures that may play indirect role in attention, including portions of temporal and parietal lobes (Mirsky, 1987). Consequently, it is apparent that the neurophysiological control of the brain functions that underlie symptoms of ADHD primarily involves those two catecholamine neurotransmitters.

Summary of Research Findings

While it is helpful to localize the brain regions that may be involved in the production of symptoms of ADHD, it is necessary to review the findings of neuropsychiatric research in order to examine whether individuals with ADHD do, in fact, present abnormalities in these areas. Brain research studies have identified both structural and functional differences in individuals with ADHD. Each of these categories needs to be reviewed separately.

Neuroanatomical Abnormalities

As reviewed by Swanson and Castellanos (2002), four major studies performed in the 1990s, all of which utilized magnetic resonance imaging (MRI) scans, consistently revealed that children with ADHD (mostly boys) exhibit smaller basal ganglia. Furthermore, a striking consistency is evident in these findings – the studies revealed a uniform decrease of about 12 percent with an effect size of about 0.75. Those studies also revealed that the cerebellum of children with ADHD was similarly smaller, and all four studies revealed said size differences in the same regions of the cerebellum (inferior posterior lobe, lobules VIII-X of the vermis). As discussed above, the basal ganglia and cerebellum play key roles in the control of motor functions. It is apparent that the findings of these studies support the hypothesis that these brain structures are involved in the production of the symptoms of hyperactivity.

Research studies have also identified significant differences in the frontal lobes. Three studies have shown that three regions of the frontal lobes – the anterior cingulate gyrus (linked to the control of executive functions), the left dorsolateral region (involved in working memory and cognitive functions), and the right frontal region (liked to alertness and focusing) – have similarly been found to be smaller in ADHD groups. Once again, significant consistency was observed between these studies, with a decrease of about 10 percent and an effect size of about 0.70 being uniformly reported (Swanson & Castellanos, 2002). Furthermore, additional findings revealed that these same regions of the frontal lobes were only smaller in individuals with ADHD, and not in participants with learning disabilities (without ADHD). Consequently, it is apparent that regions of the frontal lobes also show particular abnormalities that seems specific to individuals with ADHD.

Studies investigating the size of the corpus callosum also revealed notable findings. Although some lateral inconsistencies were revealed, two research teams reported that anterior and posterior regions of the corpus callosum were smaller in ADHD groups, and these differences were not apparent in other clinical groups (Swanson & Castellanos, 2002). Additional studies by other groups of researchers also confirmed these findings (Barkley, 2006). Thus, it is likely that abnormalities in the corpus callosum contribute to the production of the symptoms of ADHD.

Neurophysiological Abnormalities

Over the past several decades, researchers have used a variety of functional brain scan techniques to investigate brain activity in patients with ADHD. Single photon emission tomography (SPECT) scans revealed that individuals with ADHD exhibited lower than normal blood perfusion in the striatum and frontal/prefrontal regions (especially on the right side), indicating lower level of activity in those areas (Swanson & Castellanos, 2002; Barkley, 2006). These findings were supported by studies that used functional magnetic resonance imaging (fMRI). In addition, when individuals were given stimulant medications (which increase dopaminergic transmission), the blood perfusion of the striatal regions returned to normal levels.

Studies that utilized positron emission tomography (PET) scans revealed somewhat variable findings, and a number of brain areas showed underactive metabolism in the brains of individuals with ADHD, but not consistently. However, the one finding that was consistent across three different studies was that the frontal lobes, especially the left anterior region, showed significant underactivity.

Results of electroencephalogram (EEG) studies have revealed findings that are also somewhat variable, but quantitative EEG (QEEG) measures have consistently shown that individuals with ADHD exhibit increased slow-wave (theta) patterns and decreased fast-wave (beta) activity in the frontal lobes, again indicating reduced frontal activation. Evoked response potential (ERP) studies have shown smaller amplitudes that are believed to be the result of smaller pre-frontal activation. Once again, studies have shown that these deficits resolve when individuals with ADHD are given stimulant medications (Barkley, 2006).

Since Wender (1971) proposed the 'dopamine hypothesis,' investigators have suspected that ADHD symptoms are secondary, at least in part, to a deficit in the dopaminergic brain functions. Current understanding of brain function confirms that the brain structures responsible for the control of motor, executive functions, and attention are activated by catecholamine transmitters, especially dopamine and norepinephrine. In fact, recent research findings point specifically to deficits in three of the brain's four dopaminergic pathways (mesocortical, mesolimbic, and nigrostriatal), as well as the prefrontal norepinephrine pathway (Stahl, 2008). Studies of individuals with ADHD lend further credence to these hypotheses. Examination of cerebral spinal fluid reveal that children with ADHD exhibit lower levels of dopamine (Halperin *et al.*, 1997), and other studies of blood and urine metabolites similarly implicate dopamine and norepinephrine, although not consistently (Barkley, 2006). Studies with adults, using flouro-dopa PET scans, also confirm these findings and reveal that adults with ADHD exhibit lower dopaminergic activity in the frontal lobes (Ernst *et al.*, 2003).

Molecular genetic research has identified some of the genetic factors that underlie these neurotransmitter deficiencies and suggest an explanation about why individuals with ADHD exhibit lower catecholamine-related function. Deficits in dopamine transporter genes have been identified in children with ADHD and their probands. Specifically, the DAT1 gene on chromosome 5, the DRD4 gene on chromosome 11, the DRD5 gene on chromosome 16, and the DBH transporter gene have been implicated (Barkley, 2006; Swanson & Castellanos, 2002). These genetic factors likely result in reduced dopaminergic activity in key areas in the brain, including the majority of the dopaminergic system. Since dopamine is a precursor for norepinephrine, it is plausible that dopaminergic deficits also result in noradrenergic deficiency.

SUPPLEMENTS WITH ESTABLISHED EFFICACY

Although the use of many herbal and nutritional supplements has not been studied, some compounds have undergone at least some research. Moreover, since the treatment of ADHD primarily focuses on addressing symptoms in children, some of these compounds have specifically been researched in children and adolescents.

Medications that work by increasing the amount of activity in the catecholamine pathways are generally effective in addressing symptoms of ADHD. Similarly, supplements that accomplish similar changes in the brain have been shown to be effective.

Caffeine

Caffeine is a psychostimulant classified as a methylxanthine. This category also includes theophylline (commonly found in tea) and theobromine (found in chocolate). Xantine is a purine base found in most tissues and body fluids, and is converted to uric acid. Caffeine is found in many beverages. Some naturally contain caffeine in varying amounts. For example, a 5 oz cup of coffee contains 60–120 mg of caffeine, depending on the method of brewing. The same amount of tea contains only about 40 mg of caffeine (and 1 mg of theophylline). Chocolate contains up to 40 mg of caffeine per 1 oz serving (and about 200 mg of theobromine), with darker chocolate containing much more caffeine than milk chocolate. Chocolate milk contains about 35 mg of caffeine per 8 oz serving, and a cup of hot cocoa contains between 10 and 30 mg of caffeine (and about 150 mg of theobromine). Theophylline and theobromine have lesser stimulating effects than caffeine, and therefore most of the mild stimulant properties of tea and chocolate are due to their caffeine content rather than the amount of the other methylxanthines.

Caffeine is also commonly added to soft drinks. Common colas (Coke, Pepsi, etc.), and Mountain Dew contain 355 mg of caffeine per 12 oz serving, and some soft drinks are specifically marketed for their stimulant properties – Jolt contains about 700 mg of caffeine (per 24 oz), Red Bull about 250 mg (per 8 oz), and Wired about 475 mg (per 16 oz). Soft drinks usually do not list the specific amounts of caffeine, and caffeine sometimes is listed by other names – for example, it is referred as guaranine (in guarana), mateine (in mate), and theine (in tea). Thus, it is difficult for consumers to know the exact amount of caffeine that any soft drink may contain.

Caffeine is also sold in both generic and brand-name pills, including brands such as Vivarin and No-Doz. Usually, it is available in 100 mg or 200 mg tablets. In addition, small doses of caffeine are commonly added to some over-the-counter medications, including Dristan, Excedrin, Midol, and some prescription drugs commonly used to treat migraines (for example, Fiorcet).

Evidence of Efficacy

Although some studies found that caffeine was not effective in improving symptoms of ADHD (Klein, 1987), and some noted authorities recommend against its use (Barkley, 2006), there is significant evidence to the contrary. Leon (2000) reviewed the results of 19 studies that investigated the effects of caffeine on children with ADHD. The review revealed that studies consistently found at least some benefit of caffeine, and using it was better than providing no treatment at all. Positive effects included not only increased attention to task, but decreased aggression as well. In fact, in some studies reviewed, combining caffeine with prescription stimulants did not increase adverse effects but enhanced therapeutic response.

In adolescents, the use of caffeine specifically to treat symptoms of ADHD has not been studied. However, moderate intake of caffeine has been shown to help adults become better able to remain on task (Ritchie, 1975). Caffeine has also been shown to increase the speed of reaction time, and enhance the ability to perform complex, intense tasks, like performance in a flight simulator (Nehlig *et al.*, 1992). Other reviews have confirmed these findings, but also suggested that enhanced performance is evident only when there is prior evidence of fatigue and boredom (Dews, 1984). However, since the subjective experience of boredom is commonly reported by teenagers with ADHD, and it commonly is associated with difficulties in remaining on task and maintaining sustained attention, it is reasonable to expect that caffeine has some beneficial effects on reducing these problems.

In addition, caffeine has also been found to increase the ability to perform tasks that require physical exertion, such as cycling or running (Trice & Haymes, 1995). For this reason, it is banned by the International Olympics Committee (Lombardo, 1986). The mechanism by which caffeine increases physical performance is complex, but may involve increase in fatty acids that can be used as fuel by the muscles, and improvement in respiration. In fact, for over three decades, caffeine has been used to treat apnea of prematurity that is often seen in premature infants (Schmidt, 2005). It is possible that the effects of caffeine ingestion may improve oxygenation of blood, thus further contributing to its impact on vigilance and ability to sustain attention.

Pharmacodynamics

The main psychoactive effect of caffeine is evident through its inhibition of the action of adenosine. A neurotransmitter that is also found throughout most of the body, adenosine has an inhibitory function that slows metabolic activity. Its action may contribute to that of gamma aminobutyric acid (GABA) in opposing the stimulatory effects of glutamate. In fact, adenosine has been found to stabilize the function of the NMDA-type glutaminergic receptors (Fredholm *et al.*, 2001). Caffeine molecules closely resemble adenosine and occupy adenosine receptors without activating them, thus caffeine is an antagonist for adenosine. The net effect is that the inhibitory action associated with adenosine is reduced, thus providing more broad-based neuronal activation. In this manner, the pharmacodynamic action of caffeine is somewhat similar to that of modafinil (discussed in Chapter 13), which exerts its stimulant effect by inhibiting GABA, thus allowing glutamate to have a greater stimulatory effect on the brain.

In addition, adenosine acts pre-synaptically and inhibits the release of other neurotransmitters, including the catecholamines. This effect is seen on both dopamine and norepinephrine/epinephrine. By blocking adenosine, caffeine seems to increase the activation of dopaminergic receptors (Garrett & Griffiths, 1997), and causes additional release of norepinephrine and epinephrine (Bolton and Null, 1981). These effects likely contribute to caffeine's stimulant properties. However, because epinephrine is also involved in the stimulation of the limbic system's fight–flight reaction, use of caffeine sometimes results in an increase of anxiety, especially in individuals susceptible to anxiety and panic.

Pharmacokinetics

Caffeine is rapidly absorbed from the gastrointestinal tract, especially from the small intestine. When caffeine is consumed in food (for example, chocolate or a beverage), its absorption rate depends on how much food was consumed, and what other substances were consumed at the same time (for example, alcohol slows the absorption of caffeine). When used therapeutically, it is preferred to administer caffeine in tablets because they are more rapidly absorbed than caffeine ingested in food. Generally, the effects of caffeine are seen in less than an hour, and the effect lasts about 3–4 hours. However, pharmacokinetics of caffeine are dose dependent. With repeated dosing, such as is often evident in individuals who consume caffeine throughout the day, the elimination half-life is increased. There are also substantial individual differences in the rates of absorption and metabolism of caffeine, and therefore the duration of effect may be somewhat unpredictable. Still, most individuals will require at least twice per day (BID) dosing in order to address symptoms of ADHD in school and at home, and some trial and error may be necessary to maintain the effect of caffeine after school hours (for example, during homework completion), while making sure that the compound is eliminated by the body well ahead of bedtime.

Dosing

Caffeine is generally dosed by body weight. Because of its anxiety-promoting properties, low ceiling dosages have been established. In children, the recommended dose is about 2.5 mg/kg per day, and adverse effects may be seen over 300 or 400 mg per day. Since doses below 200 mg have usually been found to be clinically ineffective (Hingle, 2007), a narrow therapeutic window is available. Of course, since significant variation in metabolizing and responding to caffeine is widely reported, careful titration must be performed to determine the optimal dose for a specific patient.

Adolescents are not generally dosed by body weight. Caffeine is usually started at a dose of 200 mg every 4 hours or so for as long as the benefit of the compound is required. As with children, teens must carefully be monitored for the increase of anxiety, or interference with sleep. Generally, adverse effects on sleep are not seen in individuals who take the last dose of caffeine prior to 6:00 p.m. However, with such wide individual variation, each person's response must carefully be monitored.

Most medications require gradual increase of dose as the brain attempts to counteract the pharmacodynamic effects of the compound, and tolerance is more evident with caffeine than it is with prescription stimulants. When used at appropriate therapeutic levels, there is no appreciable tolerance observed with prescription stimulants. However, because caffeine affects adenosine, the tolerance potential is much more significant. When chronically inhibited, adenosine receptors upregulate by increasing in number, presumably to restore the equilibrium that existed prior to the administration of caffeine. Occasional use of caffeine, especially at lower doses, is not associated with significant tolerance. However, doses of 300 mg or higher result in a decrease of the stimulating effect in as little as 4 days (Evans & Griffiths, 1992). This requires careful monitoring of response in individuals who take caffeine at those (or higher) doses.

Tolerance is a sign of gradual dependence on the substance, indicating that the body has changed its function to allow for the presence of a substance in the system. Indeed, caffeine is often associated with dependence and withdrawal. Once again, wide individual differences are evident. Some individuals exhibit withdrawal effects after using as little as 100 mg of caffeine per day over an extended period of time, while others will exhibit withdrawal effects after using 600 mg of caffeine for as little as 6 days (Griffiths & Mumford, 1995). Individuals who drink coffee every day for extended periods of time usually begin to exhibit withdrawal effects after 24–28 hours, which commonly peak at 20–51 hours and last as long as 9 days (Griffiths & Mumford). The most common withdrawal effects are headaches and irritability. Interestingly, use of caffeine in pill form is not associated with tolerance and withdrawal nearly as frequently, and the vast majority of withdrawal effects are associated with the use of coffee. It is possible that other compounds in coffee are responsible for magnification of the dependence and withdrawal. However, individuals who use caffeine at doses of 300 mg or higher should be monitored for possible signs of dependence and withdrawal. One possible way to counteract some of these effects is to use caffeine intermittently – for example, only during the week and not on weekends.

Adverse Effects

Caffeine is usually well tolerated. The suppression of appetite commonly seen with psychostimulants is much less evident, although a less dramatic decrease in appetite is sometimes reported. Because the absorption of caffeine can be slowed by food, caffeine is best taken before a meal or in-between meals. Those who experience some decrease in appetite may take the compound right before breakfast and right before lunch. In this way, the clinical effect will not yet be evident and no changes in appetite will be observed during the meal.

Caffeine interferes with sleep. While this is a desirable effect when greater vigilance is sought, those who take caffeine to treat symptoms of ADHD must make sure that the last dose is taken well ahead of bedtime. Since caffeine is only available in immediate-release preparations, the last dose can easily be timed to be taken at least 4–6 hours before bedtime. Teens who take higher daily doses need to monitor their sleep response very carefully, since chronic use of caffeine in higher doses has been associated with longer half-life. For some individuals, this effect may be subtle. For example, a person may feel drowsy and therefore assume that the caffeine has been eliminated from the system. However, smaller amounts of caffeine may still interfere with sleep patterns, even if the ability to go to sleep does not seem to be affected. For example, caffeine may decrease the total amount of time spent sleeping (Brenesova et al., 1975). The sleep patterns of children and teens who take caffeine should carefully be monitored to make sure that sleep is not interfered with in any way.

Caffeine is metabolized by the cytochrome P 450 1A2 liver enzyme. This means that when caffeine is used with other medications, its plasma levels may change. Taking medications that inhibit this enzyme will result in higher levels of caffeine, while taking those that induce the enzyme will lower caffeine plasma levels. Not only medications affect this enzyme. For example, nicotine is a potent inducer of 1A2, and smokers tend to metabolize caffeine twice as fast as non-smokers (James, 1991). Children and teens who are on other medications, or teens who smoke, must carefully be monitored when given caffeine.

Caffeine users sometimes report some transient adverse effects, most common of which are nausea and relaxation of some gastrointestinal sphincter functions that may results in mild diarrhea. These effects generally resolve after a few doses. Caffeine is also a diuretic. For this reason, urinary urgency is increased when caffeine is used. Individuals will urinate more frequently, and consequently some may experience increase in dehydration. For this reason, intake of fluid should generally be increased when caffeine is being administered.

Caffeine, as all stimulants, exhibits sympathomimetic qualities that include the activation of the fight–flight mechanism involved in anxiety reactions. In fact, although caffeine's psychostimulant effects are less pronounced than those seen with prescription stimulants, its effect on anxiety is at least as significant. Thus, some patients who take caffeine begin to exhibit symptoms of anxiety. This is especially likely in individuals who present a history of anxiety symptoms. Patients with comorbid symptoms of ADHD and anxiety are likely to become more anxious on caffeine. With prescription stimulants, some patients exhibit positive response in both symptom clusters, and anxiety diminishes along with symptoms of ADHD. However, this has not been seen with caffeine, and increase in anxiety is more likely. For this reason, individuals with ADHD and symptoms of anxiety generally should not use caffeine.

The risk of developing motor tics on stimulant medications is well known. However, because caffeine's effect on brain pathways that control motor functions is less significant, the onset (or exacerbation) of tics is rarely reported with caffeine. Studies have not been performed to investigate the response of individuals with ADHD and comorbid tics. However, since caffeine is not known to exacerbate tics in the vast majority of individuals, a trial of caffeine in this population of patients may be reasonable.

Use of caffeine results in some cardiovascular effects that are similar to other psychostimulants, including small increases in pulse rate. Caffeine causes vasoconstriction in the brain, and as a result it has been found to be effective in addressing migraine headaches. For this reason, caffeine is sometimes added to migraine medications. Peripherally, however, caffeine generally causes vasodilation, thus increasing blood flow. Because caffeine is not associated with cardiac risks, the use of caffeine does not usually necessitate the kinds of cardiac function tests (for example, a baseline EKG) that are sometimes needed when patients at risk for cardiovascular problems are placed on prescription stimulants.

Because the stimulating effects of caffeine are not as significant as they are for prescription stimulants, rebound effects are rarely reported. When the compound is eliminated from the body, it is likely that symptoms of ADHD will return to unmedicated levels, but further exacerbation of the symptoms is not expected. This is one reason why caffeine has sometimes been added to a prescription stimulant, instead of augmenting the dose of the prescription medication. With higher doses of immediate-release prescription stimulants, rebound effects are more likely, since the elimination slope is very steep and the medication is eliminated rapidly. With caffeine, these effects are not commonly seen.

Although extended-release stimulants have much lower risk of rebound effects, some individuals do not respond well to the gradual release of the compound, and clinical effects may not be sufficient. Patients who seem to do best on regular-release compounds but exhibit significant rebound may try to take a lower dose of the prescription stimulant augmented with caffeine. Clinical improvement may be similar to that seen on a higher dose of the prescription stimulant, but the rebound effect may be less evident.

SUPPLEMENTS WITH LIKELY EFFICACY

Although caffeine is the only supplement that has undergone significant research and has shown consistent efficacy, some other compounds have also undergone at least some research, although results are sometimes contradictory. In addition, not all of these have been researched with children and adolescents. Clinicians must use their judgment when weighing the benefits and drawbacks of these supplements.

Omega-3 Polyunsaturated Fatty Acids

Beneficial effects of Omega-3 have been widely touted for about a decade. Indeed, the supplement has been found to stabilize mood, reduce depression, protect the brain against Alzheimer's, and reduce negative effects of low density lipoproteins (LDL), the type of fat responsible for clogging of the arteries. While much of the research about Omega-3's beneficial effects comes from studying cultures where endogenous diet is rich in the intake of Omega-3 in food (for example, by consuming fish), some evidence now exists about beneficial effects of Omega-3 supplementation.

Omega-3 supplements are generally available as caplets filled with fish oil rich in Omega-3. The pills usually contain 1000 mg, but those containing higher and lower amounts are also available. In addition, since the caplets are usually rather large, and may be difficult to swallow by some patients, other forms are also available – for example, a chewable preparation. As is the case with all supplements, there are many manufacturers, and Omega-3 supplements are sold in drug stores, supermarkets, and health food stores. Many are also available through the Internet.

Omega-3 is also sold by prescription in 1000 mg tablets that contain 465 mg of eicosapentaenoic acid (EPA) and 375 mg of docosahexanoic acid (DHA). These are approved to treat hyperlipidemia and are marketed as Lovaza (formally Omacor). They are manufactured in a process that removes mercury from the fish oil, and therefore these pills are marketed as superior to other Omega-3 supplements (which usually do not remove mercury from the fish oil): the amount of mercury contained in fish oil supplements is considered to be much lower than it is in many types of fish, since the oil is not usually derived from fish known to have high amounts of mercury. In addition, plant-based Omega-3 supplements (in flax, soybean, or canola oil), also available on the market, do not contain mercury. One potential benefit of Lovaza is that, as an FDA-approved compound, its sale and manufacture is regulated, and therefore the consumer can be more certain that Lovaza really contains the ingredients that it claims to have, in the specific amount that is advertised. Consumers must balance these benefits against the added cost of this medication and the inconvenience of seeking a prescription.

Although evidence of the effectiveness of Omega-3 fatty acids to treat symptoms of ADHD is only now emerging, the supplement is already shown to have benefits in stabilizing mood and possibly improving symptoms of depression. For this reason, children and adolescents who present with comorbid symptoms of ADHD and agitation or depression may especially be good candidates for a trial of Omega-3 supplementation.

Evidence of Efficacy

Omega-3's efficacy to treat symptoms of ADHD is not well established, and some studies reveal limited efficacy. For example, Voigt et al. (2001) found no benefit in using DHA to address symptoms of ADHD in children, and Hirayama et al. (2004) reported similar results. However, others have found more promising results. Richardson (2003) reported that children with ADHD who took a mixture of DHA, EPA, and two types of Omega-6 fatty acids experienced significant improvement in hyperactivity and impulsivity, and another, placebo-controlled, trial revealed that children who took a mixture of Omega-6 and Omega-3 fatty acids experienced decreases in inattention and disruptive behavior (Stevens et al., 2003). Another study revealed similar findings, but also found that children with ADHD, Inattentive Type responded better to Omega-3/6 than those with symptoms of hyperactivity and/or impulsivity (Johnson et al., 2009). Overall, the results of all these studies are inconsistent. At first glance, it may seem that different combinations of DHA/EPA may be responsible for the differential response in studies. However, since these fatty acids undergo significant cross-transformation in the body (as described below), it is unlikely that taking one form is likely to be better than another.

The use of Omega-3 to treat symptoms of ADHD has also been researched with teenagers. In one small study, levels of endogenous

DHA have been found to be lower in teens with ADHD (Colter *et al.*, 2008), but augmentation was not studied to see whether it had beneficial effects. Similarly, it has been hypothesized that low levels of DHA or related fatty acids are also responsible for difficulties with cognitive functioning in adults, including problems remaining on task (Richardson, 2003). As with the adolescent study, supplementation of Omega-3 was not studied whether it would be beneficial. Prior research, however, linked low levels of essential fatty acids (Omega-3/6) with low levels of monoamine metabolites in the cerebrospinal fluid (Hibbeln *et al.*, 1998b). Although this finding is correlational, some studies with children reveal that symptoms of ADHD are accompanied by such deficits. Thus, it is plausible that supplementation with essential fatty acids may have some beneficial effects for individuals with ADHD.

Pharmacodynamics

Essential Omega-3 fatty acids include a-linolenic acid (ALA), EPA, and DHA. These cannot be synthesized by the body and must be ingested from food. Following ingestion, DHA inhibits lipogenesis and stimulates oxidation. ALA, EPA, and DHA undergo downconversion and retroconversion (as described below) and contribute to the metabolism of various nutrients and lipids. This is responsible for a broad-based therapeutic effect that includes changes in cardiovascular function, decrease in triglycerides, and improvement in pulmonary function. Most of these effects are directly associated with DHA, although related fatty acids may play a contributory role.

DHA is taken up by the brain at greater rates than the other fatty acids. DHA is then incorporated into the phospholipids of cell membranes. DHA contributes to proper formation and elongation of synapses. In addition, DHA-containing phospholipids improve cell function by stabilizing the membrane fluidity and changing firing rates of neurons (Horrocks & Yeo, 1999). Thus, DHA may play a role in the synchronization of neuronal action. It can be hypothesized that poor phosphorization may be partially responsible for decreased neuronal function, and when such deficits are evident in catecholaminergic pathways that control executive functions, focusing, and self-control, symptoms of ADHD are apparent. Consequently, increasing phosphorization of cell membranes in these areas may be responsible for the beneficial effects of DHA (and other fatty acid) supplementation sometimes observed in individuals with ADHD.

Eicosanoids contribute to this process. They are localized in cells and serve as catalysts for a large number of processes, including the movement of calcium in and out of the cells (Enig & Fallon, 1999). Because calcium channels are involved in the rates of firing of brain cells, regulation of these channels changes the brain's action potential. It is possible that EPA's regulation of calcium channels may contribute to DHA's influence of cell membrane phosphorization, providing a synergistic effect on the rates of neuronal firing. When this regulation of firing affects catecholaminergic pathways, improvement in symptoms of ADHD may be observed.

Pharmacokinetics

Following ingestion, the metabolism of fatty acids begins in the small intestine by special digestive enzymes. These lipases break down fatty acids into individual chains, glycerol, and monoglycerides (glycerol with one remaining fatty acid still attached). These are then absorbed through the intestinal wall into the lymph stream. Fat molecules are then carried in the lymph system and slowly metabolized to provide gradual release of energy (Enig, 2000).

Essential fatty acids go through many conversions. ALA is converted into EPA and DHA, and these are then gradually absorbed into cell membranes. However, they also undergo complex cross-metabolism. While Omega-6, also known as linoleic acid (LA), undergoes a one-way transformation into various fatty chains, culminating in docosapentaenoic acid, ALA undergoes circular transformation that involves many steps, including the formation of EPA and DHA, and then retroconversion of EPA and DHA. It is difficult to determine how the body regulates the amounts of DHA and EPA that remain in the cells. It is likely that these are constantly transformed into each other to provide a balance of essential nutrients necessary for many metabolic processes, including membrane phosphorization.

Because ALA is converted into EPA and DHA, and EPA and DHA are retroconverted into each other, it is not necessary to purchase a specific combination of these fatty acids. Some manufacturers focus on the hypothesized benefits of DHA over EPA, or vice versa, and Omega-3 pills are available in various combinations of these components. Consumers need to keep in mind that the balance of these components in the pill is probably immaterial, since the complex conversion chains will probably result in the same balance of these nutrients in the body, regardless of the specific ratio included in the caplet.

Optimal ratio of Omega-6 to Omega-3 in the human body is estimated to be 2:1. However, it is not uncommon for individuals in westernized countries to consume diets where the two are ingested at a ratio of about 20:1. For this reason, the majority of supplements primarily focus on delivering additional amounts of Omega-3 into the body, and any amounts of Omega-6 in the tablet may be superfluous, since the common diet already includes so many foods rich in LA. When purchasing a supplement, consumers should select one that maximizes the amount of Omega-3 and minimizes the amount of Omega-6 in the preparation.

Manufacturers of Omega-3 generally advise to take the supplements with or without food. Researchers, however, have long recognized that Omega-3 fatty acids ingested in food are better absorbed than those taken in supplements. Some studies have found that Omega-3 taken without a meal is poorly absorbed. For this reason, nutritionists generally recommend to take an Omega-3 supplement as part of a meal, so that it is absorbed together with the food that is being consumed (Neville, 2006).

In order to prevent oxidation of fatty acids before they are taken up into cell membranes, antioxidants must be present. Those whose diets are rich in antioxidant foods probably consume enough of these during a meal to prevent fatty acid oxidation. However, those who consume meals low in antioxidants may need to take an antioxidant supplement – for example, tocopherol, a form of vitamin E. For this reason, some formulations of Omega-3 supplements include a small amount of tocopherol. However, instead of (or in addition to) tocopherol, some supplements also include vitamins A and/or D. Because these vitamins do not get cleared from the body, clients should be careful with these supplements because high intake of these vitamins may lead to toxicity.

Although fatty acids are metabolized and absorbed rapidly, the onset of effect is not evident for a long time. Some have reported that the onset of clinical effect is not evident for weeks, even months, and that treatment for up to 3 months is necessary to determine the eventual clinical response (Lake, 2007). This makes it difficult to dose the supplements, since clinical effects are not likely to be immediately evident.

Dosing

Omega-3 supplements are not usually dosed by body weight. In children, the recommended starting dose is 500 mg, and usually doses range up to 4000 mg/day (Bezchlibnyk-Butler & Virani, 2004). Some have found doses below 1000 mg/day to be ineffective (Lake, 2007). Because Omega-3 is generally well tolerated, gradual titration is recommended. However, the maximum dose is often determined by how many tablets the child is willing to take and whether digestive effects (for example, fish burps or a fishy taste in the mouth) prevent further increase in dose. Because response will not immediately be evident, it is difficult to determine what dose will eventually be effective.

Teens are generally dosed at 1000–4000 mg/day (Bezchlibnyk-Butler & Jeffries, 2007). Some have found doses below 2000 mg/day to be ineffective, and some adults require doses in excess of 9000 mg (Lake, 2007). As with children, dosing should gradually be increased to a maximum level that can be tolerated with minimal gastrointestinal discomfort. Again, it is difficult to determine what dose will be effective since response to the supplement may not immediately be evident.

Co-factors are necessary for metabolism of some of the fatty acids, especially EPA. Carnitine is necessary for the elongating EPA and transporting it across inner cell membranes. It is possible that some of the inconsistent findings about the efficacy of fatty acids may be secondary to carnitine deficits. For this reason, supplementation with l-carnitine has been studied and has shown promising effects in hyperactive girls with fragile X syndrome (Torrioli et al., 1999). Since humans metabolize only a portion of the necessary supply of carnitine, supplementing fatty acid therapy with l-carnitine may be helpful. L-carnitine is supplied in capsules, tablets, solution, and chewable wafer. Children may take about 250 mg of l-carnitine with fatty acids, while adults may need to take about 500 mg. These doses are generally well tolerated although a small incidence of seizures has been reported (Medical Economics, 2008a). Individuals with risk factors for seizures should consider l-carnitine supplementation only under supervision of a physician.

Adverse Effects

Omega-3 oils are generally well tolerated. The most common adverse effects involve the gastrointestinal tract, including nausea and diarrhea. Because the majority of Omega-3 supplements are sold as fish oils, some individuals experience an unpleasant, 'fishy' taste in their mouth, a 'fishy' smelling breath after a meal during which Omega-3 supplement was taken, and fishy 'burps' that may last for several hours. For this reason, some manufacturers offer 'burpless' formulas manufactured by increasing the thickness of the pill's outer coating. This allows the supplement to survive the stomach acids and dissolve when it reaches the small intestine. These have been shown to effectively reduce the above problems. Omega-3 supplements are also available in non-fish based formulas that are not associated with burps or an unpleasant taste.

Because Omega-3 supplements are oil based, there is a caloric value associated with the caplet. The exact amount varies, but generally a 1000 mg pill will contain about 20 calories. For individuals who consume a low amount, an extra 20 or 40 calories per day will probably have a minimal amount on weight. However, those on higher amounts (for example, 8000 or 9000 mg per day) must remember that they are consuming an additional 160 or 180 calories. In addition, fatty acids are high density lipoproteins (HDL) and contribute to the overall HDL levels within the body. While this is generally beneficial, those on high levels of Omega-3 supplements who also consume diets rich in HDL may experience additional increases of HDL and total cholesterol, which may not always be beneficial. Individuals who take high doses of fatty acid supplements should periodically check their cholesterol profile.

Omega-3 fatty acids are associated with an antithrombotic effect. Patients who take blood thinners (like aspirin) must be careful about taking subsequent fatty acid supplements, and should consult a physician before initiating Omega-3 therapy. In addition, some patients regularly use over-the-counter non-steroidal anti-inflammatory drugs (NSAIDs, like Advil or Motrin) to manage headaches, backaches, or similar conditions. While combining fatty acids with NSAIDs has not been shown to pose a risk, many NSAIDs have some blood thinning properties, and combining NSAIDs with fatty acids has sometimes been linked to nose bleeds and easy bruising (Medical Economics, 2008a). For this reason, those who take NSAIDs daily should probably consult a physician before initiating Omega-3 therapy.

Use of fatty acid supplements has sometimes been reported to alter glucose tolerance, especially in patients with type 2 diabetes. The mechanism of this is poorly understood, and some studies have not confirmed this finding. However, because there is a risk, children and adolescents who are diabetic and take insulin should consult their physician before starting Omega-3 treatment.

S-Adenosyl-L-Methionine (SAMe)

SAMe is a natural substance present in the body. It was discovered in 1952 by an Italian scientist, and became marketed in Europe shortly afterward, where it is considered (and regulated as) a drug. It has only been available in the US since 1999, and it is classified as a nutritional supplement. It is known by a variety of names, including ademetionine, S-adenosylmethionine, and also sometimes referred to as SAM or SAM-e. It is primarily used to treat osteoarthritis, fibromyalgia, and liver disorders. Efficacy for those applications is well established with many studies published in European journals, and it is considered to be one of the most researched nutritional supplements (Settle, 2007).

More recently, SAMe has also been shown to have potentially beneficial effects in treating symptoms of depression (as discussed in Chapter 6) and ADHD. Its impact on depression is recognized in the US and abroad, and is presumed to be secondary to pharmacodynamic effects that resemble the action of some antidepressants. These include the increase in catecholaminergic activity throughout the brain, and, consequently, benefits in treating symptoms of ADHD have also been reported.

Evidence of Efficacy

The evidence of SAMe's benefits in treating symptoms of ADHD comes primarily from the recognition that SAMe is an effective antidepressant, and studies, as well as meta-analyses, have shown that its efficacy is at least as significant as that of tricyclic antidepressants (Settle, 2007). SAMe regulates the activity of catecholaminergic pathways, including stimulation of the ones that are involved in symptoms of ADHD. Thus, the rationale seems sound, although the evidence at this time is limited.

There are a few studies that have investigated the benefit of SAMe in treating ADHD. A small, open-label study with adults found that SAMe was beneficial in reducing symptoms of distractibility and self-control (Wood et al., 1985), although the benefits were possibly secondary to improvements in mood symptoms. Another study reviewed benefits of SAMe (and other supplements) in treating ADHD and found short-term improvement (Nemzer et al., 1986), and a large, open trial follow-up with about 6000 patients has been announced but its results have not yet been disseminated (Walsh, 2003).

Unfortunately, the benefits of SAMe have been reported to only last for 2 or 3 months. It is apparent that tolerance develops, perhaps due to downregulation effects. For this reason, use of SAMe should probably be reserved for applications with those individuals who present with comorbid symptoms of depression that may be exacerbating symptoms of ADHD. In addition, SAMe has primarily been used with adults. Although no specific counterindications exist for use with children or adolescents, clinicians should be very cautious when using SAMe with young clients.

Pharmacodynamics

SAMe is a second messenger. This term refers to substances that act within cells to change some aspects of cell metabolism. In this case, SAMe is a methyl donor that contributes to dozens of reactions throughout the brain, including the synthesis of monoamine transmitters – dopamine, norepinephrine, and serotonin, among others (Settle, 2007). This action is responsible, at least in part, for its antidepressant effect, and probably underlies the reduction of symptoms of ADHD. Since functional deficits in ADHD result from underactivation of key pathways for dopamine and norepinephrine, producing additional amount of these catecholamines has potential benefits in alleviating the symptoms (as has been shown with many of the medications used to treat ADHD). Indeed, a review of European research revealed that SAMe may be involved in increasing activity in dopaminergic and serotonergic pathways (Settle).

SAMe is also involved in methylation and/or phosphorization processes that affect membrane fluidity. As such, its effects may be similar to those of Omega-3 fatty acids, where regulation of the membrane fluidity may be involved in stabilization of neurotransmitter release and neuronal firing. SAMe has been found to increase the number of receptors on the cell, increase binding to receptors, and enhance membrane fluidity (Settle, 2007). These effects likely contribute to increases in dopamine and serotonin, and further enhance its clinical effect.

Pharmacokinetics

SAMe is available in tablets. Some of these have enteric coating, and some do not. Those that are coated are a better choice because SAMe is absorbed from the small intestine, and therefore as much compound as possible should 'survive' the stomach acids and get through into the small intestine. In addition, SAMe is unstable at temperatures above freezing (0 degrees Celsius, or 32 degrees Fahrenheit). A wide variety of SAMe preparations are available on the market. Forms that have been researched for efficacy are stable at higher temperatures, but other forms are marketed for which efficacy may be questionable. Consumers should seek the form that includes SAMe paratoluene sulfonates (SAMe tosyls) because these salts have been found to be stable at room temperature. Additionally, SAMe must be kept very dry because moisture can cause hydrolysis. It is recommended that the best form to purchase is the stable formulation of SAMe tosyls that is also enteric-coated (Medical Economics, 2008a).

SAMe should be taken on an empty stomach – about 1 hour before or 2 hours after a meal. The peak is usually attained in 3–5 hours (Medical Economics, 2008a), but onset of clinical effect is not generally evident for at least 1–2 weeks (Walsh, 2003).

SAMe is metabolized by the liver but seems to have minimal effects on liver enzymes, and drug–drug interactions have not been reported with SAMe. Most of the substance is incorporated into various cells, and only a small portion is eliminated in urine (15 percent) and feces (23 percent). Thus, liver and kidney function seems to have limited effect on the metabolism and excretion of SAMe (Medical Economics, 2008a).

When SAMe is metabolized, co-factors are involved. Metabolism of SAMe to homocysteine requires the presence of vitamin B6. This pathway probably has minor (if any) effects on symptoms of ADHD, and therefore levels of vitamin B6 are less important for this specific application. SAMe is also metabolized into methionine and this pathway has greater relevance to ADHD. In order to accomplish this metabolism, folic acid and vitamin B12 are needed (Medical Economics, 2008a). Consequently, when minimal effects of SAMe supplementation are seen, vitamin B complex can be added. Since these compounds are already present in a normal diet, supplementation should be minimal and higher, focused doses of these vitamins are not recommended.

Dosing

The clinical dose of SAMe varies widely. Children should start at about 200 mg once per day (preferably in the morning) and gradually titrate at intervals of 1–2 weeks between dose increases. Teenagers and adults are generally dosed up to 2400 mg/day (Bezchlibnyk-Butler & Jeffries, 2007), although doses above 1600 mg/day have not been studied for adverse effects (Medical Economics, 2008a). Clearly, children should receive lower doses, although no specific guidelines exist for dosing children and adolescents. According to the National Center for Health Statistics (2002), the weight of an average adult male in the US is about 190 pounds (about 86 kg). Thus, the dose-to-weight ratio for adults is about 18–28 mg/kg per day. The effective ratio for children and adolescents may be similar. Clinicians are advised to 'start low and go slow' – begin minimal dose, and gradually titrate making sure that the above mg/kg ratios are not exceeded.

Adverse Effects

SAMe is generally well tolerated. Suppression of appetite and weight change are not reported. However, mild gastrointestinal upsets (nausea, diarrhea, and flatulence) may be evident at the start of treatment (Medical Economics, 2008a). These usually resolve after a week or two. Sometimes, those with higher doses experience more persistent nausea (Bezchlibnyk-Butler & Jeffries, 2007).

SAMe may interfere with sleep and some insomnia has been reported (Medical Economics, 2008a). For this reason, it is generally recommended that SAMe should be taken in the morning. Especially when used to treat symptoms of ADHD, the activating effect may be beneficial and may contribute to a reduction in distractibility.

Because SAMe is not a stimulant, it poses little risk of motor tics. However, other motor effects have rarely been reported, including some hyperactive muscle movement (Medical Economics, 2008a). When encountered, the dose should be lowered for a week or two, following which the patient may gradually be re-challenged with a higher dose, if needed.

Because SAMe does not alter liver enzymes, and does not seem to rely on any one CP450 enzyme for metabolism, drug–drug interactions are less likely. However, SAMe may have some effects on lowering lipids and improving liver function. It is also used to treat osteoarthritis and fibromyalgia. Thus, patients who already take medications to lower cholesterol, or treat osteoarthritis or fibromyalgia, should consult their physician before initiating SAMe therapy.

Although a specific 'black box' warning that applies to all antidepressants is not issued for SAMe, because of its antidepressant action, SAMe may be associated with a small increase in suicidal tendencies in those patients who present with symptoms of depression. As with any antidepressant, clinicians should carefully monitor patient response and intervene if an increase in suicidal thoughts or plans becomes evident. In addition, like all antidepressants, SAMe is also associated with a small risk of inducing hypomanic or manic symptoms (Bezchlibnyk-Butler & Jeffries, 2007), and some patients who have tendencies toward symptoms of bipolar disorder may exhibit 'switching' from depressive to manic symptoms. Once again, careful monitoring of dose/response and adverse effects is necessary.

SUPPLEMENTS WITH POSSIBLE EFFICACY

In addition to the supplements discussed above, there is some data available that suggests that other compounds may also have some efficacy in treating symptoms of ADHD. However, since the data that supports the use of the following supplements is extremely limited, clinicians should proceed with caution, and consider the use of the compounds discussed in this section as experimental.

Inositol

Inositol is an isomer of glucose and is present in high concentrations in the brain. It is part of intracellular processes mediated by second messenger systems, and may be involved in regulating the activity of monoamines (especially serotonin, with possible action on dopamine and norepinephrine) as well as other neurotransmitters. As discussed in Chapters 6 and 8, inositol has primarily shown efficacy in treating symptoms of depression (Settle, 2007) and anxiety (Bezchlibnyk-Butler & Jeffries, 2007), including anxiety-spectrum disorders such as obsessive compulsive disorder and trichotillomania. Its use in treating symptoms of ADHD is recent and scant evidence exists thus far. While some studies reported that use of inositol may aggravate symptoms of ADHD (Bezchlibnyk-Butler & Jeffries), others have found that inositol supplementation, with or without concomitant use with Omega-3 fatty acids, improved symptoms of ADHD in children (Alvarado *et al.*, 2004). At this time, inositol is probably best reserved for a cautious trial with individuals who exhibit symptoms of ADHD that are significantly exacerbated by anxiety or depression.

Inositol is available in several forms, and only some of these are appropriate for psychiatric use. These include inositol and myo-inositol. Other forms, such as inositol hexaphosphate, inositol nicotinae, and D-chiro-inositol have not been shown to have mental health effects and are used to treat cancer, vascular diseases, and insulin resistance.

Inositol is dosed at much higher levels than other supplements. Therapeutic doses usually range from 12–18 g per day, taken in divided doses (usually two to three times per day). Inositol is also available as a powder that dissolves easily in water or juice. This may be a good option for those who have difficulties swallowing pills. Dosing usually starts at 2 g twice per day, increasing to up to 6 g three times per day. Inositol can be taken with or without food. Onset of clinical effect is usually observed in 2–4 weeks.

Inositol is generally well tolerated at doses of up to 20 g per day (Settle, 2007). In children, the studied dose was 50 mg/kg per day (Alvarado *et al.*, 2004). Common adverse effects are mild and include gastrointestinal upset, such as nausea, diarrhea, and flatulence. Few studies have reviewed possible interactions between inositol and other drugs, but the supplement is considered safe to use with other medications (Settle). Because of its antidepressant effects, rare episodes of switching into mania have been reported. Patients with symptoms of agitation or depression who take inositol should carefully be monitored for signs of manic or hypomanic symptoms.

Dimethylaminoethanol and Choline

Choline (trimethylaminoethanol) is involved in the synthesis of the neurotransmitter acetylcholine. Dimethylanimoethanol is the immediate precursor of trimethylaminoethanol. Choline is involved in maintaining cell membrane integrity, and regulating of neuronal firing. Acetylcholine is an endogenous neurotransmitter that has not been directly implicated in symptoms of ADHD. However, acetylcholine is involved in motor control, and disturbance in dopamine–acetylcholine balance is a well-known mechanism that underlies significant motor side effects of many medications (for example, those seen with first-generation low-potency antipsychotics, like Thorazine and Mellaril). Thus, changes in acetylcholine activity may have some beneficial effects in improving symptoms of ADHD.

Dimethylaminoethanol, also known as dimethylethanolamine or DMAE, was once marketed in the US as Deaner but was withdrawn in 1980 because the FDA required proof for its claims of efficacy in treating symptoms of minimal brain dysfunction (Arnold, 2002). Nevertheless, several placebo-controlled trials performed in the 1960s and 1970s have shown that it was effective in improving symptoms of ADHD in children at doses of 500 mg/day or higher. Today, DMAE is not widely available, but choline supplements can be purchased from many drug stores and nutritional supplement vendors. There appears to be no difference in purchasing DMAE or choline, since one is converted to the other.

Choline is sometimes utilized with other supplements. For example, Alvarado et al. (2004) studied the joint benefits of inositol and choline, and found a combination of the two to be effective in treating symptoms of ADHD. Since choline is generally well tolerated, supplementing inositol with choline may be an option to consider for patients who are candidates for treatment with inositol.

Doses of 3 mg/day of choline have been studied with adults and produced few side effects (Medical Economics, 2008a). Usual effective doses are 425–550 mg/day for adults, and 250–350 mg/day for children. Choline is generally regarded as safe, and pregnant mothers are sometimes encouraged to take choline to aid the brain development of the fetus. The most common side effects are nausea, diarrhea, and loose stools. High doses of choline have sometimes resulted in hypotension and increases in depressive symptoms. Those who use choline jointly with inositol should stay within the lower levels of the therapeutic range for both compounds.

Pycnogenol

Pycnogenol is a generic name for a mixture of procyanidins extracted from the bark of the pine tree (*Pinus maritima*) common to the Gascogne region of France. Pycnogenol has many active compounds, primarily consisting of dimmers of catechin, and oligomers of catechin and epi-catechin. Similar compounds are also found in cocoa, chocolate, and some fruit. Their pharmacodynamic action primarily consists of antioxidant properties and possible anti-inflammatory effects. Pycnogenol may also influence the release of catecholamines (including dopamine and norepinephrine) and nitric oxide synthesis.

Some researchers reported that oxidative stress may underlie symptoms of Parkinson's disorder (Olanow, 1996), and some have hypothesized that similar factors may underlie symptoms of ADHD. For many decades, pycnogenol has been used in Europe to treat symptoms of hyperactivity. Heimann (1999) reviewed many anecdotal reports and reported a case study where supplementation with pycnogenol for 4 weeks resulted in a significant decrease in hyperactivity and impulsivity in a patient with ADHD. A subsequent trial with 61 children and adolescents with ADHD also found beneficial effects after taking 1 mg/kg of pycnogenol for one month (Trebaticka et al., 2006). Notably, the treatment effects were more significant in boys than in girls. Another study also found that the addition of pycnogenol to the treatment of ADHD with dextroamphetamine was superior to the use of dextroamphetamine alone (Medical Economics, 2008a).

Pycnogenol is generally supplied in tablets and capsules, and creams and lotions containing it are also available but have not been studied for their effectiveness. Pycnogenol is generally dosed at the ratio of 1 mg/kg, and adult doses range from 25–200 mg/day. Pycnogenol is generally well tolerated and the available literature reports no adverse effects. However, because it may produce vasorelaxation and inhibition of platelet activity, those who take blood thinners (for example, aspirin) should exercise caution.

Rhodiola

Rhodiola (*Rhodiola rosea*) is a perennial plant that grows in the US, Canada, Europe, and parts of Asia. Its root, also known as golden root, is commonly used in Asia and Europe to treat fatigue and cognitive blunting. Its pharmacology is complex and includes a large number of active compounds, such as flavonoids, monoterpernes, phenylpropanoids, triterpenes, phenolic acids, and phenylethanol derivatives. It has multiple effects, including antioxidant, anticarcinogenic, cardioprotective, and neuroendocrine properties. Its psychopharmacological effect may include agonist properties for serotonin and dopamine (perhaps secondary to monoamine oxidase inhibition), as well as influence on opioid peptides (such as beta-endorphins). Although its benefit in treating symptoms of ADHD has not been studied, rhodiola has been shown to have some antidepressant and psychostimulant effects (Shevtsov et al., 2003; Darbinyan et al., 2007). In addition, use of rhodiola concomitantly with a stimulant has shown to have additive effects (Medical Economics, 2007).

Rhodiola is usually available in capsules or tablets that usually contain 100 mg of a mixture of 3 percent rosavins and 1 percent salidroside. Although other active compounds are found in the preparation, their role is unknown, and therefore rosavins and salidrose are generally sought. Rhodiola is given in 100–200 mg per dose, usually taken two to three times per day. Dosing for children has not been studied, but no contraindications exist, and therefore a dose of 100 mg one to twice per day can cautiously be tried, and gradually titrated upward if well tolerated.

Rhodiola is presumed safe and no adverse effects have been reported in available literature. Similarly, it is not presumed to interact with prescription medications (Medical Economics, 2007). However, because of its antidepressant effects, it may pose a risk of 'switching' into manic or mixed-manic episodes in a manner that is similar to all compounds with antidepressant effects.

SUPPLEMENTS NOT LIKELY TO BE EFFECTIVE

It is not possible to review the variety of compounds that, at one time or another, have been tried to treat symptoms of ADHD and have not shown to be effective, or lack sufficient rationale about how they may affect brain action to improve distractibility, and/or hyperactivity/impulsivity. However, some of these compounds continue to be marketed, and naturopathic zealots continue to espouse the benefits of some of these supplements despite the lack of evidence of efficacy. Clinicians who seek to practice in the area of naturopathic psychopharmacology should be aware of compounds that continue to be propagated in folklore or late-night infomercials, despite evidence to the contrary.

St. John's Wort

St. John's Wort is an herb that exists in some 370 species found throughout the world, but is originally endogenous to Europe. St. John's Wort contains a plethora of active ingredients, including dozens of flavonoids and acylphloroglucinols (especially hyperforin). St. John's Wort is known to be an effective antidepressant, and hyoperforin is thought to be responsible for most of its psychoactive activity. St. John's Wort increases the amount of serotonergic activity in the brain, and for this reason it also has anxiolytic properties. In addition, it may suppress monoamine oxidase, the enzyme responsible for the breakdown of all monoamines. Thus, in addition to its serotonergic effects, it may increase the activity of norepinephrine and dopamine (Schroeder *et al.*, 2004), and some have presumed that it may have beneficial effects in treating symptoms of ADHD.

However, several studies have found that St. John's Wort failed to improve symptoms of ADHD. Studies examining its effects on symptoms of ADHD in adults have not shown a significant effect (Barkley, 2006), and placebo-controlled research on children and adolescents with ADHD rendered similar results (Weber *et al.*, 2008). Although using this herb with adults who have comorbid symptoms of depression and ADHD may be beneficial, St. John's Wort is not likely to have much positive effect on symptoms of ADHD in individuals who do not exhibit depression, agitation, or anxiety.

Vitamin Therapy

Vitamin supplementation is generally administered in one of three strategies – daily multivitamin use that supplements daily intake to meet recommended daily allowances (RDA), megavitamin cocktails that significantly exceed RDA, or focused megadoses of a single vitamin. None of these have been shown to be an effective treatment for symptoms of ADHD.

The first of those strategies may be beneficial to overall health, but has not been shown to improve symptoms of ADHD. Although supplementation of one-a-day multivitamin has been shown to improve cognitive functioning (Benton & Cook, 1991), presumed benefits exist only for those who exhibit vitamin deficiencies because of dietary deficits, and no additional benefits for individuals who consume normal, healthy diets have been shown in research (Benton & Buts, 1990). Thus, while the use of a multivitamin may help those who have poor diets, it is not a treatment to address symptoms of ADHD in children or adolescents with ADHD.

Megadose supplementation of multiple vitamins similarly has been found to be ineffective in double-blind, placebo-controlled studies that lasted up to 6 months (Arnold, 2002). A variety of combinations have been researched, but none seem to have any beneficial effects on symptoms of ADHD or learning disorders. In addition, some vitamins pose a significant risk when taken in excess. For this reason, megadoses of multivitamins are not only ineffective, they may be dangerous, especially when RDA levels of vitamins such as A or B6 are significantly exceeded. Clinicians are encouraged to advise their patients and clients against trials of such unproven and potentially dangerous methods.

Focused megadoses of specific vitamins have not been adequately studied, but no reasonable rationale has thus far emerged as to the potential efficacy of those compounds to improve symptoms of ADHD. Again, it is important to observe daily RDA limits and not exceed those for many vitamins, since adverse effects may result in a variety of problems, from neuropathic effects to liver damage. Clinicians should advise their patients and clients against these approaches.

Focus Factor

A wide variety of multivitamin compounds exists on the market that purports to treat many disorders, including ADHD. One of the best known is Focus Factor, a cocktail of some 40 compounds that primarily includes RDA doses of multivitamins, and small doses of dimethylaminoethanol (DMEA), trimethylaminoethanol (choline), and docosahexaenoic acid (DHA), as well as other herbs with unproven pharmacology or efficacy. To understand the potential benefits of this preparation, various groups of ingredients have to be examined separately.

Essentially, Focus Factor is a multivitamin. As such, it is not likely to do any harm, but is also unlikely to have any significant benefits in improving symptoms of ADHD unless the patient is on a diet that significantly restricts the intake of common nutrients. If that is the case, a drug-store multivitamin is likely to provide the same benefit at a fraction of the cost.

The second group of ingredients includes DMEA, choline, and DHA. The potential benefits of those are discussed above, separately for each of those ingredients. In order to be potentially effective, each of those needs to be given in higher doses than are included in Focus Factor, and each of those ingredients can be purchased in a local pharmacy of nutritional supplement store for a smaller price.

The final group of ingredients includes rarely used herbs, such as huperzine and vinpocetine, which are scarcely studied and have no reasonable rationale about potential benefits in treating symptoms of ADHD. Overall, while there is no evidence that Focus Factor may be harmful, there is also no evidence that most individuals derive any benefit from this compound.

Iron

Iron is a chemical element involved in the anabolism of catecholamines. Iron is present throughout the body and is converted into amino acids. The vast majority of necessary iron intake is derived from the normal diet, and many iron-rich foods are commonly consumed in meats, cereals, fruit, and vegetables. Some members of at-risk populations may require iron supplementation – for example, those who are malnourished, infants who are not breast-fed, or individuals who have lost a lot of blood. However, iron supplementation in patients who are not iron deficient is dangerous. Careful RDA limits must be observed and excess iron intake has been associated with serious toxic effects, including death. Children are especially at risk for these problems, and iron supplementation should only be undertaken under the supervision (and recommendation) of a physician (Medical Economics, 2008a).

Some studies examined the effects of iron supplementation on symptoms of ADHD. For example, Sever *et al.* (1997) found some decrease in symptoms in children with ADHD, and Burattini *et al.* (1990) found a decrease in symptoms of hyperactivity, but both studies used iron supplements with children who were initially found to exhibit iron deficiency, and iron supplementation generally has no positive effects on children with ADHD who do not exhibit iron deficiency. Since the vast majority of children and adolescents with ADHD probably do not exhibit iron deficiency, the effect of iron supplementation in this population is unknown. Given the risks of iron supplementation, clinicians should stay away from this practice unless it can be confirmed that the patient exhibits iron deficiency, and any iron supplementation should be given under close supervision of a physician.

SUMMARY

In order to help clinicians select the compounds that are appropriate given the specific cluster of symptoms evident in each patient, an algorithm was developed and is presented in Figure 5.1. This diagram takes into account the amount of research support available for each compound, as well as the specific mechanism of action of each supplement and its applicability to the treatment of ADHD and common comorbidities.

Patients with symptoms of ADHD without comorbid depression or anxiety should initially be tried on caffeine, and if insufficient response is obtained, pycnogenol may be tried (as monotherapy or adjunct). If insufficient response is evident, Omega-3 supplements may be

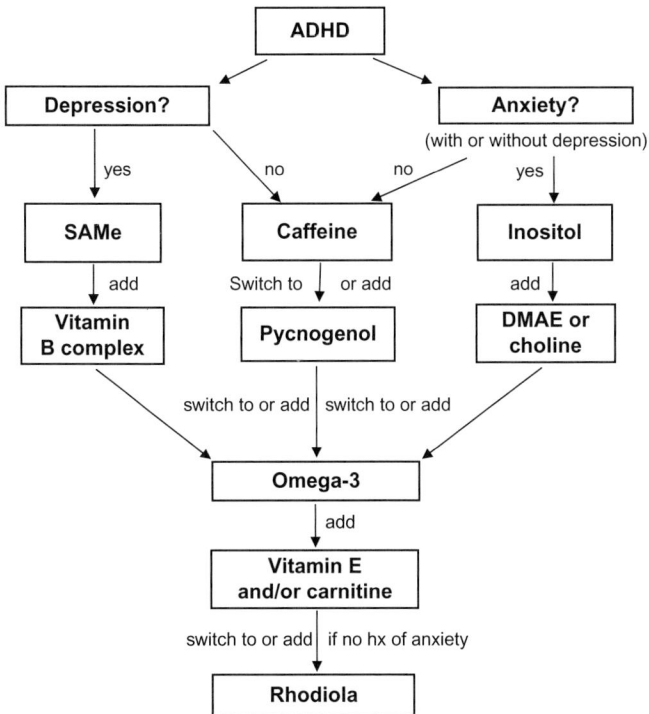

FIGURE 5.1 Algorithm for treatment of ADHD with naturopathic supplements.
© Elsevier 2009.

attempted, again as monotherapy or as adjuncts to caffeine and/or pycnogenol. If insufficient response is still evident, vitamin E and/or carnitine may be added. As a last resort, caffeine and/or pycnogenol can be discontinued and rhodiola can be tried as monotherapy or adjunct to Omega-3 (with or without vitamin E and/or carnitine).

Patients with symptoms of ADHD and comorbid depression should initially be tried on SAMe, and vitamin B complex can be added. If insufficient response is apparent, Omega-3 can be attempted, as monotherapy or adjunct to SAMe (used with or without B complex), and vitamin E and/or carnitine may also be added. As a last resort, SAMe and vitamin B complex can be discontinued and rhodiola can be tried as monotherapy or adjunct to Omega-3 (with or without vitamin E and/or carnitine).

Patients with symptoms of ADHD and comorbid anxiety (with or without comorbid depression) should initially be tried on inositol, and DMAE or choline can be added. If insufficient response is apparent, Omega-3 can be attempted, as monotherapy or adjunct to inositol (used with or without vitamin E and/or carnitine), and vitamin E and/or carnitine may also be added. Because of its potentially activating effects, patients with anxiety probably are not good candidates for rhodiola.

If multiple supplements are being administered, extreme caution must be exercised and, ideally, medical monitoring should be utilized.

Chapter 6

Depression

With contributions from Georae Letizia

Depression in children and adolescents has often been overlooked or minimized as normal mood swings that accompany developmental changes. In fact, until the past few decades, the spectrum of depressive disorders was not considered applicable to the pediatric population. Depression in children is no longer being dismissed, and researchers and clinicians now recognize it as a substantial problem affecting peer relationships, home life, academics, and physical well-being.

Although there were some documented accounts of depression in children during the 1940s and 1950s, the existence of childhood depression did not gain wide acceptance until the 1960s. It took another decade until diagnostic criteria specific to youth were established and researchers began empirical investigations (Miller, 1998). In recent years, the epidemiology, etiology, and symptoms of depression in youth have been studied more extensively and effective treatment options have been identified.

Recognizing depression in children is complicated by several factors. Self-reports usually are not obtainable with infants and toddlers. Since most young children are not able to adequately verbalize what they are feeling, clinicians and researchers must rely on information gathered from parents, teachers, and other significant adults in the child's life. Although teenagers are usually able to express their feelings, they may resist doing so and view depression as a sign of weakness. In addition, depressive symptoms may be masked by co-occurring conditions (for example, anxiety).

Depression falls within the category of mood disorders. DSM-IV-TR (APA, 2000) identifies two depressive disorders – major depressive disorder (MDD), and dysthymic disorder – and a residual diagnosis of depressive disorder not otherwise specified for those individuals who present with significant symptoms of depression but do not meet the criteria for the other two diagnoses. Depressive disorders vary from each other by symptom severity and duration. In addition, some diagnostic criteria for children and adolescents differ from those for adults.

SYMPTOMS OF DEPRESSION

For years there was disagreement over the symptoms of childhood depression. Some clinicians supported the notion that children exhibit the same symptoms as adults, while others felt that childhood depression symptoms are 'masked.' Currently, most agree that depression in youth shares some of the same symptoms as seen in adults, but the presentation of the symptoms may be significantly different. Moreover, the symptoms of depression have far reaching effects across many functional domains of the depressed youngster's life, leading to a wide range of secondary symptoms.

Core Symptoms

For children, adolescents, and adults, the necessary symptoms for a diagnosis of depression are similar; a consistently depressed mood and lack of interest in activities once deemed pleasurable. To receive a diagnosis of MDD at least one major depressive episode must have occurred, with no history of manic episodes. In contrast, dysthymia is a more chronic, low-grade depression that does not include a major depressive episode. Rarely, both MDD and dysthymia may occur simultaneously, a syndrome commonly referred to as double depression. The DSM expanded its diagnostic descriptions of depressive disorders to include some varied expressions of symptoms specific to children and adolescents, but some researchers argue that the DSM system still does not sufficiently recognize the different presentation of symptoms in youth (Weiss & Garber, 2003).

Major Depressive Disorder (MDD)

Major depressive disorder may be a single episode or recurrent. It can be mild, moderate, or severe. If symptoms resolve for at least 2 months, the condition is considered in remission. The DSM reports that the average age of onset of MDD is the mid-20s, but has been decreasing in recent years. Accordingly, in a review of the literature on pediatric depression, Stark and colleagues (2006) discuss several studies that found the age onset of MDD to fall between ages 15 and 19. In children, the incidence of depression occurs equally across both sexes. However, in adolescence the likelihood of depression in girls is double that of boys.

The distinguishing factor of MDD is the occurrence of a major depressive episode, lasting for at least 2 consecutive weeks. The features include depressed mood or loss of interest in pleasurable activities, along with at least four other symptoms – irritation, weight change, change in sleep patterns, psychomotor agitation or retardation, fatigue, feelings or worthlessness or guilt, diminished ability to concentrate, or recurrent thoughts of death. Symptoms must be severe enough to cause difficulty in daily functioning – social, occupational, or academic – and be present almost every day, for most of the day.

Although depressed adults typically display sad affect, depressed children and adolescents may present with irritable or cranky mood. Very young children are more sensitive to environmental changes and may have more frequent mood disturbances. The depressed or irritable mood they exhibit may manifest as angry outbursts and bouts of crying. With limited verbal and cognitive abilities, depressed children may use aggression as an outlet for their feelings, or they may express their symptoms through somatic complaints. Temper tantrums and behavioral problems are common in depressed children and their irritability may be carried into adolescence.

As with adults, fatigue, loss of energy, and sleep difficulties are common symptoms in pediatric depression. Children may complain that they are too tired to complète schoolwork or chores, and fatigue may lead to being primarily involved in passive activities (watching television or using the computer). Sleep difficulties may include trouble falling asleep, waking in the middle of the night and not being able to go back to sleep, and waking very early (without sufficient sleep). Instead of insomnia, hypersomnia is considered an atypical symptom, and it is more commonly seen in depressed adolescents (APA, 2000). With hypersomnia, despite excessive sleep, the adolescent may still feel tired and fatigued.

Psychomotor retardation or agitation may also be apparent. The child may seem lethargic, with slow speech and body movement; or the opposite – overactive, edgy, jumpy, and tense. Adolescents are more likely to experience psychomotor retardation, while young children tend to exhibit more agitation (APA, 2000). Changes in appetite are common, such as a decrease in the desire to eat, leading to weight loss. In contrast, some youngsters may overeat and become overweight. Across all developmental levels, a key feature of depression is impaired memory and concentration. Distractibility and foggy thinking are often reported, along with difficulty making decisions. Depressed children and adolescents are likely to exhibit a decline in school performance.

Feelings of worthlessness and a lack of competency are prevalent in depression. Low self-esteem may be accompanied by ruminations, undeserved self-blame, and an overall pessimistic attitude. Guilt may be excessive, unrealistic, and overwhelming. These traits are often more severe in children than adults (Turkington and Tzeel, 2004; Mash and Barkley, 2006; Shugert and Lopez, 2002; Kovacs, 1989). Feelings of hopelessness may become intense and lead to preoccupation with suicidal ideation. In young children, these thoughts may be expressed through bizarre or morbid play. Depressed adolescents may have recurrent thoughts of suicide and a history of suicide threats and attempts.

Dysthymic Disorder

Dysthymia is a milder form of chronic depression. Aside from an absence of a major depressive episode, many of the same symptoms seen in MDD are also present in dysthymia; but symptoms are persistent and less severe. Children may present with irritable mood as well as the general sadness seen in adults. The duration of symptoms must be at least 2 years for adults and 1 year for children, and not abate for more than 2 months during that time. As with MDD, low self-esteem, difficulty with concentration and decision making, and feelings of hopelessness are common. Although epidemiological studies are lacking, some researchers believe that dysthymia is under-diagnosed in children (Welfel and Ingersoll, 2001). Dysthymic disorder occurs with equal frequency in both sexes. According to the DSM, it may have an early onset, before the age of 21. However, Stark and colleagues (2006) reviewed several studies that set the age of first onset at 11. Atypical features are more likely to occur with early onset, and are two to three times more common in females (APA, 2000). The most frequently seen atypical features are excessive sleep, increased appetite, mood reactivity, and rejection sensitivity. With mood reactivity, positive external events can improve affect, almost immediately. In contrast, rejection sensitivity refers to a pathological perception of interpersonal rejection.

Secondary Symptoms

Depressed youth face many obstacles that can compromise their quality of life. Intra-personally, the impact of depression can be devastating. It can be equally as disturbing to interpersonal relationships, academic performance, and other areas of daily functioning.

Interpersonal relationships suffer in many ways. Depressed children may lose interest in activities once enjoyed with friends and withdraw from the social ties that could provide a buffer against depression. Isolating themselves from others reinforces a sense of loneliness. Low self-esteem and feelings of worthlessness make it difficult to cultivate new friendships, and angry, aggressive, hostile, behaviors make it hard to maintain friendships. Also, irritable children are argumentative, which may drive others away. The child will withdraw further and social skills will decline more.

Depressed children frequently have poor academic performance. Tardiness and absenteeism often coincide with lethargy, hypersomnia, and frequent somatic complaints. Inability to concentrate, distractibility, and memory problems make it difficult to pay attention and follow instructions. Low frustration tolerance can interfere with task completion. Learning is a cumulative process and as depressive symptoms continue the child is likely to fall behind academically.

A lack of adequate coping skills correlates with depression and places youth at increased risk of developing substance abuse problems. Early onset of depression carries a high probability of substance abuse (Miller, 1998). Adolescents may self-medicate, turning to drugs and alcohol as a coping mechanism. Relief is only temporary and substance abuse is likely to compound the problems.

As the child grows older, responsibilities increase. Low self-esteem and feelings of inadequacy come together to create a sense of being overwhelmed by increased expectations. Depressed teens over-generalize and exhibit tendencies to magnify the negative and minimize the positive. Perfectionistic tendencies may develop in response to excessive guilt. Overall, the depressed child or adolescent has a pessimistic outlook, which serves to reinforce their depression.

RULE-OUTS AND COMORBID DISORDERS

Co-occurring psychological disorders are common in youth. This is especially true with depression. Children who meet the criteria for one DSM diagnosis are likely to also meet criteria for one or more others, and comorbid disorders present additional challenges that must be considered in order to develop a comprehensive treatment plan. When assessing a child it is important to recognize that many of the symptoms of depression overlap with those seen in other psychological disorders. Hence, depression may mask or be masked by symptoms associated with other disorders. Another consideration is the developmental stage of the child. Patterns of comorbidity vary with age, and depressed children and adolescents often present with different symptom clusters.

When pediatric depression is identified, an accurate diagnostic picture that includes or rules out possible coexisting disorders is crucial. Comorbidity can influence the course and treatment response of both disorders. Youth who receive multiple psychological diagnoses suffer with more severe disturbances, experience greater impairment, and have poorer treatment outcomes than children with a single diagnosis. Along with comorbidity comes an increase in duration and severity of depression, and also a greater likelihood of suicidal ideation (Kovacs *et al.*, 1993). A comprehensive evaluation must consider other psychological disorders that frequently co-occur with depression.

Anxiety Disorders

Disorders along the anxiety spectrum are the most common comorbidities associated with depression. Studies report that anxiety coexists in 33–60 percent of pediatric depression cases (Hammen & Rudolph, 2003). The disorders are so interrelated that some believe they are different manifestations of the same underlying mechanism. Depression and anxiety are internalizing disorders that share the primary characteristic of a high level of distress. Many symptoms of the two disorders overlap, including tension, fear, worry, poor concentration, disruptions in sleep patterns, and changes in eating habits. The distinguishing features are anhedonia, associated with depression, and hyperarousal, seen in anxiety. When depression and anxiety co-occur, they may exacerbate each other's symptoms. For instance, excessive worry and rumination seen in depression may be intensified by the fearfulness and obsessive thinking associated with anxiety. Symptoms may also mask, or be masked by additional co-occurring disorders, such as substance abuse and disruptive disorders.

The relationship between anxiety and depression is complex. Both conditions are likely to recur and persist into adulthood. Statistically, 80 percent of children diagnosed with comorbid depression and anxiety are at risk for future anxiety episodes, whereas depression alone is not a predictor of subsequent anxiety. Conversely, children diagnosed with only anxiety have a significant risk of later being diagnosed with dysthymia.

Treatment of coexisting depression and anxiety is complicated. A full analysis of the inter-relationship of symptoms is needed in order to create a comprehensive treatment plan, and combined psychotherapy and psychopharmacology are usually recommended. However, in some cases, pharmaceutical approaches beneficial to one of the disorders may be block the effectiveness of treatment for the other, or even exacerbate the other's symptoms. For example, some antidepressants exacerbate anxiety, and some anxiolytics increase the risk of depressive symptoms. The same is true with herbal and nutritional supplements. Therefore, treatment must proceed with caution, and close monitoring is needed.

Disruptive Disorders

The Office of the Surgeon General (1999), reports that some form of disruptive behavioral disorder is present in 10.3 percent of children, ages 9–17. These disorders are frequently comorbid with depression. Between 14 and 36 percent of children diagnosed with depression also exhibit symptoms of Conduct Disorder (Kovacs *et al.*, 1988), and the overlap between depression and oppositional defiant disorder may be even higher, especially in boys (Boylan *et al.*, 2007). There is a good deal of symptom overlap among these disorders, making a differential diagnosis very difficult. Although the DSM treats depression and conduct disorders as two separate diagnostic categories, the symptoms are so intertwined that the International Classification of Diseases (ICD-10) has created a diagnostic category for Depressive Conduct Disorder (World Health Organization, 1992).

The common threads of distractibility, poor concentration, restlessness, and irritability run through ODD, CD, and depression. Each of these disorders can lead to learning problems, poor study skills, and impaired interpersonal relationships. When co-occurring, these problems are magnified.

Children often express their depression through acting out. Oppositional behavior and ill-tempered moods common in depressed youth could easily be mistaken for a disruptive disorder. A comorbid diagnosis should only be considered if the disruptive behaviors occur in the presence as well as the absence of a depressive episode. There is no consensus as to whether depression precedes or follows disruptive disorders. Comorbidity, however, is associated with increased risk of suicidality (Singer, 2006; Daviss, 2008). In addition, depressed teens with a comorbid disruptive disorder exhibit a higher risk of substance abuse, and effective treatment must address all of these problems simultaneously.

Attention Deficit Hyperactivity Disorder (ADHD)

Comorbid depression and ADHD is a common occurrence. Children and adolescents with ADHD face a risk of developing depression that is four times greater than those without the disorder, and up to 14 percent of children with dysthymia also have ADHD, although some researchers believe that it is an underestimate. Recognizing depression in youth with ADHD is difficult because many symptoms overlap, including restlessness, irritability, and poor concentration. The distinguishing features that lead to an additional diagnosis of depression are anhedonia, hopelessness, social withdrawal, psychomotor retardation, and suicidal ideation, which are atypical for ADHD alone.

With children and adolescents, depression may surface several years after the onset of ADHD. Symptoms of ADHD often create conflicts

and impairments at home, in school, and with peers that is condu-
cive to the development of depression. Children and adolescents with
comorbid depression and ADHD experience even greater impairment –
intra-personally, cognitively, and socially – and are at increased risk for
suicidal thoughts and behaviors (Singer, 2006; Daviss, 2008).

Comorbid depression and ADHD warrant pharmacotherapy that
addresses both sets of symptoms. When prescription medications are
used, bupropion, and atomoxetine may treat all symptoms simultaneously,
but often two sets of medications may be needed, one for symptoms of
ADHD, and the other for symptoms of depression. When using herbal
and nutritional supplements, one compound may not be able to address
all symptoms. Because there is little research regarding the use of multiple supplements, especially in the pediatric population, caution is needed
if such an approach will be utilized.

Adjustment and Trauma

Children and adolescents who have undergone traumatic experiences are
much more likely to exhibit a variety of difficulties, including changes
in mood, agitation, depression, and related symptoms. In addition to
emotional changes, many children and teenagers may exhibit changes in
behaviors, including acting out and difficulties with being managed.

Post-Traumatic Disorders

Children and adolescents who have been exposed to severe trauma,
such as abuse, loss of a parent, severe injury, or exposure to a major
catastrophe, may exhibit symptoms of acute stress disorder (ASD) or
post-traumatic stress disorder (PTSD). Children with ASD or PTSD will
usually exhibit substantial disturbance of overall functioning, including
anxiety and hypervigilance, sleep disturbance and nightmares (which
do not necessarily need to contain trauma-related content), reliving the
event through play (or other forms of flashbacks), and avoidance of
(and/or detachment from) trauma-related stimuli. Significant depression
often accompanies these symptoms.

When clinicians encounter children or adolescents with ASD or PTSD,
all symptom groups must be managed. Intensive psychotherapy and/or
psychiatric treatment is likely to be necessary, and depression should not
be treated in isolation. While using an antidepressant supplement may be
helpful, it is not likely to be effective unless the other symptoms are also
being addressed. Unfortunately, this will usually mean that multiple supplements will need to be used, and such cases should be approached with

extreme caution, since the use of multiple supplements has rarely been researched, especially in the pediatric population.

Adjustment Disorders

Children and adolescents who have been exposed to less severe stressful events, like family conflicts, moves, or parental separation, may experience less severe variants of emotional and behavioral disturbances. Within the DSM system, these may meet the criteria for various forms of adjustment disorder (APA, 2000), and some specific subtypes of adjustment disorder include symptoms of depression. Youngsters who experience such emotional reactions commonly benefit from counseling and psychotherapy in order to help them cope with the stressors. If depression is apparent, an adjunct use of an antidepressant supplement may be beneficial. However, clinicians should administer treatment that comprehensively focuses on helping the child or adolescent cope with the stressful events.

ETIOLOGY

As our understanding of depression has continued to evolve, its complexity has become apparent. There is no one theory of its etiology that is either comprehensive or consistently replicable, and varied presentations of depression may have different etiologies. Researchers currently recognize that the manifestations of depression are multifactorial and consist of the interplay between a combination of exogenous and endogenous variables. Some of the causal factors may trigger the activation of others. Also, several of these variables may convene in depression's maintenance, recovery delay, or relapse.

Genes affect personality and temperament, and a genetic vulnerability may predispose children to depression. Twin studies have revealed a 40 percent chance of heritability, though the likelihood of developing depression may be mediated by socio-environment factors (Sutker and Adams, 2001). A genetic relationship is presumed based on findings that children suffering with depression are 1.5–3 times more likely to have a first degree biological relative with the disorder (APA, 2000). However, the link between parent and child may also be mediated by environmental factors, such as family dysfunction.

Development of depressive disorders is probably best viewed from a diathesis-stress perspective (Zubin & Spring, 1977). With depression, it is often difficult to disentangle cause from effect. However, it appears that external stressors interact with internal vulnerabilities to promote the onset, maintenance, and recurrence of depression. Various factors overlap and may even work in concert to intensify symptoms. Internal vulnerabilities may initiate maladaptive behavioral features and external factors may activate endogenous mechanisms of depression.

As discussed in Chapter 8, in response to stress the body prepares for 'fight or flight' by activating the stress response system, primarily including the limbic system and the hypothalamic–pituitary–adrenal (HPA) axis. Hence, dysregulation of the HPA axis results in depressive symptoms that may reflect not only a response to stress, but also an attempt to adapt to excessive and prolonged stress. Contradictory symptoms of depression coincide with three unsuccessful ways of adapting to stress. First is self-preservation via hyperarousal or hypervigilance, which can manifest as agitation, anorexia, anxiety, insomnia, and reduced libido. The second is energy conservation, manifesting as fatigue, hypersomnia, overeating, psychomotor retardation, chronic inhibition of sexual behavior. The third is behavioral disengagement or adaptive learning, manifesting as anhedonia, low motivation, impairment in memory, and decreased concentration (Shelton, 2000).

Currently, it is widely accepted that the receptors for the monoamine transmitters norepinephrine and serotonin (and, to a lesser extent, dopamine) play a key role in depression, and portions of the brain regulated by these neurotransmitters are presumed to be underactive. In addition, neuroanatomical abnormalities in relevant brain structures have also been identified. These changes contribute to various symptoms of depression.

Symptoms of 'Classic' Depression

The 'classic' or 'typical' symptoms of depression include sadness, apathy, withdrawal, anhedonia, psychomotor retardation, fatigue, distractibility, memory problems, insomnia, and loss of appetite/weight. Norepinephrine and dopamine dysfunction is commonly associated with these symptoms, but it is more likely that various monoamines may be 'out of tune' with each other, thus causing the symptoms (Stahl, 2008, p. 490).

Mood depression may be linked to the underactivation of portion of the limbic system, including the amygdala, and the anterior cingulate cortex. Apathy may be the result of underactivation of the ventromedial and dorsolateral portion of the prefrontal cortex, as well as portions of the hypothalamus and the nucleus accumbens. Insomnia may involve the thalamus, hypothalamus, basal forebrain, and portions of the prefrontal cortex. Fatigue may be linked to monoamine deficiencies in the prefrontal cortex, as well as the striatum and nucleus accumbens. Psychomotor retardation is linked to motor circuits in the striatum, cerebellum, and prefrontal cortex. Loss of appetite and weight may involve the underactivation of the hypothalamus (Stahl, 2008).

Symptoms of 'Atypical' Depression

The 'atypical' symptoms of depression typically include a combination of some 'classic' symptoms, described above, with increased appetite/weight, hypersomnia, and social hypersensitivity (APA, 2000). Although not specifically included in the DSM's description of atypical features, many clinicians also include psychomotor agitation, rather than retardation, as a feature of atypical depression. Stahl (2008) makes a distinction between 'reduced positive affect' and 'increased negative affect' (p. 499), and this way of conceptualizing depression may be useful. The former may be characteristic of classic symptoms of depression, while the latter may be descriptive of many atypical features.

Increased negative affect is likely secondary to norepinephrine and serotonin dysfunction. Agitation and anger may be associated with over-activation of portion of the limbic system, including the amygdala. As discussed in Chapter 8, such overactivation also underlies symptoms of anxiety and may be one reason why anxiety and depression co-occur in many cases. Further psychomotor activation may be associated with the overactivation of motor circuits in the striatum, cerebellum, and prefrontal cortex. As discussed above, hypersomnia may involve the thalamus, hypothalamus, basal forebrain, and portions of the prefrontal cortex, and the neurophysiological changes may be in the opposite direction to that associated with insomnia. Increase in appetite and weight may involve the overactivation of the hypothalamus (Stahl, 2008).

Summary of Research Findings

In order to investigate the above etiological hypotheses, brain-imaging studies have been performed for several decades. It is not possible to review, in detail, the plethora of findings that have been obtained from the many studies, but this section summarizes the most salient neuroanatomical and neurophysiological abnormalities that many brain imaging studies have identified.

Neuroanatomical Abnormalities

Through the use of Magnetic Resonance Imaging (MRI), researchers have been investigating the abnormalities in brain structure that are associated with depression. Hippocampal volume loss is perhaps the most frequently reported neuroanatomical abnormality associated with depression (Drevets, 2001). For example, Neumeister *et al.* (2004) found that recurrent MDD is associated with hippocampal volume loss in the posterior hippocampus. It is more likely to occur in those exposed to early life stressors, such as children who have been severely abused (Savitz & Drevets, in press). Indeed, hippocampal volume reduction has been reported in children and young adults with MDD (MacMaster *et al.*, 2008; Lange & Irle, 2004). In addition, longitudinal studies that followed depressed subjects over several years found that those with low hippocampal volume were less likely to be in remission 1 year later and more likely to have further reductions in hippocampal volume at the 3 year mark (Savitz & Drevets).

Other brain changes have also been documented. For example, reductions in the size of the amygdala and the prefrontal cortex have also been shown (Leonard & Myint, 2009). Depressed patients show a reduction in the thickness in the right (but not left) cortical gray matter, especially including the inferior and middle frontal gyri, somatosensory and motor cortices, dorsal and inferior parietal regions, the inferior occipital gyrus, and posterior temporal cortex. Even more importantly, studies of people with a family history of major depression similarly revealed a 28 percent reduction in the thickness of gray matter in these areas, whereas people with no known risk of depression did not reveal those changes (Peterson *et al.*, 2009). Such findings lend further credence to the hypothesis of genetic vulnerability for depression.

Neurophysiological Abnormalities

Neurotransmitter deficiency has long been expected to be a contributory factor in symptoms of depression. While the original theories focused on the importance of norepinephrine and serotonin, today it is widely accepted that dopamine also plays a role. Earliest evidence for the involvement of these monoamines came from the recognition that monoamine oxidase inhibitors (MAOIs), medications that increase the levels of all monoamines, improve symptoms of depression, and reserpine, a medication that depletes catecholamines, has been shown to induce depression. In addition, all antidepressants currently on the market reduce symptoms of depression by increasing brain levels of serotonin, norepinephrine, and dopamine, in various combinations.

There is further evidence of monoamine deficiencies in people with a history of depression. Leonard (1986) reviewed results of decades of research and concluded that norepinephrine and serotonin deficiencies are well documented in MDD. More recently, Neumeister *et al.* (2004) induced tryptophan (a precursor for serotonin) depletion in people with a history of MDD and normal controls. Tryptophan depletion induced a return of depressive symptoms in patients with history of MDD, but not in normal controls. In addition, tryptophan depletion was associated with an increase in regional cerebral glucose utilization in the orbitofrontal cortex, medial thalamus, anterior and posterior cingulate cortices, and ventral striatum in patients with a history of MDD but not in controls. Thus, these results may reveal vulnerabilities in the serotonergic system in a circuit that probably plays a key role in the pathogenesis of MDD. Interestingly, the results were associated with various increases in neuronal firing, suggesting that a depletion of a neurotransmitter does not necessarily result in the underactivation of relevant brain regions. This may be relevant to the pathogenesis of atypical symptoms of depression described in the previous section.

PET scans reveal results that identify the brain areas that may be involved in the symptoms of depression. Milak *et al.* (2005) found that depressed mood correlated with metabolism in the cingulate gyrus, thalamus, and basal ganglia, and sleep disturbance correlated with metabolism in the limbic system and basal ganglia. Furthermore, loss of motivation (apathy) was negatively correlated with metabolism in parietal and superior frontal cortical areas. In addition, similar findings were obtained from adolescents with depression. Forbes *et al.* (2009) revealed that depressed teens exhibited underactivation of the striatal and caudate regions of the brain (associated with the expression of positive affect), and overactivation of the dorsolateral and medial prefrontal cortex (associated with emotional reactivity).

Increased reactivity of the amygdala to negative stimuli has consistently been shown in patients with MDD by studies that utilized a variety of brain scan methods. Patients with MDD repeatedly demonstrated increased changes after negative stimuli, and changes in baseline levels before stimuli were presented, suggesting hypersensitivity to stimulation. In addition, similar changes were also evident in first-line relatives of patients with MDD. For example, healthy individuals with a family history of MDD exhibited mood depression and greater amygdala activation in response to fearful faces (see Savitz & Drevets, in press, for a review).

The HPA axis is a neuroendocrin system that has a vital role in the stress response through the increased production of corticotropin releasing factor (CRF) by the hypothalamus. An exaggerated stress response results in increased cortisol levels, which, in turn, are associated with depression. In response to increased CRF, the pituitary secretes adrenocorticotropic hormone (ACTH), causing a release of cortisol in the adrenal gland (Shelton, 2000). Consequently, dysregulation of the HPA axis may result in either over or under response to stress.

Some research has started to look at different changes in the HPA axis associated with different presentations of depression. Antonijevic (2008) found that the nature and extent of the HPA axis alterations and sleep architecture changes are associated with distinct subtypes of depression. For example, an increase in HPA activity, and associated increases in corticotropin-releasing hormone (CRH) and an impaired negative feedback via glucocorticoid receptors, was mostly evident in patients with 'classic' symptoms of depression, including melancholic presentation of symptoms (as per description in APA, 2000, p. 419). These patients also revealed most evident sleep-EEG alterations, including disrupted sleep, low amounts of deep sleep, and short REM sleep latency. In contrast, patients with atypical features revealed reduced activity of the HPA axis and noradrenergic neurons ascending from the locus coeruleus, and less significant REM sleep alterations. These findings may explain the different symptom presentation in different patients with depression.

SUPPLEMENTS WITH ESTABLISHED EFFICACY

Depression is the one area of psychopharmacology where naturopathic compounds have been studied the most. Although the majority of research has been done with adult patients, results of some studies confirm that the efficacy seen with adults is similarly obtained with children and adolescents.

Medications that work by increasing the amount of activity in the catecholamine pathways, especially noradrenergic and serotonergic, are generally effective in addressing symptoms of depression. Similarly, supplements that accomplish similar changes in the brain have been shown to be effective.

St. John's Wort

St. John's Wort (*Hypericum perforatum*) is an herb that exists in some 370 species found throughout the world, but is originally endogenous to Europe. It is sometimes also known as Tipton's Weed or Klamath weed. It is available in a variety of preparations, including capsules, liquid, oils, and raw herb to be brewed as tea. St. John's Wort contains a plethora of active ingredients, including flavonoids, naphthodianthrones, phloroglucinols, phenolic acids, terpenes, and xanthones (Spinella, 2001).

These exert a variety of psychoactive effects, and several of these are described below.

The use of St. John's Wort has a long history and it is widely accepted across Europe as first line treatment for depression. In Germany, between 1993 and 2003, the number of prescriptions for it tripled (Butterweck, 2003). In the past decade, St. John's Wort has also been experiencing increased popularity in the United States.

Evidence of Efficacy

Of all herbal supplements, St. John's Wort is the one that has been researched most extensively and there is strong support for its efficacy in reducing depressive symptoms, especially for treating mild to moderate severity of symptoms. Dozens of placebo-controlled studies been performed, and meta-analyses of these are also available. For example, a meta-analysis of 15 studies revealed that about twice as many patients who took the herb improved as compared to placebo, and that the improvement was evidenced by a 50 percent or greater drop in severity of symptoms (Nierenberg *et al.*, 2002). Similarly, a meta-analysis of randomized trials comparing the efficacy of St. John's Wort with prescription antidepressants revealed that the herb was at least as effective, and in some trials even more so. In addition, there were fewer drop-outs in the herb-treated groups because the herb was better tolerated than prescription antidepressant medications (Nierenberg *et al.*). Another review also revealed similar efficacy to prescription antidepressants, including amitriptyline, imipramine, maprotyline, and fluoxetine, and when combined with valerian, St. John's Wort has been shown to be similarly effective to diazepam and desipramine (Medical Economics, 2007). St. John's Wort for treatment of severe depression, however, has not received the same empirical support (Hypericum Depression Trial Study Group, 2002). Thus, it is clear that St. John's Wort is a good option to treat symptoms of depression that are of mild to moderate severity.

In Europe, the herb is also used with children and adolescents, although research studies supporting this use are more limited. One observational trial revealed St. John's Wort was effective in treating symptoms of depression in children 12 years of age or younger, and doses of 300–900 mg/day were tolerated with minimal side effects (Hübner & Kirste, 2001). Reduction of symptoms was rapid, and a significant number of the children showed response in as little as 2 weeks. In another study, 33 children and adolescents (aged 6–16 years) were treated with a dose of up to 900 mg/day and revealed significant improvement after 2 months of treatment, and the herb was also well tolerated (Findling *et al.*, 2003), and a similar study with adolescents confirmed these results (Simeon *et al.*, 2005). Although these results are preliminary, it is apparent that the efficacy of St. John's Wort in children and adolescents may be similar to its efficacy in adults, and the herb is tolerated with minimal side effects.

Pharmacodynamics

St. John's Wort appears to share some of the same pharmacological effects as many prescription antidepressants – it appears to act on serotonin, dopamine, norepinephrine, noradrenaline, GABA, and glutamate (Medical Economics, 2007; Chatterjee *et al.*, 1998; Stahl, 2008). The mechanism of action of St. John's Wort is very complex. Because the plant contains so many active ingredients, only some of these have been researched with regard to their pharmacodynamic properties, and various constituents appear to account for different effects of the herb. The three main constituents that have been investigated for their antidepressant qualities are hypericin, amentoflavone, and hyperforin (Spinella, 2001). Hypericin appears to act as a monoamine reuptake inhibitor and may increase synaptic levels of serotonin, norepinephrine, and dopamine (Spinella). Pseudohypericin appears to add to this effect and works as a monoamine oxidase inhibitor (MAOI), but its MAOI activity is weak and is not likely to account for its efficacy in symptom reduction. Another constituent, amentoflavone, has been shown to significantly inhibit serotonin receptors (Medical Economics) and may also act as an agonist at GABA benzodiazepine receptors.

More recently, hyperforin has been the focus of study and may significantly contribute to St. John's Wort's clinical effects. Hyperforin may act as an inhibitor of catechol-O-methyl transferase (COMT), another enzyme that breaks down monoamines (Spinella, 2001), but it also has been suggested that its mechanism may involve blocking reuptake of serotonin, dopamine, and noradrenaline, and hyperforin may also act on GABA and glutamate (Muller, 2005; Chatterjee *et al.*, 1998). Procyanidins may also act at BAGA receptors, and flavonoids may act on opioid mu and kappa receptors (Spinella). All in all, it is likely that various constituents are responsible for the antidepressant properties of St. John's Wort, and utilizing the whole plant with its multiple constituents has a synergistic effect (Butterweck, 2003; Spinella, 2001).

Pharmacokinetics

A 300 mg tablet of St. John's Wort is absorbed from the gastrointestinal tract and the most active ingredients are lipophyllic, aiding its absorption. Hyperforin reaches maximum plasma levels in about 3 hours, and hypericin reaches these levels in about 4 hours. Half-life for hyperforin is about 9 hours, but the half-life for hypericin is much longer and may reach 24 hours (Spinella, 2001). Long-term dosing of 300 mg three times per day (TID) revealed that steady state was reached after 4 days of treatment (Spinella, 2001).

St. John's Wort utilizes the CYP450 enzyme system for metabolism, but the exact pathways have not been identified thus far (Medical Economics, 2007; Chatterjee *et al.*, 1998; Stahl, 2008). However, the herb exerts significant effects on liver metabolism. While the ingestion of the herb appears to induce liver metabolism, perhaps by inducing P-glycoprotein, hyperforin has also been found to significantly induce CYP 3A4 enzyme (Lee *et al.*, 2007). Because this enzyme is responsible for the metabolism of many medications, the use of St. John's Wort with prescription medications should generally be avoided.

Dosing

For adults, the standard dose is 300 mg, and because of hyperforin's short half-life, the herb must be taken three times per day (TID). Usually, it is recommended that standardized extracts with 0.3 percent hypericin should be used (Medical Economics, 2007). In children, the usual starting dose in 150 mg TID, and the dose is gradually increased until about 900 mg/day in teenagers, although lower doses in younger children, and higher doses in mature teens may be needed. In some cases, adults need doses of 1800 mg/day (Bezchlibnyk-Butler & Jeffries, 2007), and similar range is reported for the pediatric population (Bezchlibnyk-Butler & Virani, 2004).

Adverse Effects

St John's Wort is generally well tolerated and minimal side effects are reported. Sometimes, gastrointestinal irritation, nausea, constipation, and feeling of uncomfortable fullness has been reported (Medical Economics, 2007). Usually, taking the compound with food may reduce these difficulties. Fatigue and/or restlessness has also been reported in some cases (Spinella, 2001). Frequent urination has also been reported.

Photosensitivity has been reported with the use of this compound. This means that some individuals who take the herb become more sensitive to sunlight and may easily experience sunburns. The mechanism of this problem is attributed to increased sensitivity to ultraviolet waves (UVA and UVB). Patients who take St. John's Wort should be monitored for this reaction and, if one is observed, use of sun blocking sunscreens will be necessary. For children and adolescents who spend a lot of time outside, this problem must especially be monitored.

St. John's Wort is contraindicated during pregnancy due to evidence of damage to reproductive cells (Medical Economics, 2007). Female adolescents who take St. John's Wort and are suspected of being sexually active must be advised of this risk, and should use contraception to prevent pregnancy. However, oral contraceptives are metabolized by the same CYP3A4 pathway that is induced by St. John's Wort, and breakthrough bleeding and pregnancy have been reported as a result of the increased metabolism of oral contraceptives (Lee et al., 2007). Sexually active females must be aware of this risk and utilize other forms of birth control.

Cardiovascular effects have been reported in a minority of patients, and these may include swelling and an increase in heart rate. Even more importantly, a small risk of hypertension appears to be present in some patients. Although MAOI activity appears to be a minor component of this herb's pharmacodynamics, it may pose some risk that is similar to prescription MAOI medications. Patients who take MAOIs must avoid products that contain tyramine, because decreased regulation of the MAO enzymes may lead to excess levels of noradrenaline, causing unsafe levels of blood pressure. Foods rich in tyramine include most aged food products, including cheese and aged meats, and tyramine-rich food products are plentiful in the typical American and European diet. The exact degree of this risk is not yet known, and thus far only one case has been reported that presented with a hypertensive crisis potentially due to St. John's Wort (Medical Economics, 2007). However, clinicians should use caution and monitor the blood pressure of patients who take St. John's Wort (especially after meals), at least in the initial phases of treatment.

Perhaps the greatest risk associated with the use of St. John's Wort is its effect on the liver, and the resultant potential for significant drug interactions. Generally, St. John's Wort should not be utilized whenever patients take prescription medications. Of particular concern are protease inhibitors, anticoagulants, anticonvulsants, antiretrovirals, immunosuppressants, cardiovascular drugs, and anticancer drugs (Lee et al., 2007; Medical Economics, 2007). This list is by no means exhaustive. Usually, a 14 day washout period is often recommended when stopping or starting St. John's Wort.

Although a specific 'black box' warning that applies to all antidepressants is not issued for St. John's Wort, because of its antidepressant action, St. John's Wort may be associated with a small increase in suicidal tendencies in those patients who present with symptoms of depression. As with any antidepressant, clinicians should carefully monitor patient response and intervene if an increase in suicidal thoughts or plans becomes evident. In addition, like all antidepressants, St. John's Wort is also associated with a small risk of inducing hypomanic or manic symptoms (Bezchlibnyk-Butler & Jeffries, 2007), and some patients who have tendencies toward symptoms of bipolar disorder may exhibit 'switching' from depressive to manic symptoms. Once again, careful monitoring of dose/response and adverse effects is necessary.

S-Adenosyl-L-Methionine (SAMe)

After St. John's Wort, SAM-e is the most commonly used nutritional supplement for treating depression. It was discovered in 1952 by an Italian scientist, and became marketed in Europe shortly afterward, where it is considered (and regulated as) a drug. It has only been available in the US since 1999, and it is classified as a nutritional supplement. It is known by a variety of names, including ademetionine, S-adenosylmethionine, and also sometimes referred to as SAM or SAM-e. It is primarily used to treat osteoarthritis, fibromyalgia, and liver disorders. Efficacy for those applications is well established with many studies published in European journals, and it is considered to be one of the most researched nutritional supplements (Settle, 2007).

While St. John's Wort is regarded as effective in treating mild to moderate depression, SAMe has been shown to be effective in dysthymia as well as more severe depression, including MDD (Mischoulon, 2007). More rapid onset of effect and low side-effect profile also add to its appeal.

Evidence of Efficacy

During the 1970, 1980s, and 1990s, 39 studies, including 25 controlled studies, investigated the efficacy of SAMe and confirmed its benefit in treating symptoms of depression (Settle, 2007). Bressa (1994) discussed results of meta-analyses of placebo-controlled studies, and reported that the studies consistently reveal that SAMe is far superior to placebo, outperforming placebo by a margin that is wider than seen in many placebo-controlled studies of prescription medications. Pancheri et al. (1997) reviewed another meta-analysis and confirmed that SAMe is superior to placebo by a margin that is at least equal to tricyclic antidepressants (TCAs), and one study found SAMe to be superior in efficacy to TCAs. In addition to these early studies, more recent, larger, and well-controlled studies revealed similar results. Pancheri *et al.* (2002) studied 293 patients with non-psychotic, moderately severe depression and found SAMe as effective as imipramine. Similarly, Delle Chiaie *et al.* (2002) studied 576 patients with non-psychotic MDD and again found SAMe as effective as imipramine, but with fewer adverse effects. In a recent meta-analysis, Mischoulon (2007) reported that patients treated with SAMe often report faster inset of effects than patients treated with pharmaceutical antidepressants, with some subjects responding in a few days and most responding within 2 weeks. Mischoulon also found support for using SAMe adjunctively with TCAs, and the combination hastened the onset of symptom reduction when compared to TCAs administered as monotherapy. Brown *et al.* (2002) reviewed studies of SAMe co-administered with TCAs and discovered evidence of therapeutic response with only one-third the TCA dosage. In addition, for treatment resistant patients who show partial or no response to SSRIs, research reviewed by Mischoulon reveals that SAMe augmentation significantly improved efficacy.

Thus far, very limited evidence exists for the effectiveness in the pediatric population. Schaller and Bazzan (2004) reported case studies of children, aged 8–16 years, with MDD that responded well to the use of SAMe. The dosage ranged from 400–800 mg/day, and in one case, SAMe was discontinued after a few weeks, and the mood symptoms relapsed. After SAMe was restarted, remission was again evident. All individuals tolerated the supplement well, although one teenager started to experience slight tremor and anxiety on a dose of 1800 mg/day before his dose was reduced, and he eventually revealed good response on 1200 mg/day with no adverse effects. Although these findings are preliminary, they seem to confirm the results of many research studies that has revealed SAMe to be effective with adults. Consequently, there is good reason to suggest a cautious trial of SAMe for children and adolescents with significant symptoms of depression.

Pharmacodynamics

SAMe is a second messenger. This term refers to substances that act within cells to change some aspects of cell metabolism. In this case, SAMe is a methyl donor that contributes to dozens of reactions throughout the brain, including the synthesis of monoamine transmitters – dopamine, norepinephrine, and serotonin, among others (Settle, 2007). This action is responsible, at least in part, for its antidepressant effect. Since functional symptoms of depression may result from underactivation of key pathways for norepinephrine and dopamine, producing additional amount of these catecholamines has potential benefits in alleviating the symptoms (as has been shown with many of the medications used to treat depression). Indeed, a review of European research revealed that SAMe may be involved in increasing activity in dopaminergic and serotonergic pathways (Settle). In addition, SAMe may also block reuptake of monoamines, leading to increased availability of serotonin, norepinephrine, and dopamine (Schatzberg *et al.*, 2007).

SAMe is also involved in methylation and/or phosphorization processes that affect membrane fluidity. As such, its effects may be similar to those of Omega-3 fatty acids, where regulation of the membrane fluidity may be involved in stabilization of neurotransmitter release and neuronal firing. SAMe has been found to increase the number of receptors on the cell, increase binding to receptors, and enhance membrane fluidity (Settle, 2007). These effects likely contribute to increases in dopamine and serotonin, and further enhance its clinical effect.

Pharmacokinetics

SAMe is available in tablets. Some of these have enteric coating, and some do not. Those that are coated are a better choice because SAMe is absorbed from the small intestine, and therefore as much compound as possible should 'survive' the stomach acids and get through into the small intestine. In addition, SAMe is unstable at temperatures above freezing (0 degrees Celsius, or 32 degrees Fahrenheit). A wide variety of SAMe preparations are available on the market. Forms that have been researched for efficacy are stable at higher temperatures, but other forms are marketed for which efficacy may be questionable. Consumers should seek the form that includes SAMe paratoluene sulfonates (SAMe tosyls) because these salts have been found to be stable at room temperature. Additionally, SAMe must be kept very dry because moisture can cause hydrolysis. It is recommended that the best form to purchase is the stable formulation of SAMe tosyls that is also enteric coated (Medical Economics, 2008a).

SAMe should be taken on an empty stomach – about 1 hour before or 2 hours after a meal. The peak is usually attained in 3–5 hours (Medical Economics, 2008a). In adults, there is a sex difference in plasma concentration, with women attaining three to six times the value of men. Whether this same effect is seen in children and adolescents is not known. Onset of clinical effect is not generally evident for at least 1–2 weeks (Walsh, 2003).

SAMe is metabolized by the liver but seems to have minimal effects on liver enzymes, and drug–drug interactions have not been reported with SAMe. Most of the substance is incorporated into various cells, and only a small portion is eliminated in urine (15 percent) and feces

(23 percent). Thus, liver and kidney function seems to have limited effect on the metabolism and excretion of SAMe (Medical Economics, 2008a).

When SAMe is metabolized, co-factors are involved. Metabolism of SAMe to homocysteine requires the presence of vitamin B6. This pathway probably has minor (if any) effects on symptoms of ADHD, and therefore levels of vitamin B6 are less important for this specific application. SAMe is also metabolized into methionine and this pathway has greater relevance to ADHD. In order to accomplish this metabolism, folic acid and vitamin B12 are needed (Medical Economics, 2008a). Consequently, when minimal effects of SAMe supplementation are seen, vitamin B complex can be added. Since these compounds are already present in a normal diet, supplementation should be minimal, and higher, focused doses of these vitamins are not recommended.

Dosing

The clinical dose of SAMe varies widely. Children should start at about 200 mg once per day (preferably, in the morning) and gradually titrate at intervals of 1–2 weeks between dose increases. Teenagers and adults are generally dosed up to 2400 mg/day (Bezchlibnyk-Butler & Jeffries, 2007), although doses above 1600 mg/day have not been studied for adverse effects (Medical Economics, 2008a). Clearly, children should receive lower doses, although no specific guidelines exist for dosing children and adolescents. According to the National Center for Health Statistics (2002), the weight of an average adult male in the US is about 190 pounds (about 86 kg). Thus, the dose-to-weight ratio for adults is about 18–28 mg/kg per day. The effective ratio for children and adolescents may be similar. Clinicians are advised to 'start low and go slow' – begin minimal dose, and gradually titrate making sure that the above mg/kg ratios are not exceeded.

Adverse Effects

SAMe is generally well tolerated. Suppression of appetite and weight change are not reported. However, mild gastrointestinal upsets (nausea, diarrhea, and flatulence) may be evident at the start of treatment (Medical Economics, 2008a). These usually resolve after a week or two. Sometimes, those with higher doses experience more persistent nausea (Bezchlibnyk-Butler & Jeffries, 2007). SAMe may interfere with sleep and some insomnia has been reported (Medical Economics, 2008a). For this reason, it is generally recommended that SAMe should be taken in the morning, although some studies reviewed above reported success in twice per day (BID) dosing. Rarely, motor side effects have been reported, including some hyperactive muscle movement (Medical Economics). When encountered, the dose should be lowered for a week or two, following which the patient may gradually be re-challenged with a higher dose, if needed.

Because SAMe does not alter liver enzymes, and does not seem to rely on any one CP450 enzyme for metabolism, drug–drug interactions are less likely. However, SAMe may have some effects on lowering lipids and improving liver function. It is also used to treat osteoarthritis and fibromyalgia. Thus, patients who already take medications to lower cholesterol, or treat osteoarthritis or fibromyalgia, should consult their physician before initiating SAMe therapy.

Like St. John's Wort, SAMe may be associated with a small increase in suicidal tendencies in those patients who present with symptoms of depression. As with any antidepressant, clinicians should carefully monitor patient response and intervene if an increase in suicidal thoughts or plans becomes evident. In addition, like all antidepressants, SAMe is also associated with a small risk of inducing hypomanic or manic symptoms (Bezchlibnyk-Butler & Jeffries, 2007), and some patients who have tendencies toward symptoms of bipolar disorder may exhibit 'switching' from depressive to manic symptoms. Once again, careful monitoring of dose/response and adverse effects is necessary.

SUPPLEMENTS WITH LIKELY EFFICACY

In addition to supplements discussed above, some other compounds have also undergone at least some research, although results are sometimes contradictory. In addition, these have not sufficiently been researched with children and adolescents. Clinicians must use caution when using these supplements.

Omega-3

Omega-3 is an essential fatty acid that does not occur naturally in the body and must be taken in through diet. Natural sources are fish, walnuts, flaxseed, soybeans, and canola oil. There are also food products that have been enriched with Omega-3, such as eggs, yogurt, and milk. Beneficial effects of Omega-3 have been widely reported in research literature, the supplement has been found to stabilize mood (as discussed in Chapter 7), protect the brain against Alzheimer's, and reduce negative effects of low density lipoproteins (LDL), the type of fat responsible for clogging of the arteries. While much of the research about Omega-3's beneficial effects comes from studying cultures where endogenous diet is rich in the intake of Omega-3 in food (for example, by consuming fish), some evidence now exists about beneficial effects of Omega-3 supplementation.

Omega-3 supplements are generally available as caplets filled with fish oil rich in Omega-3. The pills usually contain 1000 mg, but those containing higher and lower amounts are also available. In addition, since the caplets are usually rather large, and may be difficult to swallow by some patients, other forms are also available – for example, a chewable preparation. As is the case with all supplements, there are many manufacturers, and Omega-3 supplements are sold in drug stores, supermarkets, and health food stores. Many are also available through the Internet.

Omega-3 is also sold by prescription in 1000 mg tablets that contain 465 mg of eicosapentaenoic acid (EPA) and 375 mg of docosahexanoic acid (DHA). These are approved to treat hyperlipidemia and are marketed as Lovaza (formally Omacor). They are manufactured in a process that removes mercury from the fish oil, and therefore these pills are marketed as superior to other Omega-3 supplements (which usually do not remove mercury from the fish oil): the amount of mercury contained in fish oil supplements is considered to be much lower than it is in many types of fish, since the oil is not usually derived from fish known to have high amounts of mercury. In addition, plant-based Omega-3 supplements (in flax, soybean, or canola oil), also available on the market, do not contain mercury. One potential benefit of Lovaza is that, as an FDA-approved compound, its sale and manufacture is regulated, and therefore the consumer can be more certain that Lovaza really contains the ingredients that it claims to have, in the specific amount that is advertised. Consumers must balance these benefits against the added cost of this medication and the inconvenience of seeking a prescription.

Deficiencies of Omega-3 have been implicated in various types of depression, including MDD, Seasonal Affective Disorder, pregnancy related depression, and other subclinical depressions (Lin & Su, 2007). Some have suggested that the rising rates of depressive disorders closely correlate with decreasing dietary intake of Omega-3 – as the consumption of fish has steadily decreased in the western diet, there has been a corresponding increase in the incidences of various forms of depression, while rates of depression remain low in Asian countries where far more fish is consumed (Lake, 2007). In addition, depressed people exhibit lower concentrations of Omega-3 in their blood, but this association may or may not be clinically relevant. It has also been suggested that the ration of

Omega-3 to Omega-6 is paramount. The western diet has shifted toward greater Omega-6 consumption, and excessive omega-6 intake coupled with decreased omega-3 consumption may lead to an unhealthy omega-6 to omega-3 ratio, while less Omega-6 and more Omega-3 may be supportive of better physical and mental health (Simopoulos, 2002).

Evidence for Efficacy

Much of what we know of Omega-3 supplementation for relief of depressive symptoms comes from studies conducted with adults. Almost 30 years ago, Rudin (1981) published a series of case reports that reported mood improvement in patients taking Omega-3 supplements (flaxseed oil). Since, a number of studies have been performed, some of which followed the randomized, placebo-controlled design, and research findings suggest a benefit in treating depression with Omega-3 supplements, although a few studies have been contradictory (Lake, 2007). For example, Puri et al. (2002) reported sustained improvement over a 9 month period in patients treated with 4 g/day, and several other studies reported similar results, although the required doses sometimes reached over 9 g/day (Lake). All of the patients tolerated the supplement well and adverse effects were minimal. However, another study failed to replicate these results at 2 g/day (Marangell et al., 2003). It is possible that higher doses are required to improve symptoms of depression. As adjunctive therapy, when added to a traditional antidepressant regimen for patients suffering with recurrent or treatment resistant unipolar depression, Omega-3 proved to be a beneficial add on, with significant response evident in only 3 weeks (Nemets et al., 2002).

Benefits of using Omega-3 with children are only recently beginning to be researched. In one pilot study Nemets et al. (2006), found that depressed children, ages 6–12, showed more than a 50 percent reduction in symptoms, and 4 out of 10 met the criteria for remission. They also noted that there were no adverse reactions reported. This preliminary finding needs to be replicated but it offers hope that Omega-3 supplements may be as effective in children and adolescents as they appear to be for adults.

Pharmacodynamics

Essential Omega-3 fatty acids include a-linolenic acid (ALA), eicosapentaenoic acid (EPA), and docosahexaenoic acid (DHA). Following ingestion, DHA inhibits lipogenesis and stimulates oxidation. ALA, EPA, and DHA undergo downconversion and retroconversion (as described below) and contribute to the metabolism of various nutrients and lipids. This is responsible for a broad-based therapeutic effect that includes changes in cardiovascular function, decrease in triglycerides, and improvement in pulmonary function. Most of these effects are directly associated with DHA, although related fatty acids may play a contributory role.

DHA is taken up by the brain at greater rates than the other fatty acids. DHA is then incorporated into the phospholipids of cell membranes. DHA contributes to proper formation and elongation of synapses. In addition, DHA-containing phospholipids improve cell function by stabilizing the membrane fluidity and changing firing rates of neurons (Horrocks & Yeo, 1999). Thus, DHA may play a role in the synchronization of neuronal action. It can be hypothesized that poor phosphorization may be partially responsible for decreased neuronal function, and when such deficits are evident in catecholaminergic pathways, symptoms of depression may be apparent. Consequently, increasing phosphorization of cell membranes in these areas may be responsible for the beneficial effects of DHA (and other fatty acids) in reducing depression.

Eicosanoids contribute to this process. They are localized in cells and serve as catalysts for a large number of processes, including the movement of calcium in and out of the cells (Enig & Fallon, 1999). Because calcium channels are involved in the rates of firing of brain cells, regulation of these channels changes the brain's action potential. It is possible that EPA's regulation of calcium channels may contribute to DHA's influence of cell membrane phosphorization, providing a synergistic effect on the rates of neuronal firing. When this regulation of firing affects catecholaminergic pathways, improvement in symptoms of depression may be observed.

Pharmacokinetics

Following ingestion, the metabolism of fatty acids begins in the small intestine by special digestive enzymes. These lipases break down fatty acids into individual chains, glycerol, and monoglycerides (glycerol with one remaining fatty acid still attached). These are then absorbed through the intestinal wall into the lymph stream. Fat molecules are then carried in the lymph system and slowly metabolized to provide gradual release of energy (Enig, 2000).

Essential fatty acids go through many conversions. ALA is converted into EPA and DHA, and these are then gradually absorbed into cell membranes. However, they also undergo complex cross-metabolism. While Omega-6, also known as linoleic acid (LA), undergoes a one-way transformation into various fatty chains, culminating in docosapentaenoic acid, ALA undergoes circular transformation that involves many steps, including the formation of EPA and DHA, and then retro-conversion of EPA and DHA. It is difficult to determine how the body regulates the amounts of DHA and EPA that remain in the cells. It is likely that these are constantly transformed into each other to provide a balance of essential nutrients necessary for many metabolic processes, including membrane phosphorization.

Because ALA is converted into EPA and DHA, and EPA and DHA are retroconverted into each other, it is not necessary to purchase a specific combination of these fatty acids. Some manufacturers focus on the hypothesized benefits of DHA over EPA, or vice versa, and Omega-3 pills are available in various combinations of these components. The balance of these components in the pill is probably immaterial, since the complex conversion chains will probably result in the same balance of these nutrients in the body, regardless of the specific ratio included in the caplet.

Optimal ratio of Omega-6 to Omega-3 in the human body is estimated to be $2:1$. However, it is not uncommon for individuals in westernized countries to consume diets where the two are ingested at a ratio of about $20:1$. For this reason, the majority of supplements primarily focus on delivering additional amounts of Omega-3 into the body, and any amounts of Omega-6 in the tablet may be superfluous, since the common diet already includes so many foods rich in LA. When purchasing a supplement, consumers should select one that maximizes the amount of Omega-3 and minimizes the amount of Omega-6 in the preparation.

Manufacturers of Omega-3 generally advise to take the supplements with or without food. Researchers, however, have long recognized that Omega-3 fatty acids ingested in food are better absorbed than those taken in supplements. Some studies have found that Omega-3 taken without a meal is poorly absorbed. For this reason, nutritionists generally recommend to take an Omega-3 supplement as part of a meal, so that it is absorbed together with the food that is being consumed (Neville, 2006).

In order to prevent oxidation of fatty acids before they are taken up into cell membranes, antioxidants must be present. Those whose diets are rich in antioxidant foods probably consume enough of these during a meal to prevent fatty acid oxidation. However, those who consume meals low in antioxidants may need to take an antioxidant supplement – for example, tocopherol, a form of vitamin E. For this reason, some formulations of Omega-3 supplements include a small amount of tocopherol. However, instead of (or in addition to) tocopherol, some supplements also include vitamins A and/or D. Because these vitamins do not get cleared from the body, clients should be careful with these supplements because high intake of these vitamins may lead to toxicity.

Although fatty acids are metabolized and absorbed rapidly, the onset of effect is not evident for a long time. Some have reported that the onset of clinical effect is not evident for weeks, even months, and that treatment for up to 3 months is necessary to determine the eventual clinical response (Lake, 2007). This makes it difficult to dose the supplements, since clinical effects are not likely to be immediately evident.

Dosing

Omega-3 supplements are not usually dosed by body weight. In children, the recommended starting dose is 500 mg, and usually doses range up to 4000 mg/day (Bezchlibnyk-Butler & Virani, 2004). Some have found doses below 1000 mg/day to be ineffective (Lake, 2007). Because Omega-3 is generally well tolerated, gradual titration is recommended. However, the maximum dose is often determined by how many tablets the child is willing to take and whether digestive effects (for example, fish burps or a fishy taste in the mouth) prevent further increase in dose. Because response will not immediately be evident, it is difficult to determine what dose will eventually be effective.

Teens are generally dosed at 1000–4000 mg/day (Bezchlibnyk-Butler & Jefries, 2007). Some have found doses below 2000 mg/day to be ineffective, and some adults require doses in excess of 9000 mg (Lake, 2007). As with children, dosing should gradually be increased to a maximum level that can be tolerated with minimal gastrointestinal discomfort. Again, it is difficult to determine what dose will be effective since response to the supplement may not immediately be evident.

Co-factors are necessary for metabolism of some of the fatty acids, especially EFA. Carnitine is necessary for the elongating EFA and transporting it across inner cell membranes. It is possible that some of the inconsistent findings about the efficacy of fatty acids may be secondary to carnitine deficits. For this reason, supplementation with l-carnitine has been studied and has shown promising effects (Torrioli *et al.*, 1999), although some studies have not found this to be true (Fokkema *et al.*, 2005). Since humans metabolize only a portion of the necessary supply of carnitine, supplementing fatty acid therapy with l-carnitine may be helpful. L-carnitine is supplied in capsules, tablets, solution, and chewable wafer. Children may take about 250 mg of l-carnitine with fatty acids, while adults may need to take about 500 mg. These doses are generally well tolerated although a small incidence of seizures has been reported (Medical Economics, 2008a). Individuals with risk factors for seizures should consider l-carnitine supplementation only under supervision of a physician.

In addition, some studies have shown that a form of carnitine, acetyl-l-carnitine (ALC) facilitates fat metabolism and stimulates protein and phospholipid synthesis (Settle, 2007). Even more importantly, there is some research that supplementation with ALC, as monotherapy, improves symptoms of depression (Bella *et al.*, 1990), and some have found that it was especially effective in reducing more severe symptoms (Tempesta *et al.*, 1987). Doses ranged from 1500–3000 mg/day, usually taken three times per day (TID). Thus, it may be effective to augment treatment with Omega-3 by adding ALC, starting at 500 mg/day and gradually increasing to 1–3 mg/day in divided doses (Settle).

Adverse Effects

Omega-3 oils are generally well tolerated. The most common adverse effects involve the gastrointestinal tract, including nausea and diarrhea. Because the majority of Omega-3 supplements are sold as fish oils, some individuals experience an unpleasant, 'fishy' taste in their mouth, a 'fishy' smelling breath after a meal during which Omega-3 supplement was taken, and fishy 'burps' that may last for several hours. For this reason, some manufacturers offer 'burpless' formulas manufactured by increasing the thickness of the pill's outer coating. This allows the supplement to survive the stomach acids and dissolve when it reaches the small intestine. These have been shown to effectively reduce the above problems. Omega-3 supplements are also available in non-fish based formulas that are not associated with burps or an unpleasant taste.

Because Omega-3 supplements are oil based, there is a caloric value associated with the caplet. The exact amount varies, but generally a 1000 mg pill will contain about 20 calories. For individuals who consume a low amount, an extra 20 or 40 calories per day will probably have a minimal amount on weight. However, those on higher amounts (for example, 8000 or 9000 mg per day) must remember that they are consuming an additional 160 or 180 calories. In addition, fatty acids are high density lipoproteins (HDL) and contribute to the overall HDL levels within the body. While this is generally beneficial, those on high levels of Omega-3 supplements who also consume diets rich in HDL may experience additional increases of HDL and total cholesterol, which may not always be beneficial. Individuals who take high doses of fatty acid supplements should periodically check their cholesterol profile.

Omega-3 fatty acids are associated with an antithrombotic effect. Patients who take blood thinners (like aspirin) must be careful about taking subsequent fatty acid supplements, and should consult a physician before initiating Omega-3 therapy. In addition, some patients regularly use over-the-counter non-steroidal anti-inflammatory drugs (NSAIDs, like Advil or Motrin) to manage headaches, backaches, or similar conditions. While combining fatty acids with NSAIDs has not been shown to pose a risk, many NSAIDs have some blood thinning properties, and combining NSAIDs with fatty acids has sometimes been linked to nose bleeds and easy bruising (Medical Economics, 2008a). For this reason, those who take NSAIDs daily should probably consult a physician before initiating Omega-3 therapy.

Use of fatty acid supplements has sometimes been reported to alter glucose tolerance, especially in patients with type 2 diabetes. The mechanism of this is poorly understood, and some studies have not confirmed this finding. However, because there is a risk, children and adolescents who are diabetic and take insulin should consult their physician before starting Omega-3 treatment.

Vitamin B9

The B family of vitamins contains eight vitamins that play important physiological functions in the body. These include B1 (thiamine), B2 (riboflavin), B3 (niacin), B5 (pantothenic acid), Vitamin B6 (pyridoxine), B7 (biotin), B9 (folic acid), and B12 (cobalamins). B vitamins are involved in cellular metabolism and, like all other vitamins, must be obtained from the diet.

Vitamin B9 (folate) has particularly been implicated in symptoms of depression. Low blood concentrations of folate have been found in depressed individuals (Young, 2007), and a drop in folate levels may occur after the onset of depression, and decreased folate levels are also associated with a longer course of depression and greater severity of symptoms (Morris et al., 2008). Low folate levels are also predictive of poor response to antidepressant medications (Kemper & Shannon, 2007), depressed individuals who had previously remitted are more likely to relapse when their folate levels are low (Papakostas et al., 2004).

Folate is found in green leafy vegetables, fortified foods such as cereal and bread, fruit, and organ meats. Folic acid is a synthetic form of folate. Although foods high in folate are plentiful in the western diet, folate can be inactivated through cooking and processing, and folate deficiency is presumed to be the most frequently occurring vitamin deficiency (Berriman, 2004). Supplemental folate, usually in the form of folic acid, is available in a wide variety of doses, ranging from tens of micrograms to several milligrams per capsule. Folate, as opposed to folic acid, is also available, but is usually more expensive and no credible studies thus far have proven benefit of one over the other. Consequently, there appears to be no valid reason to buy the more expensive ingredient.

Evidence of Efficacy

Benefits of folate to treat depression have been researched for decades. In a retrospective survey of studies performed prior to 1970, Carney and Sheffield (1970) found that psychiatric patients who received folate supplementation exhibited better recovery and shorter time in the hospital. In a long-term, double-blind study, Coppen et al. (1986) found that patients randomized to a group receiving 200 mcg/day of folate exhibited significant improvement in their levels of depression as compared to a group receiving placebo. In addition, Godfrey et al. (1992) found that depressed outpatients with normal levels of folate prior to onset of treatment improved as significantly as patients taking amitryptiline (a TCA).

Several studies have also researched the use of folate as an adjunct to augment treatment with a prescription antidepressant. Coppen and Bailey (2000) studied 127 patients with MDD who were treated with fluoxetine (an SSRI), and randomized them to a group augmented with folate and another augmented with placebo. Results revealed that patients receiving fluoxetine and folate improved more significantly than those receiving fluoxetine alone, and this difference was especially notable in women. Similar results were reported by Alpert et al. (2002) who also found that supplementation with folate in addition to an SSRI revealed greater improvement in symptoms of depression. In their recent review, Morris et al. (2008) found support for adding folate to fluoxetine, desmethylimipramine, and Venlafaxine, and improvement was noted even in those patients who were previously partial responders or non-responders to the medications.

Folate supplementation to treat depression has not been studied in children or adolescents. Some children are born with a genetic disorder characterized by deficiency in methylenetetrahydrofolate reductase (MTHFR), a folate metabolizing enzyme responsible for catabolism of methionine, and the result often is hyperhomocysteinemia, a disorder that contributed to serious cardiovascular risks and is considered a major cause of pediatric heart attacks and strokes (Garoufi et al., 2006). Consequently, folate supplements have safely been used in children who are shown to be folate deficient. Consequently, given folate's safety and the amount of data that supports its use in adults, a cautious trial of folate supplementation in children and adolescents with depression may be a reasonable treatment alternative.

Pharmacodynamics

The mechanism of action of folate is not fully understood. Folate plays a role in the metabolism of SAMe, a transmethylating agent that has been shown to improve symptoms of depression when taken as a supplement (as described earlier in the chapter). Thus, increasing levels of folate may increase levels of SAMe. In addition, folate breaks down homocystein, which appears in high levels in depressed individuals (Folstein *et al.*, 2007), and the breakdown of homocystein also plays a role in the generation of SAMe.

Pharmacokinectics

Folic acid is absorbed through the small intestine and should generally be taken on an empty stomach, since the bioavailability is significantly decreased when the supplement is taken with food (Medical Economics, 2008a). Folate is metabolized in the liver and its metabolites are excreted through the kidneys. The amount that remains in systemic circulation is gradually absorbed into various body tissues. Folate does not seem to affect liver metabolism in any way.

Dosing

Dietary reference intakes (DRI) for folate have been established and range from 150 mcg/day in infants to 400 mcg/day in adults. In addition, upper intake levels (UL) have also been established and range from 300 mcg/day for infants to 800 mcg/day for adults (Medical Economics, 2008a). The dosage used in research varies greatly and ranges from 200 mcg/day to 50 mg/day (Settle, 2007). A dosage of 1 mg/day is considered safe for children (Kemper & Shannon, 2007), but higher doses have also been used with no adverse effects. It seems sensible to recommend that doses above 1 mg/day in children should only be used under monitoring by a medical professional.

To avoid masking a deficiency of vitamin B12, folate should be taken with vitamin B12 dosed around the DRI levels (Settle, 2006), which range from 0.9 mcg/day in infants to 2.4 mcg/day in adults (Medical Economics, 2008a). This may also provide additional benefit, since preliminary research has shown that supplementation with vitamin B12 seems to also reduce symptoms of depression (Coppen & Bolander-Gouaille, 2005). In fact, some research has also shown that supplementation with other B vitamins may reduce symptoms of depression. Benton *et al.* (1995) found that supplementation with 10 times DRI levels of vitamin B2 and B6 was associated with improvement in mood, and low levels of B1 have also been associated with depression (Settle, 2007). Consequently, it may be best to supplement with folate as part of a B complex vitamin regimen that does not exceed 10 times DRI for any of the B vitamins.

Adverse Effects

Folate is generally well tolerated. Mild side effects may include skin flushing, rash, changes in sleep patterns, and gastrointestinal discomfort. These are rare and usually not consistently replicated (Medical Economics, 2008a).

Although folate does not affect liver enzymes, supplementation with this vitamin nevertheless has been found to alter the metabolism of several medications, including some anticonvulsants. In addition, some medications may interfere with folate levels, including non-steroidal anti-inflammatory drugs (NSAIDs), like ibuprofen, and pancreatic enzymes (Medical Economics, 2008a). Generally, supplementation with folate, especially at higher doses, should not be performed when the patient is taking any medications unless the combination is monitored by a medical professional.

Folate has not been associated with any increase in suicidal tendencies; however, perhaps because of its antidepressant tendencies, supplementation with folate may carry a small risk of inducing hypomanic symptoms, and case reports exist that are suggesting of some patients developing hypomanic symptoms (Settle, 2007). As with all supplements, careful monitoring of dose/response and adverse effects is necessary.

Inositol

Inositol is an isomer of glucose and is present in high concentrations in the brain. It was once classified as part of the B vitamin group and was designated vitamin B8, but was then found to be synthesized by the human body and was declassified as a vitamin. Inositol is found in many foods, including high-bran cereals, fruit, nuts, and beans. Inositol is available in several forms, and only some of these are appropriate for psychiatric use. These include inositol and myo-inositol. Other forms, such as inositol hexaphosphate, inositol nicotinae, and D-chiro-inositol have not been shown to have mental health effects and are used to treat cancer, vascular diseases, and insulin resistance.

Supplemental inositol is available in capsules of various strengths, generally ranging from 500–1000 mg. Inositol powder is also available. In the 1970s, Barkai et al. (1978) found that depressed individuals had significantly lower levels of inositol in cerebral spinal fluid (CSF) than that of non-depressed people. Since that time, inositol has been researched as a treatment for symptoms of depression.

Evidence of Efficacy

Both open-label and controlled studies have revealed inositol's efficacy in improving symptoms of depression. In an open 4 week study, Levine *et al.* (1993) found that 6 g/day of inositol was effective in reducing symptoms of depression. Subsequent double-blind, placebo-controlled study similarly revealed that up to 12 g/day of inositol was effective in reducing symptoms of depression, but effects were not seen until about 4 weeks of treatment, and the improvement in symptoms was much greater in females than in males. Upon discontinuation of treatment, half of the subjects relapsed into depression. In a review of controlled studies, Levine *et al.* (1999) concluded that inositol appears to exhibit efficacy that is similar to serotonergic antidepressants (SSRIs). However, a subsequent study found that adding inositol to treatment with SSRIs did not produce beneficial results (Levine *et al.* 1999). In all of the studies, patients tolerated the supplement well and side effects were minimal.

Unfortunately, to date, no studies have been performed to investigate the efficacy of inositol to treat depression in children and adolescents, and therefore clinicians must attempt to extrapolate to the pediatric population the results from studies performed with adults. Because inositol is generally well tolerated and few risks have been identified, clinicians may cautiously attempt a trial of this nutraceutical with pediatric patients.

Pharmacodynamics

The mechanism of action of inositol is not fully understood. Inositol may be involved in neurotransmitter synthesis and is a precursor to the phosphatidylinositol (PI) cycle, an important intracellular second messenger system. By changing the PI cycle, inositol may exert intracellular changes that are similar to those seen when a post-synaptic receptor is activated, but without the need to activate that receptor. Thus, it may 'fool' the cell into thinking that it is activated (Belmaker *et al.*, 2002). Consequently, it may be involved in regulating the activity of monoamines (especially serotonin, with possible action on dopamine and norepinephrine) as well as other neurotransmitters.

Pharmacokinetics

Inositol is absorbed from the small intestine. It is hypothesized that inositol is metabolized to phosphatidylinositol and then converted to phosphatylinositol-4,5-bisphosphate, which is a precursor to second-messenger molecules. Unfortunately, little else is known about the pharmacokinetics of inositol, and time to peak and elimination half-life have not been established. Thus far, no effect on liver metabolism has been identified.

Dosing

Although there is no recommended daily intake for inositol, the average daily dietary intake is estimated to be about 1 g/day (Medical Economics, 2008a). Inositol is dosed at much higher levels than other supplements. Therapeutic doses usually range from 12–18 g/day, taken in divided doses (usually two to three times per day). Inositol is also available as a powder that dissolves easily in water or juice. This may be a good option for those who have difficulties swallowing pills. Dosing usually starts at 2 g twice per day, increasing to up to 6 g three times per day (Settle, 2007). Inositol can be taken with or without food. Onset of clinical effect is usually observed in 2–4 weeks.

Adverse Reactions

Inositol is generally well tolerated at doses of up to 20 g/day (Settle, 2007). In children, the studied dose (for ADHD, as discussed in Chapter 5) was 50 mg/kg per day (Alvarado *et al.*, 2004). Common adverse effects are mild and may include gastrointestinal upset, such as nausea, diarrhea, and flatulence. Rarely, an increase in blood glucose levels has been observed (Belmaker *et al.*, 2002). At high doses, there are rare reports of decreased peripheral nerve conduction (Settle). The supplement is considered safe to use with other medications, but few studies have investigated such combinations.

Inositol is contraindicated during pregnancy because it may induce uterine contractions (Settle, 2007). Female adolescents who take inositol and are suspected of being sexually active must be advised of this risk, and should use contraception to prevent pregnancy.

Like St. John's Wort and SAMe, inositol may be associated with a small increase in suicidal tendencies in those patients who present with symptoms of depression. As with any antidepressant, clinicians should carefully monitor patient response and intervene if an increase in suicidal thoughts or plans becomes evident. In addition, like all antidepressants, inositol is also associated with a small risk of inducing hypomanic or manic symptoms, and case reports exist of patients 'switching' from depressive to manic symptoms (Potter *et al.*, 2009). Careful monitoring of dose/response and adverse effects is necessary.

SUPPLEMENTS WITH POSSIBLE EFFICACY

In addition to supplements discussed in the above two sections, a few other compounds may also have some efficacy in treating symptoms of depression. However, since the data that supports the use of the following supplements is extremely limited, clinicians should proceed with caution, and consider the use of the compounds discussed in this section as experimental.

Tryptophan and 5-Hydroxytryptophan

Tryptophan, also referred to as L-tryptophan, is an essential amino acid. Of all essential amino acids, it is the one that is least abundant. It is a protein with many functions in the body, and it is a building block for many endogenous substances. It is also a precursor for serotonin. Consequently, it has been researched as a hypnotic and an antidepressant.

Supplementation with tryptophan has been attempted for many years, and studies report inconsistent results. Because it competes to cross the blood–brain barrier, levels of tryptophan seem to be unpredictable and the response does not appear to be uniform. However, a modified version of tryptophan, 5-hydroxytryptophan (5-HTP) appears to cross the blood–brain barrier less competitively and seems to show more promise in results of research studies.

Several open and controlled studies reveal potential efficacy. Van Hiele (1980) reported that more than half of patients with refractory depression responded favorably to 5-HTP and nearly half exhibited complete recovery when treated with 50–600 mg/day over several months. Byerley and Risch (1985) reviewed results of additional open and placebo-controlled studies and reported that 29–69 percent of subjects responded favorably to treatment with 5-HTP. Efficacy of 5-HTP has also been compared to treatment with prescription antidepressants. Angst et al. (1977) found that 5-HTP was as effective as TCAs, and Poldinger et al. (1991) found that 5-HTP was as effective as SSRIs. These results reveal that 5-HTP may be a promising treatment for depression. Unfortunately, thus far, the use of 5-HTP has not been researched in children or adolescents.

In neurons, tryptophan is converted into 5-HTP, which is then further converted to serotonin (5-hydroxytryptamine, or 5-HT). Theoretically, supplementation with either should increase levels of serotonin in the brain, but because of the blood–brain barrier competition mentioned above, supplementation with 5-HPT seems to increase synaptic levels of serotonin more effectively (Settle, 2007). Increase in serotonergic activity is associated with the antidepressant effects of medications such as SSRIs and some TCAs, and consequently the pharmacodynamics of the antidepressant mechanism of 5-HTP may involve similar effects of serotonergic activity agonism, although 5-HTP seems to accomplish this by increasing the availability of the precursor, rather than the reuptake inhibition mechanism utilized by prescription antidepressants (SSRIs and TCAs).

Following ingestion, tryptophan is absorbed from the small intestine and metabolized in the liver. However, 5-HTP is more easily transformed into serotonin in the small intestine, and therefore to prevent this effect, carbidopa is sometimes taken with 5-HTP to delay its demabolism. The portions not synthesized during first pass effect enter systemic circulation and become distributed to the brain and other tissues. The half-life of tryptophan and 5-HTP is presumed to be very short due to its rapid conversion into serotonin, and appears unrelated to the duration of the clinical effect, since antidepressant action is likely due to the increase in serotonin.

Tryptophan tablets are generally available in tablets and capsules with dosages ranging from 50–1000 mg, and 5-HTP is dosed similarly. Because research studies identified a very wide range of effective dose, trial and error is likely to be necessary to determine the appropriate dose for a specific patient. Children and adolescents should begin with a dosage of 50–100 mg and the dose should gradually be titrated until clinical response is evident. Doses above 1000 mg/day should only be used under medical supervision.

Tryptophan and 5-HTP are usually well tolerated, although some patients may exhibit daytime drowsiness, dizziness, and dry mouth. At higher doses, additional problems with nausea, lack of appetite, and headaches may become evident (Medical Economics, 2007). Because tryptophan and 5-HTP may exert sedative effects, concurrent use of other compounds that exert similar effects (for example, alcohol) should be avoided.

Tryptophan and 5-HTP are associated with a small risk of cardiac dysfunctions. Because tryptophan is converted into serotonin in the brain as well as peripherally, increases in serotonin may become evident in tissues and muscles, including the heart. When taken with carbidopa, these effects are not seen (Xu et al., 2002).

Tryptophan and 5-HTP need to be used cautiously with patients who have been diagnosed with diabetes or exhibit family history of diabetes. One of tryptophan's metabolites, xanthurenic acid, has been found to have a diabetogenic effect in animals. Although no cases in humans have been reported, caution should be exercised.

Phenylalanine and Phenylethylamine

Phenylalanine is an amino acid found in mother's milk and a number of foods, including meat, poultry, fish, cottage cheese, lentils, peanuts, and sesame seeds. Phenylalanine is an essential nutrient, but some individuals are born with a genetic disorder, phenylketonuria (PKU), that prevents them from metabolizing phenylalanine, and, if untreated, phenylalanine accumulates in the body, becomes converted into phenylpyruvate, and the individual usually develops seizures, brain damage, and mental retardation. PKU is usually treated by arranging the diet to avoid foods high in phenylalanine. Structurally, phenylalanine is closely related to dopamine, epinephrine (adrenaline), and tyrosine. Phenylalanine is converted into tyrosine, which then becomes converted into catecholamine neurotransmitters. Consequently, supplementation with phenylalanine has been presumed to have antidepressant effects.

Phenylethylamine (PEA) is metabolized from phenylalanine. It is a neurotransmitter and a hormone, and may act as a neuromodulator for catecholamines. PEA increases extracellular levels of dopamine and modulates noradrenergic transmission. PEA also antagonizes GABA(B) receptors, suppressing their inhibitory effects. Thus, along with phenylalanine, supplementation with PEA has been presumed to have antidepressant effects.

Supplementation with phenylalanine has been recommended for decades (Growdon *et al.*, 1977), although few controlled studies exist to investigate claims of effectiveness. It has also been presumed to be beneficial in the pediatric population (Zeisel, 1986). After reviewing a number of studies, Sabelli (2002) concluded that the antidepressant effect of phenylalanine was weak but potentially useful, especially as an adjunct to prescription antidepressants.

PEA has been researched somewhat more extensively. For example, Fisher *et al.* (1972) found that depressed patients excreted lower levels of PEA in their urine, and since that time these results have been replicated many times, in urine as well as in blood plasma (Sabelli, 2002). Supplementation with PEA has also been shown to be effective in a few small studies, and PEA was shown to be effective even in patients who failed to respond to prescription antidepressants (Sabelli). However, few controlled studies have been performed and the use of PEA has not been researched in the pediatric population.

When used to treat depression in adults, phenylalanine was generally dosed at 1–10 g/day. This translates to a range of 11.6–116 mg/kg/day. Those who desire to attempt supplementation of phenylalanine with children or adolescents should begin at the low end of this range and gradually increase the dose, carefully monitoring response and side effects. PEA is generally dosed at 10–60 mg/day in adults, which translates to about 0.1–0.7 mg/kg/day. Once again, this range can be used to adjust the dose if a trial of PEA is desired in pediatric patients. Pharmacokinetics of phenylalanine or PEA have not been established.

In research studies, phenylalanine and PEA have been well tolerated with very few adverse effects, and no effects of nausea, fatigue, sleep changes, or cardiovascular effects have been observed. Both PEA and phenylalanine have been found to be activating and the supplements should generally be given in the morning. Despite these activating effects, however, no 'switching' into manic or hypomanic states has been reported.

Rhodiola

Rhodiola (*Rhodiola rosea*) is a perennial plant that grows in the US, Canada, Europe, and parts of Asia. Its root, also known as golden root, is commonly used in Asia and Europe to treat fatigue and cognitive blunting. Its pharmacology is complex and includes a large number of active compounds, such as flavonoids, monoterpernes, phenylpropanoids, triterpenes, phenolic acids, and phenylethanol derivatives. It has multiple effects, including antioxidant, anticarcinogenic, cardioprotective, and neuroendocrine properties. Its psychopharmacological effect may include agonist properties for serotonin and dopamine and norepinephrine (perhaps secondary to monoamine oxidase inhibition), as well as influence on opioid peptides (such as beta-endorphins) and nicotinic receptors for acetylcholine. Importantly, it may also act on cellular membrane and improve the ability of serotonin and catecholamine precursors to cross the blood–brain barrier (Saratikov & Krasnov, 1987). Thus, it may be beneficial to augment treatment with tryptophan/5-HTP and/or phenylalanine/PEA with rhodiola.

Rhodiola has been shown to have antidepressant and psychostimulant effects. Saratikov and Krasnov (1987) reviewed the results of a number of studies that showed that patients with asthenia (fatigue, decline in work capacity, trouble falling asleep, poor appetite, irritability, and headaches) responded favorably to rhodiola at doses of 50 mg three times per day (TID). Treatment durations ranged from 10 days to 4 months, and in studies up to 64 percent of cases exhibited significant improvement. More recently, similar results have been reported by Shevtsov *et al.* (2003) and Darbinyan *et al.* (2007).

Rhodiola is usually available in capsules or tablets that usually contain 50–100 mg of a mixture of 3 percent rosavins and 1 percent salidroside. Although other active compounds are found in the preparation, their role is unknown, and therefore rosavins and salidrose are generally sought. Rhodiola is given in doses of 50–200 mg per dose, usually taken two to three times per day. Dosing for children has not been studied, but no contraindications exist, and therefore a dose of 50 mg once to twice per day can cautiously be tried, and gradually titrated upward if well tolerated.

Rhodiola is presumed safe and no adverse effects have been reported in available literature. Similarly, it is not presumed to interact with prescription medications (Medical Economics, 2007). However, because of its antidepressant effects, it may pose a risk of 'switching' into manic or mixed-manic episodes in a manner that is similar to many compounds with antidepressant effects.

Ginger

Ginger (*Zingiber officinale*) is a tropical perennial that grows in Asia, west Africa, and the Caribbean. Ginger is well known as a spice, but its medicinal uses date back thousands of years. Ancient Greeks and Romans imported ginger from Asia, and it was known in China in the fourteenth century bc (Spinella, 2001). It is even mentioned in the Koran as a divine drink. More recently, it is recognized in the world for a variety of medicinal properties, including antiemetic, anti-inflammatory, antimicrobial, antioxidant, antithrombotic, cardiotonic, and antimigraine effects, and it is approved by Germany's Commission E as a treatment for loss of appetite, travel sickness, and dyspepsia (Medical Economics, 2007).

Ginger has several active constituents, including aromatic ketones and terpenoids, and some of these may have anxiolytic and antidepressant properties. These psychoactive properties may be secondary to the inhibition of 5HT3 receptors, as well as eicosanoid inhibition that results in greater GABA activity. GABA conductance may further be increased by inhibition of arachnoid acid metabolites (Spinella, 2001). In addition, abnormally higher levels of cortisol are found in many patients with major depression, and levels of cortisol reduced in patients with depression after ginger supplementation (Piccirillo *et al.*, 1994). Since new antidepressant drugs are being developed that target this pathway of symptom production (Stahl, 2008), it is possible that supplementation with ginger may offer some benefits.

Ginger supplements are available in tablets and capsules ranging from 100–1000 mg. Chewable tablets are also available, and liquid and tea bags preparations may be obtained. Generally, the use of tablets and capsules is recommended because it is easier to control the dosage. In some studies, higher doses of ginger taken on an empty stomach were associated with the development of ulcers, and therefore it is recommended to take ginger supplements with a meal. Very little is known about pharmacokinetics of ginger, but animal studies suggest that following absorption and systemic distribution, it is rapidly cleared. However, serum binding was equally rapid, especially for one of the gingerol ketones (Spinella, 2001). At least some of the constituents of ginger are metabolized by the liver, and cross-metabolism of some of the constituents into others also seems evident (Spinella).

When used to treat nausea, dyspepsia, motion sickness, or arthritis, dosage generally range from 0.5–4 g/day. This can be converted to approximately 5.8–46.5 mg/kg/day. Children and adolescents should be dosed toward the lower end of this ratio, and gradually titrated while monitoring response and adverse effects. According to available data, ginger has a very wide therapeutic window and lethal doses have been reported to range from 250–680 mg/kg (Medical Economics, 2007). It is clear that the clinical range is a tiny fraction of this dose.

In doses listed above, ginger is generally well tolerated and adverse effects are rare. Some patients experience mild gastrointestinal distress, flatulence, bloating, and heartburn. In higher doses, some patients have experienced dermatitis, cardiac arrhythmias, and central nervous system depression.

According to Germany's Commission E, ginger is contraindicated during pregnancy. However, research studies failed to reveal any difficulties of malformations in the fetus, and ginger is sometimes used as an effective remedy for morning sickness (Medical Economics, 2007).

The use of ginger with some medications should be avoided. Concurrent use with anticoagulants may increase the risk of bleeding, and therefore the use of the supplement with any medications that decrease platelet aggregation should only be done under monitoring by medical professionals.

Chromium

Chromium is an essential nutrient involved in glucose and lipid metabolism. It is a trace mineral found in many sources of food, including beef, chicken, eggs, wheat germ, spinach, some fruit, and some seafood (like oysters). Supplemental chromium is available in tablets and capsules generally ranging up to 200 mcg.

Some research findings suggest that chromium supplementation may be effective in reducing symptoms of depression. McLeod et al. (1999) published several single-case reports of patients with dysthymia who improved after supplementation with 200–400 mcg/day of chromium for up to 4 weeks. In all cases, the supplementation resulted in a complete or nearly complete resolution of symptoms. Similarly, McLeod and Golden (2000) reported cases of eight patients with symptoms of depression who responded to 400–600 mcg/day of chromium. Once again, in all cases the therapy resulted in complete or nearly complete remission of symptoms, and the two patients who continued to take chromium supplements for 15 months revealed no relapse. In addition, Davison et al. (2003), in a small, double-blind, placebo-controlled trial, found that patients receiving 600 mcg/day of chromium exhibited significant improvement and all but one had a remission of symptoms by the end of 8 weeks of treatment. In all of these trials, chromium supplementation was well tolerated. Chromium supplementation has not been researched with children or adolescents, and those who desire to try this approach with pediatric patients must exercise much caution.

Several theories have been forwarded about chromium's pharmacodynamics, especially regarding its antidepressant effects. Enhanced insulin sensitivity may facilitate greater noradrenergic and serotonergic activity. In animal studies, chromium increases serum and brain levels of noradrenaline, tryptophan, serotonin, and melatonin. In addition, chromium may downregulate post-synaptic serotonin receptors, particularly of the 2 A type (Franklin & Odontiatis, 2003). At this point, all of these effects are hypothesized and have not been sufficiently researched.

Following ingestion, a small portion of chromium is absorbed and is bound to transferrin and albumin. It is then distributed to various tissues in the body, and depending on the compartment, its half-life ranges from 1 day to about 12 weeks, but turnover may be as slow as 1 year (Medical Economics, 2008a). Most of the ingested dose is excreted in the feces, and absorbed portion is excreted through the kidneys. Chromium should not be taken with meals that contain foods with high levels of phytic acid (unleavened bread, raw beans, seeds, nuts, grains, and soy) because these decrease the absorption of chromium (Medical Economics).

Dietary reference intake (DRI) levels range from 11 mcg/day for infants to 35 mcg/day for adults (Medical Economics, 2008a). Upper intake levels have not been established. In research with adults, clinical doses range up to 600 mcg/day, or about 7 mcg/kg/day. Doses for children must be much lower, but no ranges have been established. Clinicians should begin with the lowest dose possible and gradually titrate to a level that does not exceed the mcg/kg/day ratio for adults.

At low levels, chromium is well tolerated. Some may experience initial insomnia, so the supplement may be given in the morning. Some patients have also revealed vivid dreams that resolved after 2 weeks of treatment (Settle, 2007). Mild side effects may also include psychomotor activation and slight tremor.

At high doses (above 1 mg/day) a variety of adverse reactions has been reported, including contact dermatitis and renal failure in a small number of cases (Settle, 2007). Single cases of anemia, thrombocytopenia, hemolysis, and liver dysfunction have also been reported. Those with hypoglycemia should exercise caution because chromium may further lower blood glucose levels (Medical Economics, 2008a).

There are few reported drug interactions, but patients who take beta-blockers (a type of blood pressure medication) may experience higher levels of HDL cholesterol levels after chromium use. In addition, ascorbate may increase the absorption of chromium, possibly leading to excessive plasma levels of chromium, and consequently the use of vitamin C should generally be avoided with chromium supplements.

SUPPLEMENTS NOT LIKELY TO BE EFFECTIVE

It is not possible to review all compounds that have been speculated to treat symptoms of agitation and mania. However, some of these compounds are sometimes marketed to treat symptoms of schizophrenia and psychosis, despite the lack of evidence of efficacy. In addition to being ineffective, some of these compounds may actually be dangerous when used at high doses. Clinicians who seek to practice in the area of naturopathic psychopharmacology should be aware of these compounds and the potential risks that they may pose.

Dehydroepiandrosterone

Dehydroepiandrosterone (DHEA) is a natural substance produced in the brain, as well as the adrenal glands and the gonads. DHEA, and its major metabolite, dehydroepiandrosterone-3-sulfate (DHEAS) are the most abundant steroids circulating in the human body. DHEA is metabolized to various hormones, including testosterone and estrogen. In the brain, DHEA is classified as a neurosteroid and may act as a modulator of GABA A and glutamate NMDA receptors (Medical Economics, 2008a).

DHEA has been investigated as a pharmacological compound for many decades, and has been shown to have some efficacy in the treatment of lupus, asthmatic attacks, and severe burns. Supplementation with DHEA or DHEAS has been attempted in the treatment of symptoms of depression in adults, and some studies have reported promising results (Wolkowitz & Reus, 2002).

Use of DHEA should be cleared with a medical professional. DHEA is usually contraindicated in children and adolescents, and use of the compound in this population should generally be avoided (Medical Economics, 2008a). Supplementation with DHEA has been associated with significant adverse effects, including dermatological problems, hirsutism and voice changes in women (which may be permanent), cardiovascular problems, hepatitis, insulin resistance, and manic symptoms. In addition, males who use DHEA may have an increased risk of prostate cancer (Medical Economics). Consequently, the risks of DHEA supplementation, especially with children and adolescents, significantly outweigh any presumed benefits, and clinicians should avoid using this compound with pediatric patients.

Iron

Iron is a chemical element involved in the anabolism of catecholamines. Iron is present throughout the body and is converted into amino acids. The vast majority of necessary iron intake is derived from the normal diet, and many iron-rich foods are commonly consumed in meats, cereals, fruit, and vegetables. Some members of at-risk populations may require iron supplementation – for example, those who are malnourished, infants who are not breast-fed, or individuals who have lost a lot of blood. However, iron supplementation in patients who are not iron deficient is dangerous. Careful RDA limits must be observed and excess iron intake has been associated with serious toxic effects, including death. Children are especially at risk for these problems, and iron supplementation should only be undertaken under the supervision (and recommendation) of a physician (Medical Economics, 2008a).

Some studies examined the effects of iron supplementation on symptoms of depression, but results are primarily evident in women, especially those who are shown to be iron deficient (Medical Economics, 2008a). In addition, children who are iron deficient also show symptoms of fatigue and attentional difficulties, so treatment of these children with iron supplements may be warranted. Since the vast majority of children and adolescents do not exhibit iron deficiency, the effect of iron supplementation in this population is non-existent. Given the risks of iron supplementation, clinicians should stay away from this practice unless it can be confirmed that the patient exhibits iron deficiency, and any iron supplementation should be given under close supervision of a physician.

Serine

Serine is non-essential amino acid supplied from food or synthesized by the body from a number of metabolites, including glycine. Serine is found in soybeans, nuts (especially peanuts, almonds, and walnuts), eggs, chickpeas, lentils, meat, and fish (especially shellfish). Serine is produced by the body when insufficient amounts are ingested. It is metabolized from ketones and glycine, and retroconversion with glycine also occurs.

As with most amino acids, when food is ingested that contains serine, the molecule is extracted in the small intestine and absorbed into circulation. There, it travels through the body, crosses the blood–brain barrier, and enters neurons, where it gets metabolized into glycine and many other molecules. Thus, the amount of serine in cells is regulated through these metabolic processes. If too little is ingested, more serine is converted from various sources. When too much is ingested, only a portion is converted to glycine, and the remainder is metabolized into folate and many other proteins.

As with all precursors, only a limited amount of serine is converted to glycine, and supplementation seems to be of limited value. Although non-peer reviewed sources list it as effective in treatment of a variety of symptoms of psychological disorders (especially, depression and anxiety), there is no empirical research to support these claims. Thus, although supplementation with serine is not associated with significant adverse effects, benefits are unlikely, and therefore clinicians are advised to avoid using serine supplements.

SUMMARY

In order to help clinicians select the compounds that are most likely to be effective, an algorithm was developed and is presented in Figure 6.1. Patients should initially try one of two most researched compounds, St. John's Wort and SAMe. Because the former has been researched with the pediatric population a little more extensively, it seems prudent to start treatment with St. John's Wort, but if insufficient response is evident, patient may be switched to SAMe.

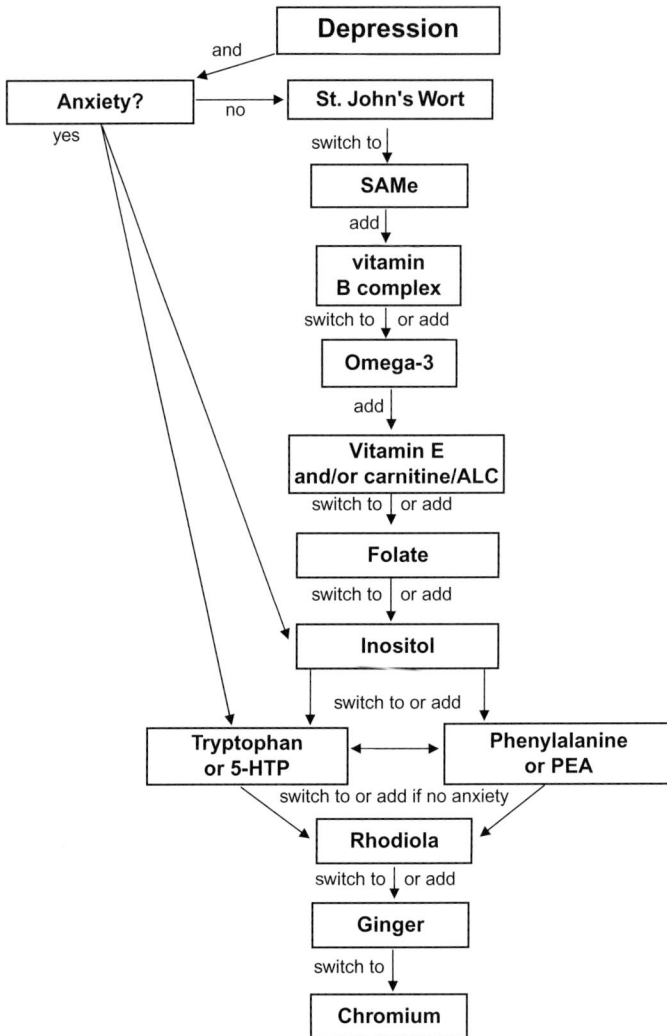

© Elsevier 2009.

FIGURE 6.1   Algorithm for treatment of depression with naturopathic supplements.
© Elsevier 2009.

If these compounds are not sufficiently effective, Omega-3 can be attempted, as monotherapy or adjunct to St. John's Wort or SAMe (used with or without B complex), and vitamin E and/or carnitine/acetyl-l-carnitine (ALC) may also be added. Folate levels may be boosted to further improve antidepressant effects, but clinicians need to impose limits on the intake of all forms of vitamin B, especially if a B complex supplement is also being used to augment the response to SAMe. Alternatively, inositol may be used as monotherapy or adjunct to St. John's Wort, SAMe (with or without vitamins B), or Omega-3 (with or without vitamin E and/or carnitine/ALC). Treatment with inositol may be especially indicated for patients who present symptoms of depression with some comorbid symptoms of anxiety.

If the above combinations are not effective, additional compounds may cautiously be tried, although their use is considered experimental. Monoamine precursors tryptophan/5-HTP or phenylalanine/PEA can be attempted, and either may be augmented with rhodiola (if patient exhibits no symptoms of anxiety). Ginger may also be added to this combination. Finally, supplementation with chromium may carefully be attempted.

If multiple supplements are being administered, extreme caution must be exercised and, ideally, medical monitoring should be utilized.

Chapter 7

Mania and Agitation

Until recently, bipolar disorder in children and adolescents has largely been overlooked, and bipolar disorder was thought to occur almost exclusively in adults. Although some researchers urged recognition of the fact that bipolar disorder also exists in children and adolescents (Garber, 1984), Biederman was one of the first to sufficiently call attention to the fact that bipolar disorder may be more common in children and adolescents than was previously recognized (Biederman *et al.*, 1996). At this time, it is widely accepted that bipolar disorder does occur in children and adolescents, although some feel that nowadays it is diagnosed too frequently in this population (Hammen & Rudolph, 2003), especially in the United States. However, epidemiological studies from abroad confirm that any variant of bipolar disorder is present in about 1 percent of children (Verlhurst *et al.*, 1997), a rate that is similar in adults (APA, 2000).

One reason for the disagreement in prevalence is that bipolar disorder in the juvenile population presents symptom profiles that are different from those commonly seen in adults. Indeed, bipolar I characterized by 'classic' mania seems quite rare in children and adolescents (Hammen & Rudolph, 2003). Instead, children and adolescents with bipolar disorder are much more likely to exhibit variants where major depressive symptoms are interspersed with hypomanic episodes (bipolar II disorder), or full-blown mania is characterized by agitation, rather than classic elation (mixed mania).

SYMPTOMS OF PEDIATRIC BIPOLAR DISORDER

Core symptoms of bipolar disorder include a wide range of disturbances, including changes in mood, self-control, and various aspects of physical functioning, including sleep, psychomotor agitation, and changes in speech patterns. Variants particularly common in children and adolescents are described herein.

Core Symptoms

As stated above, clinicians must remember that manic symptoms commonly present in adults with bipolar disorder are rarely evident in children and adolescents. In the 'classic' presentation full-blown mania, mood is elevated, self-esteem may be inflated, grandiosity is evident, speech becomes rapid and pressured, and the need for sleep may be decreased. Although this profile of symptoms sometimes occurs in adolescents, it is rare, and it is even more rare in prepubertal children. Instead, other variants of mania and hypomania are much more common.

Bipolar I Disorder with Mixed Mania

When symptoms of a mixed episode are present, aspects of both manic and depressive features are evident at the same time. Instead of elevated mood, inflated self-esteem, and a decreased need for sleep, symptoms of agitation are much more likely to be evident in children and adolescents. These commonly include significant psychomotor agitation and loss of control. Indeed, children and adolescents with bipolar disorder often exhibit high levels of aggression and violence, including destruction of property and violent assaults, including episodes of hitting parents, teachers, and other caretakers. These symptoms may be accompanied by racing thoughts and a flight of ideas. At the same time, symptoms of depression are also evident, including depression, low self-esteem, irritation, sadness and tearfulness, anhedonia, sleep disturbance (usually, insomnia), inability to concentrate, and, in some cases, suicidality (thoughts, plans, or suicidal behaviors). Some clinicians qualitatively describe this mental state as highly agitated depression.

In severe cases, additional disturbances in cognition may be evident, including psychotic symptoms. These may include auditory and/or visual hallucinations, and delusional thinking. While the exact prevalence of psychosis in children and adolescents with bipolar disorder has not been established, by some accounts about one-third to one-half of adolescents with bipolar disorder present with psychotic symptoms (Faraone *et al.*, 1997). The incidence of psychosis in prepubertal children with bipolar disorder has not been clearly established, but it is considered somewhat more rare. When psychotic features are present, the disorder is usually harder to treat, and the severity of the other symptoms (for cxample, agitation and violence) may be more significant.

Bipolar II Disorder

Bipolar disorder may occur in children or adolescents without full-blown mania. Instead, a variant with significant depressive and hypomanic symptoms may be evident. In such a presentation, periods of depressed mood, psychomotor retardation, anhedonia, sadness and tearfulness, sleep disturbance (usually, insomnia), fatigue, diminished ability to concentrate, and suicidality may be interspersed with impulsivity, agitation, psychomotor agitation, flight of ideas, and loss of self-control, although the severity of these hypomanic symptoms appears less intense and full-blown mania does not develop. This variant is especially common in children and adolescents (American Academy of Child & Adolescent Psychiatry (AACAP), 1997). Because this variant is especially associated with completed suicides, clinicians should monitor individuals with this variant of bipolar disorder very closely.

Rapid Cycling

The progression of symptom episodes should also be examined. While bipolar disorder in adults may be diagnosed when a manic episode is evident without history of a major depressive episode, this presentation is rare in the juvenile population. Instead, children and adolescents who present manic symptoms (usually, in a mixed-manic presentation) are more likely to present a history of major depressive episodes. In addition, the pattern of switching between the depressive and manic episodes must be examined. In adults, most commonly the depressive and/or manic phase will last several months. In children and adolescents, the cycling between these episodes may occur much more frequently, and rapid cycling is more likely (Child and Adolescent Bipolar Foundation Work Group, 2005).

Secondary Symptoms

Children and adolescents who present with significant depression, agitation, and loss of self-control face many obstacles that can compromise their quality of life. Their family life is usually impacted and juveniles with symptoms of bipolar disorder usually have intense conflicts with parents and siblings. Because they tend to be violent, parents become very distraught and authorities may become involved when police are called in response to major episodes (or threats) of violence. After these outbursts, they may experience much guilt and remorse, which may further exacerbate their symptoms of depression, possibly increasing suicidal tendencies.

Depressed children and adolescents strain their interpersonal relationships. When depressed, they withdraw from others, isolate, and increase their sense of loneliness. Because they are often angry, irritable, and easily agitated, their outbursts alienate peers and make it hard to maintain friendships. They are often described as unpredictable, and peers tend to shy away from maintaining close relationships with children and adolescents who present with symptoms of bipolar disorder.

Children with bipolar disorder exhibit serious difficulties in school. Depressive symptoms cause tardiness, absenteeism, inability to concentrate, distractibility, and memory problems, resulting in poor academic performance. Low frustration tolerance further interferes with task completion. During times of significant agitation and limited self-control, children and adolescents with bipolar disorder exhibit significant acting out that may include substantial aggression and violence. As a result, it often becomes hard to maintain these children and adolescents in regular education settings, and many attend special education placements.

In social settings, youth with bipolar disorder often become involved in alternative culture. Their feelings of depression and apathy often cause them to reject social norms and standards, and their impulsivity and agitation limits their judgment and increases their potential for acting out. Particularly during times of agitation, adolescent with symptoms of bipolar disorder tend to become involved in mischief, and may participate in acts of violence. Indeed, youth with bipolar disorder is more likely to commit crimes and become involved in substance abuse (Biederman *et al.*, 2000). Adolescents may turn to drugs to self-medicate, or to satisfy their thirst for stimulation and high-risk activities.

RULE-OUTS AND COMORBID DISORDERS

Co-occurring psychological disorders are common in youth with bipolar disorder. In fact, most have at least one other psychological disorder. Comorbid disorders present additional challenges that must be considered in order to develop a comprehensive treatment plan. When assessing a child it is important to recognize that many of the symptoms overlap and co-occurring disorders may mask each other's symptoms.

Depression

When a diagnosis of bipolar disorder is being considered, symptoms must be assessed to determine whether both depressive and manic symptoms are evident. To diagnose bipolar disorder, presence of at least one manic or hypomanic episode must be documented. When the manic symptoms include features of 'classic' mania, such as pressure speech, decreased need for sleep, and increased pleasure seeking behaviors, diagnosis of mania can usually be established rather easily. However, as discussed above, such cases are rare in children and adolescents, and hypomanic and mixed-manic presentation is much more common. Since agitation is particularly common during these episodes, and since agitation may also be a feature of major depressive episodes (as discussed in Chapter 6), clinicians must determine whether there are additional symptoms that are not already accounted for in the diagnosis of depression.

The DSM criteria for a hypomanic episode include the presence of a 'distinct period of persistently elevated, expansive, or irritable mood… that is clearly different from the usual nondepressed mood' (APA, 2000, p. 368). The DSM further provides examples of symptoms, and those particularly including characteristics of 'classic' episodes of mania, with lesser severity. Thus, it is evident that to be diagnosed with bipolar disorder based on the hypomanic criteria, there must be presence of *distinct* periods of alternating mood disturbance characterized by vacillations between major depressive symptoms and hypomanic episodes that are similar in character to 'classic' symptoms of mania. Consequently, distinguishing hypomanic and depressive episodes may be relatively straightforward, since most of the symptoms do not overlap.

Differentiating mixed-mania from depression may be more difficult. A mixed episode is often characterized by irritation and psychomotor agitation, and usually symptoms of 'classic' mania are absent. At the same time, criteria must be met for a major depressive episode, which may include symptoms of irritable mood and psychomotor agitation. In addition, both disorders may include the presence of psychosis during severe mood disturbance. Clearly, an overlap between these descriptions is evident. Determining whether a major depressive episode also includes symptoms of mixed mania usually involves a judgment call about the severity of the agitation. When patients exhibit major depressive symptoms accompanied by significant psychomotor activation, severe agitation (which may include violent outbursts), and impulsivity, a mixed episode may be present. In those cases, use of a mood stabilizer and an antidepressant is usually necessary. On the other hand, when the depressive symptoms are predominant and psychomotor agitation and irritability do not appear to cause violent outbursts and significant restlessness, it is more likely that all symptoms are part of a major depressive episode. In those cases, use of an antidepressant may be sufficient.

Attention Deficit Hyperactivity Disorder (ADHD)

In children and adolescents, bipolar disorder most commonly occurs together with ADHD, and 60–90 percent of youth with bipolar disorder also exhibit significant symptoms of ADHD (Spence *et al.*, 2001).

Because symptoms of these two disorders overlap so closely, it may be hard to distinguish them. Children and adolescents with ADHD may be impulsive, restless, distractible, unmotivated to perform in school, and often exhibit limited self-control and explosive behaviors. However, over and above these problems, bipolar disorder also presents symptoms of mood disturbance, periods of depression, agitation, and flight of ideas that is more severe than that associated with hyperactivity and impulsivity. In addition, children and adolescents with ADHD are generally much more violent than children and adolescents with ADHD alone. Thus, when these additional problems are present, it is likely that symptoms of bipolar disorder are evident.

When symptoms of both disorders are present, clinicians needs to consider whether to assign both diagnoses, or whether symptoms of bipolar disorder already subsume symptoms of ADHD. No consensus currently exists about this issue. While some authorities recommend assigning both diagnosis and treating both disorders as separate entities (for example, AACAP, 1997), others maintain that symptoms of bipolar disorder do not require an additional diagnosis of ADHD, since manic or hypomanic symptoms already account for the distractibility and impulsivity evident in youngsters with ADHD (Sachs & Lafer, 1998). With regard to psychopharmacological interventions, when symptoms of both disorders appear present, it is probably most prudent to begin treating symptoms of ADHD with the use of mood stabilizers (and, possibly, with adjunctive antidepressants). When manic, hypomanic, and/or depressive symptoms are brought under control, it will become evident whether residual symptoms of ADHD still remain. If so, these can then be addressed with additional compounds.

Anxiety Disorders

Symptoms of anxiety often coexist with symptoms of bipolar disorder. Anxiety is a common feature of manic symptoms, especially in the midst of a mixed episode. This anxiety may present as chronic restlessness, tension, and a non-specific 'sense of doom' that one feels day to day. This may be accompanied by social discomfort, fear of separation from parents and caretakers, and apprehension in many situations. When mania and anxiety co-occur, they may exacerbate each other's symptoms. For instance, excessive worry and rumination seen in anxiety disorders may be intensified by the restlessness and agitation associated with manic or hypomanic symptoms. Symptoms may also mask, or be masked by, additional co-occurring disorders, such as substance abuse and disruptive disorders.

Because the relationship between anxiety and mania is complex, clinicians must consider whether both disorders are present, or the manic/hypomanic symptoms already account for the evident anxiety. Generally, if symptoms of anxiety are only present during mood disturbance, and go away when mood improves, two diagnoses are not needed and symptomatic anxiety was likely an associated feature of the mood disturbance. In those cases, treating the mood disturbance is likely to diminish both symptom clusters.

Conversely, when symptoms of anxiety appear independent of mood disturbance and seem to exist even during times when mood improves, a separate anxiety disorder likely is evident. In those situations, it is prudent to start with the symptom cluster that is most impairing the patient at the time (which, usually, will be the mood disturbance), and any residual symptoms of anxiety should be addressed when the mood improves.

Disruptive Disorders

Because symptoms of mania or hypomania in children and adolescents so commonly include agitation and loss of control, youngsters with bipolar disorder often exhibit problems with the law and sensation seeking behaviors that violate rules and social standards. Since children and adolescents often express their feelings through acting out, argumentativeness and temper tantrums may be secondary to mood disturbance, in which case a comorbid diagnosis of conduct disorder or oppositional disorder is not needed. However, if acting out occurs in times when mood disturbance does not seem apparent, it is possible that bipolar disorder and a disruptive disorder are simultaneously present. In those cases, both symptom groups will need to be addressed, although it is probably best to begin treatment by addressing symptoms of the mood disorder, since it is likely to exacerbate disruptive behaviors. When mood disturbance diminishes, remaining symptoms will be easier to address behaviorally.

Adjustment and Trauma

Children and adolescents who have undergone traumatic experiences are much more likely to exhibit a variety of difficulties, including mood disturbance, agitation, and aggression. Clinicians should try to assess whether these symptoms are secondary to a mood disorder, or whether they are entirely the result of a traumatic reaction.

Post-Traumatic Disorders

Children and adolescents who have been exposed to severe trauma may exhibit symptoms of acute stress disorder (ASD) or post-traumatic stress disorder (PTSD). Youngsters with ASD or PTSD will usually exhibit substantial anxiety and hypervigilance, sleep disturbance and nightmares (which do not necessarily need to contain trauma-related content), reliving the event through play (or other forms of flashbacks), and avoidance of (and/or detachment from) trauma-related stimuli. Significant depression often accompanies these symptoms. When these symptoms accompany aggression and mood disturbance, and when it can be verified that the onset of the symptoms occurred after the trauma, it is likely that a post-traumatic reaction, rather than a mood disorder, is responsible for the symptoms.

When clinicians encounter children or adolescents with ASD or PTSD, all symptom groups must be managed. Intensive psychological and pharmacological treatment is likely to be necessary, and mood disturbance should not be treated in isolation. While using a mood stabilizer may be helpful, it is not likely to be effective unless the other symptoms are also being addressed. Unfortunately, this will usually mean that multiple supplements will need to be used, and such cases should be approached with extreme caution, since the use of multiple supplements has rarely been researched, especially in the pediatric population.

Adjustment Disorders

Children and adolescents who have been exposed to less severe stressful events may experience an adjustment disorder. This diagnosis is characterized by less extreme variants of emotional and behavioral disturbances. Youngsters who experience such emotional reactions commonly benefit from counseling and psychotherapy in order to help them cope with the stressors. If mood disturbance is apparent, an adjunct use of a mood stabilizer may be beneficial. However, clinicians should administer treatment that comprehensively focuses on helping the child or adolescent cope with the stressful events.

ETIOLOGY

The etiology of bipolar-spectrum disorders is more complex than that of most psychiatric disorders, perhaps with the exception of schizophrenia. As discussed above, in the vast majority of cases, symptoms of bipolar disorder include dimensions of depression and mania or hypomania. Thus, etiology of this disorder must include explanations of both groups of symptoms. Since the etiology of symptoms of depression was discussed in detail in Chapter 7, this chapter will focus on the etiology of symptoms of manic-spectrum mood disturbance.

Symptoms of 'Classic' Mania

Understanding the nature of brain dysfunction in manic episodes is complicated by the wide breadth of symptoms. As may be expected, this implies that many different brain regions may be involved in producing such mood disturbance. The thalamus and hypothalamus mediate a number of important psychological and physiological functions, including sleep. Individuals with classic symptoms of mania often exhibit a decrease in the need for sleep. Thus, it is presumed that thalamic and hypothalamic overstimulation interferes with normal sleep cycles and results in hyperstimulation, thus decreasing the perception of the need for sleep. Dysfunction of the basal forebrain further contributes to these problems (Stahl, 2008). Neurochemically, it is presumed that increased levels of catecholamines may be responsible for this disturbance, although changes in the glutamate–GABA balance in the brain may also be involved.

Portions of the nigrostriatal and mesolimbic brain pathways regulate thoughts and impulse control. When thought processes become disturbed and racing thoughts are evident, overstimulation of the nucleus accumbens may be responsible for these changes, and overactivation of this pathway is usually evident when symptoms become severe enough to include psychosis. Associated brain areas may also become involved, including portions of the anterior frontal lobes and the orbitofrontal cortex (Stahl, 2008). This disturbance is also implicated in the grandiosity and pressured speech that also characterizes classic manic episodes. Once again, catecholaminergic disturbances, or changes in the glutamate–GABA equilibrium may be responsible for these problems.

Symptoms of Mixed Episodes

Dysregulation of the nigrostriatal pathway is implicated in resulting in restlessness and psychomotor agitation. In this case, since the function of this pathway is the regulation of motor impulses, it is presumed that a decrease in the activation of this pathway may be responsible for impulsivity and hyperactivity, and decreases in levels of catecholamines (especially, dopamine) are usually implicated in impulsivity and hyperactivity (as discussed in Chapter 5). However, it is possible that overactivation of this pathway may also result in increased agitation and higher motor output (Stahl, 2008).

When significant anger is evident, including explosiveness and violence, the amygdala and the hippocampus may be involved in producing such mood disturbance. Indeed, some individuals who exhibit mixed-manic symptoms also report comorbid anxiety. Since amygdala is involved in producing symptoms of anxiety, it seems that it is likely that the amygdala may be hyperactivated during mixed-manic disturbances. These changes may be the result of excess catecholamine activity (especially, norepinephrine), or a disturbance in the glutamate–GABA balance.

Summary of Research Findings

While it may be helpful to conceptually localize the brain regions that may be involved in the production of various symptoms of manic disturbances, it is necessary to examine whether the findings of neuropsychiatric research reveal abnormalities consistent with the above hypotheses.

Neuroanatomical Abnormalities

Studies with adults have revealed few structural brain differences in individuals diagnosed with bipolar disorders, and the size of various brain portions usually does not differ between those with the disorder and normal controls. Although not all brain imaging studies confirmed this finding, it is generally accepted that the brains of individuals with bipolar disorder reveal greater densities of white matter, particularly in the prefrontal region (Houenou et al., 2007). Similar findings have also been obtained in research studies that examined brain differences in children and adolescents with this disorder (Lyoo et al., 2002; Pillai et al., 2002). Although the exact significance and functional implications are not known, it is possible that this increase in axonal connections is associated with the greater, and possibly less coordinated, neuronal firing usually associated with this disorder.

In addition, it is apparent that the degree of this abnormality is correlated with the length and severity of manic episodes. Houneou and colleagues (2007) specifically identified the axonal connections between the left subgenual cingulate and the amygdalo-hippocampal complex as core regions of this network. Using diffusion tensor tractography, they identified a significantly increased number of reconstructed fibers in this area, suggesting that alternating mood episodes may gradually produce greater and greater abnormalities. Similarly, Adler et al. (2006) found that individuals with bipolar disorder reveal a loss of bundle coherence in prefrontal white matter, and suggested that this loss of coherence may contribute to prefrontal cortical pathology associated with bipolar disorder. These findings may explain the phenomenon of 'kindling' (initially identified in epilepsy) associated with many (but not all) patients with bipolar disorder – each manic episode makes the patient more vulnerable to future manic episodes, and later episodes are less likely to require an environmental trigger than earlier episodes (Post, 2007).

Neurophysiological Abnormalities

Studies that utilize functional imaging to investigate brain activity in patients with bipolar disorders are more rare. Although monoaminergic overactivity is widely associated with symptoms of mania, few studies have been able to show this disturbance. Part of the difficulty in researching this disorder may lie in the need to study individuals while in the midst of a manic phase, and because of the nature of the disturbance, performing brain scans is usually impractical, and when manic symptoms resolve, those patients may return to normal brain function and imaging studies may not reveal abnormalities when symptoms are not present.

Some studies, however, are beginning to identify differences in brains of patients with bipolar disorders that continue to be evident even when patients are asymptomatic at the time. For example, using functional magnetic resonance imaging (fMRI), Altshuler *et al.* (2005) showed that patients with a history of bipolar disorder exhibited underactivity in areas associated with inhibitory brain functions, especially the orbitofrontal cortex. During a 'stop-signal' experimental task, which required inhibition of an urge, normal controls exhibited significant increase in activity in this brain area, while patients with a history of bipolar disorder revealed essentially unchanged activity in this area during baseline and the no-go task. These differences may be related to altered membrane phospholipid metabolism in the frontal lobes and basal ganglia, and Cecil *et al.* (2002) reported lowered choline levels within the orbital frontal gray matter in adolescents and young adults with bipolar disorder during a manic phase.

In addition, studies using magnetic resonance spectroscopy imaging (MRSI) are also beginning to reveal promising results. Port *et al.* (2004) identified a 'chemical fingerprint' of the relative distribution of neurotransmitters in portions of the brain involved in the production of manic symptoms, the basal ganglia, and the anterior cingulate gyrus. The scan analyzed metabolites of five neurotransmitters and produced a graph that illustrated region-by-region variations between patients with bipolar disorder and sex-matched healthy volunteers. In addition, the scans were also able to accurately predict different mood states – manic, depressed, or euthymic. Similar studies have also been also performed with children and adolescents. For example, Davanzo *et al.* (2003) were able to differentiate youngsters with bipolar disorder from those with intermittent explosive disorder by comparing MRSI scan results. It is apparent that this new technique shows much promise in identifying the neuropathology behind the symptoms of bipolar disorder.

Additional support for the neurotransmitter overactivity hypothesis comes from the examination of mechanisms of action of medications that are effective in reducing manic symptoms. Lithium is still considered the first-line medication of choice for treatment of 'classic' mania. Examination of the pharmacodynamic effects of lithium reveals that its clinical effects are primarily exerted by changing intracellular functions that reduce membrane permeability, and therefore action potential is decreased and neuronal firing is slowed (Stahl, 2008). Other medications that exert mood stabilizing effects are anticonvulsants and atypical antipsychotics. Anticonvulsants primarily work by altering the glutamate–GABA balance toward less stimulation (by increasing GABA and/or decreasing glutamate). Interestingly, lithium also decreases levels of norepinephrine, but seems to increase levels of dopamine and serotonin (Janicak *et al.*, 2006). Some of the anticonvulsant mood stabilizers similarly affect these neurotransmitters, with less intracellular effects. The most recent medications approved as mood stabilizers, atypical antipsychotics, reduce levels of dopamine and serotonin. Thus, it is apparent that reducing neuronal firing appears to have antimanic effects, although the role of dopamine and serotonin is more complex, various mood stabilizing medications alter the activity of these neurotransmitters in opposite directions.

SUPPLEMENTS WITH LIKELY EFFICACY

Unfortunately, at this time it is apparent that no naturopathic supplements have consistently revealed efficacy in research studies to reduce symptoms of mania and agitation, and therefore no compounds at this time should be considered to have established efficacy in treating symptoms of mania and agitation. However, some compounds are beginning to show promise, even though more research is needed. The best documented pharmacodynamic effect associated with mood stabilization is the overall decrease in neuronal excitation and associated decreases in neuronal firing. This reduction in overall brain stimulation is accomplished by several prescription medications, and naturopathic compounds that exert similar effects in the brain appear most likely to be effective in treating symptoms of mania and agitation. Conversely, those compounds that exert more specific action on various neurotransmitters appear to be less effective.

Omega-3 Polyunsaturated Fatty Acids

Effects of Omega-3 were previously discussed in Chapters 5 and 6. Omega-3 fatty acids, including both eicosapentaenoic acid (EPA) and docosahexanoic acid (DHA), have been presumed to have many beneficial effects, including mood stabilization, protection against dementias (especially, Alzheimer's), and reducing risks associated with low density lipoproteins' (LDL) artery clogging effects.

Omega-3 supplements are generally available as caplets filled with fish oil rich in Omega-3. The pills usually contain 1000 mg, but those containing higher and lower amounts are also available. In addition, since the caplets are usually rather large, and may be difficult to swallow by some patients, other forms are also available – for example, a chewable preparation. As is the case with all supplements, there are many manufacturers, and Omega-3 supplements are sold in drug stores, supermarkets, and health food stores. Many are also available through the Internet.

Omega-3 is also sold by prescription in 1000 mg tablets that contain 465 mg of eicosapentaenoic acid (EPA) and 375 mg of docosahexanoic acid (DHA). These are approved to treat hyperlipidemia and are marketed as Lovaza (formally Omacor). They are manufactured in a process that removes mercury from the fish oil, and therefore these pills are marketed as superior to other Omega-3 supplements (which usually do not remove mercury from the fish oil): the amount of mercury contained in fish oil supplements is considered to be much lower than it is in many types of fish, since the oil is not usually derived from fish known to have high amounts of mercury. In addition, plant-based Omega-3 supplements (in flax, soybean, or canola oil), also available on the market, do not contain mercury. One potential benefit of Lovaza is that, as an FDA-approved compound, its sale and manufacture is regulated, and therefore the consumer can be more certain that Lovaza really contains the ingredients that it claims to have, in the specific amount that is advertised. Consumers must balance these benefits against the added cost of this medication and the inconvenience of seeking a prescription.

Evidence of Efficacy

Omega-3's efficacy to treat symptoms of bipolar disorder has been researched over the past two decades, and a number of case studies and some small placebo-controlled clinical trials have revealed beneficial effects (Lake, 2007). For example, Stoll *et al.* (1999) found that an Omega-3 supplement, with a 2 : 1 ratio of EPA : DHA, dosed about 9 g/day, was effective in reducing rates of relapse into a manic episode for a small group of adult men and women with bipolar disorder. The authors further performed open-label studies with more than 150 adults with bipolar disorder and reported similar efficacy (Stoll & Locke, 2002). Although another, similar, study failed to document efficacy, it is apparent that the participants only exhibited symptoms of depression (Post *et al.*, 2003).

Omega-3 supplements may be particularly well suited for individuals who present symptoms of agitation and violence. Some researchers reported that low plasma levels of DHA were associated with increased tendencies toward violence (Hibbeln *et al.*, 1998a; Hibbeln *et al.*, 1998b), and a placebo-controlled study with school students revealed lower levels of aggression at times of stress in the group of students that took DHA supplements (Hamazaki *et al.*, 1996). Another placebo-controlled trial revealed similar results in patients diagnosed with borderline personality disorder (Zanarini & Frankenburg, 2003). Omega-3 supplements have also been found to be effective in reducing violent behaviors among prisoners (Gesh *et al.*, 2002). It is likely, then, that effects of Omega-3 supplementation may be particularly beneficial among individuals who exhibit symptoms of mixed episodes, commonly characterized by agitation and significant levels of aggression.

The use of Omega-3 to treat symptoms of bipolar disorder in the pediatric population has also been researched in a few small studies. In one prospective study, Omega-3 supplements, with 7 : 1 ratio of EPA : DHA, were found to be effective in significantly reducing manic symptoms in half of the children diagnosed with bipolar disorder, with no adverse effects (Wozniak *et al.*, 2007). Effectiveness was noted in individuals receiving 2 g or more, but doses beyond 2 g were not associated with greater improvement. Additional, small studies also revealed that supplementation with Omega-3 may improve symptoms of bipolar disorder, and participants improved despite exhibiting different variants of bipolar disorder, including bipolar I and bipolar II (Potter *et al.*, 2009). Although these findings are preliminary, they offer some support for beneficial effects of supplementation with essential fatty acids in youth with bipolar disorder. Because these supplements are generally well tolerated and risks are low, it is reasonable to recommend a trial of these supplements.

Pharmacodynamics

Essential Omega-3 fatty acids include a-linolenic acid (ALA), eicosapentaenoic acid (EPA), and docosahexanoic acid (DHA). These cannot be

synthesized by the body and must be ingested from food. Following ingestion, DHA inhibits lipogenesis and stimulates oxidation. ALA, EPA, and
DHA undergo downconversion and retroconversion (as described below)
and contribute to the metabolism of various nutrients and lipids. This is
responsible for a broad-based therapeutic effect that includes changes in
cardiovascular function, decrease in triglycerides, and improvement in
pulmonary function. Most of these effects are directly associated with
DHA, although related fatty acids may play a contributory role.

DHA is taken up by the brain at greater rates than the other fatty
acids. DHA is then incorporated into the phospholipids of cell membranes. DHA contributes to proper formation and elongation of synapses. In addition, DHA-containing phospholipids improve cell function
by stabilizing the membrane fluidity and changing firing rates of neurons (Horrocks & Yeo, 1999). Thus, DHA may play a role in the synchronization of neuronal action. It can be hypothesized that poor
phosphorization may be partially responsible for uncoordinated neuronal firing and functional imbalances whereas some brain areas are
overstimulated (for example, the nucleus accumbens, the thalamus,
the hypothalamus, and the amygdala), while others are underactive
(for example, the orbitofrontal cortex). Thus, regulation of membrane
fluidity may have beneficial effects in stabilizing neuronal firing and
decreasing the symptoms of mania and agitation (Stoll & Locke, 2002).

Eicosanoids contribute to this process. They are localized in cells and
serve as catalysts for a large number of processes, including the movement of calcium in and out of the cells (Enig & Fallon, 1999). Because
calcium channels are involved in the rates of firing of brain cells, regulation of these channels changes the brain's action potential. It is possible that EPA's regulation of calcium channels may contribute to DHA's
influence of cell membrane phosphorization, providing a synergistic
effect on the rates of neuronal firing. Again, this regulation of neuronal
excitation may be responsible for the improvement in manic and mixed-
manic symptoms associated with the use of Omega-3 supplements.

Pharmacokinetics

Following ingestion, the metabolism of fatty acids begins in the small
intestine by special digestive enzymes. These lipases break down fatty
acids into individual chains, glycerol, and monoglycerides (glycerol
with one remaining fatty acid still attached). These are then absorbed
through the intestinal wall into the lymph stream. Fat molecules are then
carried in the lymph system and slowly metabolized to provide gradual
release of energy (Enig, 2000).

Essential fatty acids go through many conversions. ALA is converted into EPA and DHA, and these are then gradually absorbed into cell membranes. However, they also undergo complex cross-metabolism. While Omega-6, also known as linoleic acid (LA), undergoes a one-way transformation into various fatty chains, culminating in docosapentaenoic acid, ALA undergoes circular transformation that involves many steps, including the formation of EPA and DHA, and then retro-conversion of EPA and DHA. It is difficult to determine how the body regulates the amounts of DHA and EPA that remain in the cells. It is likely that these are constantly transformed into each other to provide a balance of essential nutrients necessary for many metabolic processes, including membrane phosphorization.

Because ALA is converted into EPA and DHA, and EPA and DHA are retroconverted into each other, it is not necessary to purchase a specific combination of these fatty acids. Some manufacturers focus on the hypothesized benefits of DHA over EPA, or vice versa, and Omega-3 pills are available in various combinations of these components. Consumers need to keep in mind that the balance of these components in the pill is probably immaterial, since the complex conversion chains will probably result in the same balance of these nutrients in the body, regardless of the specific ratio included in the caplet.

Optimal ratio of Omega-6 to Omega-3 in the human body is estimated to be $2:1$. However, it is not uncommon for individuals in westernized countries to consume diets where the two are ingested at a ratio of about $20:1$. For this reason, the majority of supplements primarily focus on delivering additional amounts of Omega-3 into the body, and any amounts of Omega-6 in the tablet may be superfluous, since the common diet already includes so many foods rich in LA. When purchasing a supplement, consumers should select one that maximizes the amount of Omega-3 and minimizes the amount of Omega-6 in the preparation.

Manufacturers of Omega-3 generally advise to take the supplements with or without food. Researchers, however, have long recognized that Omega-3 fatty acids ingested in food are better absorbed than those taken in supplements. Some studies have found that Omega-3 taken without a meal is poorly absorbed. For this reason, nutritionists generally recommend to take an Omega-3 supplement as part of a meal, so that it is absorbed together with the food that is being consumed (Neville, 2006).

In order to prevent oxidation of fatty acids before they are taken up into cell membranes, antioxidants must be present. Those whose diets are rich in antioxidant foods probably consume enough of these during a meal to prevent fatty acid oxidation. However, those who consume meals low in antioxidants may need to take an antioxidant supplement – for example, tocopherol, a form of vitamin E. For this reason, some formulations of Omega-3 supplements include a small amount of tocopherol. However, instead of (or in addition to) tocopherol, some supplements also include vitamins A and/or D. Because these vitamins do not get cleared from the body, clients should be careful with these supplements because high intake of these vitamins may lead to toxicity.

Although fatty acids are metabolized and absorbed rapidly, the onset of effect is not evident for a long time. Some have reported that the onset of clinical effect is not evident for weeks, even months, and that treatment for up to 3 months is necessary to determine the eventual clinical response (Lake, 2007). This makes it difficult to dose the supplements, since clinical effects are not likely to be immediately evident.

Dosing

Omega-3 supplements are not usually dosed by body weight. To treat symptoms of mania or agitation in children, the recommended starting dose is 500 mg, and usually doses range up to about 4000 mg (4 g) per day (Potter et al., 2009). Some have found doses below 1000 mg/day to be ineffective (Lake, 2007). Because Omega-3 is generally well tolerated, gradual titration is recommended. However, the maximum dose is often determined by how many tablets the child is willing to take and whether digestive effects (for example, fish burps or a fishy taste in the mouth) prevent further increase in dose. Because response will not immediately be evident, it is difficult to determine what dose will eventually be effective.

Teens are generally dosed closer to 4000 mg/day, and some have found doses below 2000 mg/day to be ineffective (Lake, 2007). Since some adults require doses in excess of 9000 mg, teenagers may need to be dosed higher than 4 g/day, depending on their size and weight. As with children, dosing should gradually be increased to a maximum level that can be tolerated with minimal gastrointestinal discomfort. Again, it is difficult to determine what dose will be effective since response to the supplement may not immediately be evident.

Co-factors are necessary for metabolism of some of the fatty acids, especially EFA. Carnitine is necessary for the elongating EFA and transporting it across inner cell membranes. It is possible that some of the inconsistent findings about the efficacy of fatty acids may be secondary to carnitine deficits. For this reason, supplementation with l-carnitine has been studied and has shown promising effects in hyperactive girls with fragile X syndrome (Torrioli *et al.*, 1999). Since humans metabolize only a portion of the necessary supply of carnitine, supplementing fatty acid therapy with l-carnitine may be helpful. L-carnitine is supplied in capsules, tablets, solution, and chewable wafer. Children may take about 250 mg of l-carnitine with fatty acids, while adults may need to take about 500 mg. These doses are generally well tolerated although a small incidence of seizures has been reported (Medical Economics, 2008a). Individuals with risk factors for seizures should consider l-carnitine supplementation only under supervision of a physician.

Adverse Effects

Omega-3 oils are generally well tolerated. The most common adverse effects involve the gastrointestinal tract, including nausea and diarrhea. Because the majority of Omega-3 supplements are sold as fish oils, some individuals experience an unpleasant, 'fishy' taste in their mouth, a 'fishy' smelling breath after a meal during which Omega-3 supplement was taken, and fishy 'burps' that may last for several hours. For this reason, some manufacturers offer 'burpless' formulas manufactured by increasing the thickness of the pill's outer coating. This allows the supplement to survive the stomach acids and dissolve when it reaches the small intestine. These have been shown to effectively reduce the above problems. Omega-3 supplements are also available in non-fish based formulas that are not associated with burps or an unpleasant taste.

Because Omega-3 supplements are oil based, there is a caloric value associated with the caplet. The exact amount varies, but generally a 1000 mg pill will contain about 20 calories. For individuals who consume a low amount, an extra 20 or 40 calories per day will probably have a minimal amount on weight. However, those on higher amounts (for example, 8000 or 9000 mg per day) must remember that they are consuming an additional 160 or 180 calories. In addition, fatty acids are high density lipoproteins (HDL) and contribute to the overall HDL levels within the body. While this is generally beneficial, those on high levels of Omega-3 supplements who also consume diets rich in HDL may experience additional increases of HDL and total cholesterol, which may not always be beneficial. Individuals who take high doses of fatty acid supplements should periodically check their cholesterol profile.

Omega-3 fatty acids are associated with an antithrombotic effect. Patients who take blood thinners (like aspirin) must be careful about taking subsequent fatty acid supplements, and should consult a physician before initiating Omega-3 therapy. In addition, some patients regularly use over-the-counter non-steroidal anti-inflammatory drugs

(NSAIDs, like Advil or Motrin) to manage headaches, backaches, or similar conditions. While combining fatty acids with NSAIDs has not been shown to pose a risk, many NSAIDs have some blood thinning properties, and combining NSAIDs with fatty acids has sometimes been linked to nose bleeds and easy bruising (Medical Economics, 2008a). For this reason, those who take NSAIDs daily should probably consult a physician before initiating Omega-3 therapy.

Use of fatty acid supplements has sometimes been reported to alter glucose tolerance, especially in patients with type 2 diabetes. The mechanism of this is poorly understood, and some studies have not confirmed this finding. However, because there is a risk, children and adolescents who are diabetic and take insulin should consult their physician before starting Omega-3 treatment.

Lecithin

Lecithin is a naturally occurring fatty substance referred to as phospholipid. Although the term lecithin is sometimes used generically to refer to a wide variety of lipids (including choline and glycine), it is most commonly associated with phosphatidylcholine, a precursor for choline. It is approved by the FDA as an emulsifier and added to many food products. It is also naturally found in several foods, including egg yolks, soybeans, nuts, and whole grains, as well as in organ meats. Because lecithin is not considered an essential nutrient, no recommended daily allowance (RDA) has been established. Generally, dietary intake of lecithin ranges from 1–5 g/day, but some have proposed that current trends toward low-fat diets may be producing lecithin deficits (Potter et al., 2009).

As a supplement, lecithin is generally sold in capsules, liquid, and granulated forms. Most supplements sold in health food stores have been shown to contain only low levels of pure lecithin. Because lecithin used in research is rather pure (usually, 90 percent of pure lecithin), consumers are advised to check for the amount of pure lecithin contained in the specific formulation, and seek forms with as much pure lecithin as possible.

Evidence of Efficacy

Lecithin has been researched as naturopathic treatment for a variety of conditions, and is also covered in Chapter 10 of this book. Its benefits in treating symptoms of mania have been investigated in a few studies, performed over the past three decades. Thus far, all studies have consistently revealed good efficacy and no contradictory findings have been reported. For example, Cohen et al. (1980), in an open trial, reported that patients admitted to a psychiatric hospital with bipolar disorder were treated with lecithin supplements of varying purity – from about 50 percent pure to about 90 percent pure – as adjunct to lithium. Those treated with 90 percent pure lecithin, at dose of 30 g/day improved rapidly, and most showed worsening of symptoms upon withdrawal of the supplement. In a follow up, Cohen *et al.* (1982) reported similar findings obtained in a double-blind, placebo-controlled trial of psychiatric inpatients in a manic phase. Lecithin resulted in significant improvement compared with placebo and was noted to have a clear therapeutic effect in almost all participants. Additional anecdotal and case reports similarly reveal the supplement's benefits in addressing symptoms of bipolar disorder, particularly mania (for example, Gold, 1993; Golan, 1995). Interestingly, although lecithin is involved in the metabolism of choline, similar results have not been shown with choline supplementation, and use of lecithin produces more beneficial results (Wurtman *et al.*, 1977).

There have been fewer trials of lecithin in children and adolescents with bipolar disorder. Schreier (1981) reported the case of a 13-year-old manic girl who did not respond to prescription mood stabilizers but respond well to 15–23/day of 90 percent pure lecithin monotherapy. She attained a remission that lasted at least 13 months. Other case reports also suggest lecithin's effectiveness in the pediatric population (for example, Walsh, 2000). Since lecithin is generally well tolerated and adverse effects are rare, it appears sensible to recommend a cautious trial for pediatric patients with manic or mixed-manic symptoms.

Pharmacodynamics

Lecithin (phosphatidylcholine) is a precursor for choline. As such, it is involved in the synthesis of the neurotransmitter acetylcholine, and levels of lecithin correlate with levels of choline and acetylcholine. Consequently, one presumed mechanism of action of lecithin is the increase in the synthesis, release, and availability of acetylcholine. However, lecithin is also involved in complex intracellular processes, including the regulation of cellular membrane permeability. As discussed above, patients with bipolar disorder reveal altered membrane phospholipid metabolism, and low choline levels within the orbital frontal gray matter have been found in patients with manic symptoms. Thus, supplementation with lecithin apparently stabilizes the membrane and changes action potential.

Pharmacokinetics

Little is known about the pharmacokinetics of lecithin. Following ingestion, the lipid is absorbed from the small intestine and may enter the lymph system, as well as systemic blood circulation. It is taken up by cell membranes and becomes involved in a number of metabolic processes, including the conversion of acetylcholine.

Lecithin is absorbed and metabolized rapidly, and some patients report very rapid onset of effect (within an hour, especially in higher doses). In empirical studies, effect was seen within about a week. The half-life of lecithin is unknown, and the supplement has been dosed in varying regimens, from once to three times per day.

Dosing

Lecithin supplements are not usually dosed by body weight. To treat symptoms of mania or agitation in children, the recommended starting dose is about 1000 mg, gradually titrated upward if well tolerated. Little is known about effective doses for children, and an effective dose for adolescents has been reported to vary from 15–23 g/day (Potter *et al.*, 2009). Since response is expected within a few days, the dose can gradually be titrated in accordance with response and onset of any adverse effects. No upper limit for lecithin ingestion has been established, but dosage in adults has not been studied beyond 30 g/day.

When purchasing lecithin supplements, it is very important to seek out those with maximum phosphatidylcholine and minimum choline content. In some patients, choline supplementation has been associated with the onset of depressive symptoms (Walsh, 2000). Conversely, such a result has not been reported with lecithin supplementation (Potter *et al.*, 2009). In addition, studies have used supplements that contain 90 percent of pure lecithin. Thus, the range of 15–23 g/day of the supplement reported by Potter *et al.* (2009) can be converted to about 13.5 to about 21 g/day of pure lecithin. If supplements are purchased with lower percentage of pure lecithin, actual dose will probably need to be adjusted so that dose of pure lecithin stays within this range. Unfortunately, if supplements with low percentage of lecithin are used, this means that high doses of other ingredients will also be taken, and these can have unpredictable effects (especially if choline is also included in the supplement). Consumers need to proceed very cautiously when increasing dose of supplements with low percentage of pure lecithin.

Adverse Effects

Lecithin is generally well tolerated. Since most commercially available lecithin is derived from soy, those who are allergic to soy or its byproducts should not take lecithin. Otherwise, few adverse effects are reported, except for mild gastrointestinal symptoms, such as looser stools, or transient nausea. Higher doses of lecithin (at 25 g/day or more) have been associated with acute gastrointestinal distress, sweating, salivation, and anorexia (Potter *et al.*, 2009), although these are most often evident in supplements with a high percentage of choline. Supplements with little choline and 90 percent of pure lecithin are generally well tolerated, even at doses of 30 g/day (Cohen *et al.*, 1980).

SUPPLEMENTS WITH POSSIBLE EFFICACY

In addition to the supplements discussed above, there is some data available that suggests that other compounds may also have some efficacy in treating symptoms of mania and agitation. However, since the data that supports the use of the following supplements is extremely limited, clinicians should proceed with caution, and consider the use of the compounds discussed in this section as experimental.

Melatonin

As discussed in Chapter 9, melatonin is a neurotransmitter and a hormone, primarily released in the pineal gland to regulate circadian cycles and the onset of sleep. In addition, melatonin has been proposed to affect mood and has been presumed to offer some benefits in treating symptoms of bipolar disorder. In particular, bipolar disorder with rapid cycling has been proposed to be associated with unstable circadian rhythms (Leibenluft *et al.*, 1997). Some studies reported that patients with bipolar disorder have lower baseline levels of melatonin and increased melatonin suppression, but these results have not been replicated in other studies (Potter *et al.*, 2009). There is conflicting evidence regarding the efficacy of melatonin in the treatment of bipolar disorder. Bersani and Alessandra (2000) reported that a trial of melatonin, used to improve sleep in patients with bipolar disorder, also exhibited a significant decrease in the severity of manic symptoms. On the other hand, Leibenluft *et al.* (1997) were not able to replicate these results. Robertson and Tanguay (1997) reported that a 10-year-old boy diagnosed with treatment-resistant bipolar disorder responded rapidly to a trial of melatonin 3 mg nightly, with recurrence of sleep problems and other symptoms of mania when melatonin was discontinued after 1 month. Thus, it is apparent that use of melatonin may be helpful in some cases of bipolar disorder where severe sleep disturbance is evident.

There is no established dose range for melatonin in the treatment of bipolar disorder, and usual doses range from 0.3–5 mg/day. Doses above

5 mg may not contribute additional beneficial effect (Bezchlibnyk-Butler & Jeffries, 2007), and doses above 3 mg for longer periods of time may require medical supervision (Medical Economics, 2008a). Melatonin supplements derived from animals should be avoided. The supplement should generally be given at night, and morning administration may delay the onset of evening sleepiness by delaying the phase of the circadian rhythms (Zhdanova & Friedman, 2002). Melatonin is generally well tolerated. The most common side effects include drowsiness, headache, dizziness, and nausea. More rare effects include abdominal cramps, irritability, reduced alertness, confusion, vomiting, and hypotension. More detailed discussion of melatonin is provided in Chapter 9.

Magnesium

Magnesium is an essential mineral element with a wide range of physiological functions. It is presumed to be involved in a wide range of biological processes, including production of cellular energy and synthesis of proteins. Magnesium is abundant in the human body and plays a major role in regulating the activity of ATP and RNA. Hundreds of enzymes are dependent on magnesium in order to function. It may also be involved in a number of psychological processes regulated by membrane stability and nerve conduction, although its exact role in these processes has not yet been identified.

Supplementation with magnesium has been found to reduce neuronal excitation, and magnesium may antagonize calcium (Medical Economics, 2008a). Consequently, it has been hypothesized that magnesium supplementation may be effective in stabilizing mood. Some studies suggested beneficial effects of magnesium in stabilizing mood swings associated with premenstrual syndromes (Facchinetti et al., 1991), and therefore more broad applications in stabilizing mood have been hypothesized (Durlach et al., 1994). To date, however, these have not been investigated.

Magnesium supplements are generally available as tablets and capsules. Its pharmacokinetics are not well established, but absorption depends on amount of intake – doses below 100 mg are usually absorbed up to about 70 percent, while doses that approach 1000 mg may only be absorbed at a rate of less than 15 percent. Thus, the absorption seems regulated by the amount that can be tolerated by the body. Excess magnesium is excreted by the kidneys, and therefore individuals with compromised kidney function should not attempt magnesium supplementation without medical supervision. Recommended Daily Allowance (RDA) values for magnesium have been established, and range from about 30 mg/day for infants to about 400 mg/day for adults. RDA for boys and girls ages 9 through 13 years is established at 240 mg/day, and RDA for teenagers ranges from 360 mg/day for girls to 410 mg/day for boys. It is recognized, however, that treatment of specific disorders may require doses above this range (Medical Economics, 2008a).

Magnesium supplements are usually well tolerated at doses that do not exceed the RDA. The most common adverse reactions, usually seen at doses approaching or exceeding 350 mg, are abdominal effects, including stomach cramping, diarrhea, and nausea. Taking the supplements with food reduces the risk of these effects. Those who consume diets high in oxalic acid (spinach, sweet potatoes, rhubarb, and beans) may exhibit lower rates of absorption of magnesium. The supplement should generally be avoided with antibiotics (especially tetracycline) since it may interfere with the absorption of the drug.

Theanine

Theanine, also known as L-theanine, is a non-protein amino acid mainly found naturally in green tea (*Camellia sinensis*) and some mushrooms (*Boletus badius*). Theanine is related to glutamine, is speculated to increase levels of GABA, serotonin, and dopamine. Theanine may also interact with Kainate and NMDA receptors for glutamate. Theanine has been available in Japan as a nutritional supplement marketed to reduce stress, produce feelings of relaxation, and improve mood (Kimura *et al.*, 2007). Recently, theanine has also been marketed in the US.

Mood stabilizing effects are presumed but not well documented. In animal studies, theanine has been shown to stimulate GABA (A) receptors (Egashira *et al.*, 2007), and oppose caffeine stimulation (Kakuda *et al.*, 2000). Studies in humans are more rare. Supplementation with theanine has been shown to produce relaxing effects (Juneja *et al.*, 1999), and improve stress tolerance (Kimura *et al.*, 2007). In addition, these mood calming effects appear to be produced without sedation (Ellinoy *et al.*, 2007). Consequently, theanine may have mood stabilizing effects, but its efficacy in stabilizing symptoms of bipolar disorder has not been researched. In addition, use of theanine for any purpose has not been studied in children and adolescents. Use in this population is considered experimental and clinicians using theanine with pediatric patients must proceed with much caution.

Theanine supplements are generally available as tablets and capsules in doses between 50 and 200 mg. Although theanine is present in most green teas, the amount is unpredictable. Generally, two to three cups of green tea may contain between 30 and 50 mg of theanine (Medical Economics, 2008a), but this depends on the specific leaves being used and the brewing method. For this reason, it is best to avoid using theanine in tea when clinical effects are desired. Its pharmacokinetics are not well established, but theanine appears to be absorbed from the small intestine. Theanine crosses the blood–brain barrier and may be taken up by the cells via a sodium-coupled active transport process. No guidelines about effective dosage ranges have been established.

Theanine supplements are usually well tolerated and no adverse effects have been reported thus far. However, pregnant and nursing mothers should avoid using the supplement.

Taurine

Taurine is a non-protein organic amino sulfonic acid mainly found naturally in meat, fish, eggs, and milk. Humans also produce it from cysteine, but infants and children do so in much lower amounts, and some children lack the enzyme necessary for its metabolism. For this reason, taurine is added to most baby foods, as it is presumed to be necessary for normal retinal and brain development. Taurine has membrane stabilizing effects and consequently it has been presumed to be involved in regulating neurotransmission. It has well-documented hypotensive effects, and may even be effective as an anticonvulsant (Medical Economics, 2008a). Consequently, some have presumed that it may be effective in stabilizing mood (Balch, 2006), but these effects are poorly documented and generally speculative. Taurine has also been added to some energy drinks, but its energy-promoting effects have not been proven and are widely disputed.

Taurine is absorbed from the small intestine and enters the brain through sodium and chloride dependent transport systems. In the cell, taurine may keep potassium and magnesium inside the cell while keeping sodium out. Thus, it may affect neuronal firing. Remaining taurine is conjugated to form the bile salts and is excreted into bile, where it is transported to the duodenum to take part in the metabolism of various lipids. Excess taurine is excreted by the kidneys.

Taurine supplements are generally available as tablets and capsules and clinical doses range from 500 mg/day to 3 g/day in adults (Medica Economics, 2008a). Balch (2006) recommends a dosage of 500 mg three times per day (TID) to treat symptoms of bipolar disorder. Taurine supplements are usually well tolerated and no adverse effects have been reported thus far. However, pregnant and nursing mothers should only use the supplement under medical supervision.

SUPPLEMENTS NOT LIKELY TO BE EFFECTIVE

It is not possible to review all compounds that have been speculated to treat symptoms of agitation and mania. However, some of these compounds are sometimes marketed to treat symptoms of bipolar disorder, despite the lack of evidence of efficacy. In addition to being ineffective, some of these compounds may actually exacerbate mood disturbance. Clinicians who seek to practice in the area of naturopathic psychopharmacology should be aware of these compounds and the potential risks associated with using them to treat symptoms of mania or agitation.

Inositol

Inositol was previously discussed in Chapters 5 and 6. It is an isomer of glucose and is present in high concentrations in the brain. It is part of intracellular processes mediated by second-messenger systems, and may be involved in regulating the activity of monoamines (especially serotonin, with possible action on dopamine and norepinephrine) as well as other neurotransmitters. It has primarily been shown to be effective in the treatment of depression and anxiety, with some possible efficacy in treating symptoms of ADHD. Because of its antidepressant qualities, some have hypothesized that it may also be beneficial in treating symptoms of bipolar disorder. However, research has shown that individuals in the midst of manic phases actually show an *excess* of intracellular inositol (Potter *et al.*, 2009), and lithium, an effective mood stabilizer, may exert its clinical effect, in part, by lowering brain levels of inositol or blocking its effects (Agranoff & Stephen, 2001), although some have reported contradictory findings (Belmaker *et al.*, 1996).

Inositol may not only be ineffective, it may exacerbate the symptoms of mania. Because of its antidepressant effects, episodes of switching into mania have been reported (Potter *et al.*, 2009). It is apparent that patients who exhibit symptoms of depression may benefit from supplementation with inositol, but inositol is not a mood stabilizer and should not be used for this purpose. Those with symptoms of mixed mania may benefit from its use (as an antidepressant, as described in Chapter 6), but will require a mood stabilizer to address the manic portion of the symptoms.

S-Adenosyl-L-Methionine (SAMe)

Like inositol, SAM-e was discussed in the previous two chapters. SAMe is a natural substance present in the body. It is primarily used to treat osteoarthritis, fibromyalgia, and liver disorders, and has also been shown to have potentially beneficial effects in treating symptoms of depression and ADHD. SAMe is a second messenger involved in dozens of reactions throughout the brain, including the synthesis of monoamine transmitters – dopamine, norepinephrine, and serotonin. This action is responsible, at least in part, for its antidepressant effect. SAMe is also involved in methylation and/or phosphorization processes that affect membrane fluidity. As such, its effects may be similar to those of Omega-3 fatty acids, where regulation of the membrane fluidity may be involved in stabilization of neurotransmitter release and neuronal firing. However, unlike Omega-3 lipids, SAMe has been found to *increase* the number of receptors on the cell, *increase* binding to receptors, and *enhance* membrane fluidity (Settle, 2007). Thus, these effects are likely to increase overall firing, especially in monoaminergic pathways, and therefore SAMe is not likely to be effective in treating symptoms of mania or severe agitation.

Indeed, although SAMe has been shown to be an effective antidepressant, like all antidepressants, SAMe is also associated with a risk of inducing hypomanic or manic symptoms (Bezchlibnyk-Butler & Jeffries, 2007). Potter *et al.* (2009) suggest that presence of manic symptoms is a contraindication for the use of SAMe, unless a mood stabilizer is also used. It is apparent that patients who exhibit symptoms of depression may benefit from supplementation with SAMe, but SAMe is not a mood stabilizer and should not be used for this purpose. Those with symptoms of mixed mania may benefit from its use (as an antidepressant, as described in Chapter 6), but will require a mood stabilizer to address the manic portion of the symptoms.

Glycine

Glycine is an amino acid commonly found in proteins. It is synthesized in the body from serine, another proteinogenic amino acid naturally synthesized within cells. As one of the 20 most common amino acids found in proteins, it serves multiple metabolic functions, but some of it is also released into synapses as a neurotransmitter. Like glutamate and GABA, glycine is present in the nervous system and is an important building block for many chemical processes. As a neurotransmitter, it binds to several families of ionotropic and metabotropic receptors, but its primary inhibitory action seems to be the result of regulating chloride channels in a manner similar to the action of GABA. These effects are primarily seen in the spinal cord. In the brain, the effects of glycine are less predictable. For example, it seems to be involved in regulating glutamatergic neurotransmission at the NMDA glutamate ionotropic receptors that are involved in opening calcium channels and causing rapid depolarization of the post-synaptic cell. Thus, glycine may be an alosteric modulator for glutamate, and consequently it has been hypothesized to be useful in addressing symptoms of mania.

Although increase in glycine function may result in inhibitory effects, glycine seems to have varying effects in different parts of the brain, and supplementation with glycine has sometimes resulted in excitatory effects (Medical Economics, 2008a). For this reason, the effects of glycine supplementation are unpredictable and administration of glycine supplements is not likely to produce beneficial effects in patients with mania or severe agitation.

Vitamins

The role of vitamins and minerals in healthy mood has also been hypothesized for many decades, but very few studies exist that support their efficacy, especially in the pediatric population. Kaplan *et al.* (2007) reviewed much available data about the efficacy of vitamins in regulating mood. The analysis reviewed evidence of deficiency of vitamins and nutrient in patients with depression, as well as the use of nutritional supplements to improve mood disturbance. Only the B group of vitamins, especially thiamine (B1), pyridoxine (B6), folate (B9), and cobalamin (B12) had some data to support their role in treatment of depression, especially as an adjunct to other treatments. However, there is no support for the use of any vitamins to treat symptoms of mania. In addition, some vitamins pose a significant risk when taken in excess. For this reason, megadoses of multivitamins are not only ineffective, they may be dangerous, especially when RDA levels of vitamin A or B6 are significantly exceeded. Clinicians are encouraged to advise their patients and clients against trials of such unproven and potentially dangerous methods.

SUMMARY

In order to help clinicians select the compounds that are appropriate given the specific type of manic symptoms evident in each patient, an algorithm was developed and is presented in Figure 7.1. This diagram takes into account the amount of research support available for each compound, as well as the specific mechanism of action of each supplement and its applicability to the treatment of each type of manic symptoms.

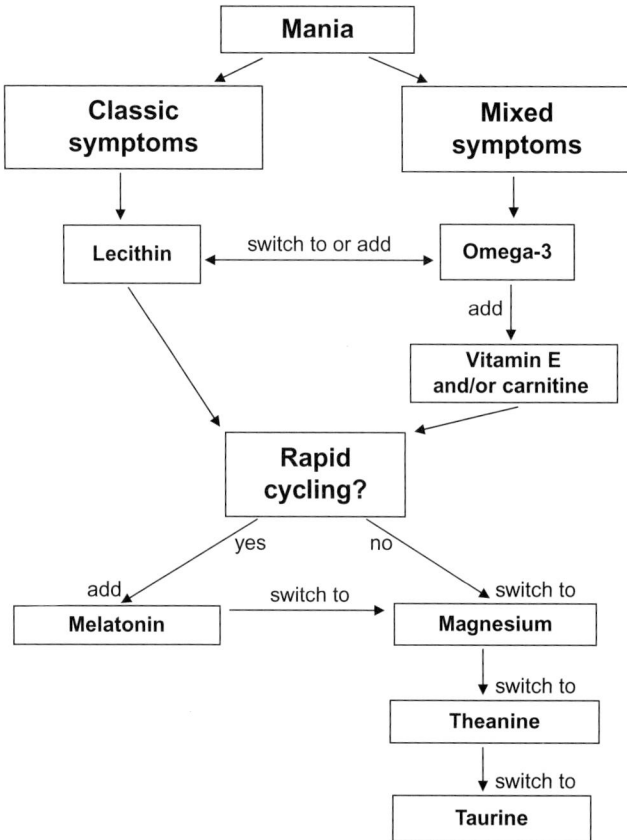

FIGURE 7.1 Algorithm for treatment of mania with naturopathic supplements.
© Elsevier 2009.

Patients with symptoms of classic mania should initially be tried on lecithin, and if insufficient response is obtained, Omega-3 may be tried (as monotherapy or adjunct), with an addition vitamin E and/or carnitine if needed. If symptoms persist, and patient exhibits a history of rapid cycling, melatonin may be added. If this combination is ineffective, lecithin should be discontinued, and magnesium can be added to Omega-3 (with or without vitamin E and carnitine), with or without melatonin. Theanine or taurine can also be substituted for magnesium in this combination, but clinicians should generally avoid using theanine, taurine, magnesium, and lecithin with each other (in any combination) without medical supervision.

Patients with symptoms of mixed mania should initially be tried on Omega-3, with an addition vitamin E and/or carnitine if needed. If insufficient response is obtained, lecithin may be tried as monotherapy or adjunct. If symptoms persist, and patient exhibits a history of rapid cycling, melatonin may be added. If this combination is ineffective, lecithin should be discontinued, and magnesium can be added to Omega-3 (with or without vitamin E and carnitine), with or without melatonin. Theanine or taurine can also be substituted for magnesium in this combination, but clinicians should generally avoid using theanine, taurine, magnesium, and lecithin with each other (in any combination) without medical supervision.

Chapter 8

Anxiety Disorders

As with depression, anxiety in the pediatric population has often been overlooked or minimized as normal childhood experiences. Currently, it is recognized that anxiety disorders in children and adolescents can cause substantial impairment and negatively affect their social, familial, educational, and developmental functioning, and may also affect their physical well-being. Point prevalence for any anxiety disorder in the pediatric population has been estimated to be between 3 and 5 percent (Foa *et al.*, 2005), and up to 20 percent of children and adolescents exhibit significant subclinical or clinical symptoms of anxiety (Albano *et al.*, 2003). Without treatment, most of the symptoms continue into adulthood, and risk for additional disorders, like depression and alcohol/substance abuse, increases (Bittner *et al.*, 2007). It is important to recognize and treat these disorders as early as possible, since successful treatment is likely to improve adoptive functioning as well as overall psychological, social, and physical development.

Recognizing anxiety in children may be obscured by expectations about what constitutes normal functioning. While it is expected for very young children to exhibit stranger anxiety and difficulties sleeping alone, by the time the child reaches school age, these should long disappear. However, some parents and professionals may consider the continued presence of these problems to be an extension of normal childhood experiences. Unfortunately, doing so often delays recognition that such behaviors are no longer developmentally appropriate and likely signal a developing anxiety disorder.

SYMPTOMS OF ANXIETY

While adults may experience a wide range of anxiety disorders, this chapter will concentrate on those anxiety disorders that are most common in children and adolescents. Most commonly, children experience separation anxiety disorder (SAD) where developmentally inappropriate anxiety occurs when the child is separated from the home or the primary caretaker. Some children and adolescents also experience generalized anxiety disorder (GAD), where daily functioning is characterized by persistent and excessive worry. Obsessive compulsive disorder (OCD) impairs functioning because persistent obsessions cause anxiety that is temporarily relieved by compulsions that often occupy a major portion of the day. Finally, some types of phobias are especially common during childhood.

Core Symptoms

For children, adolescents, and adults, the necessary symptoms for diagnosis of an anxiety disorder are similar; and usually include anxiety, fear, and hyperarousal that may be situational or may be present for most of the day. Usually, the following diagnoses are mutually exclusive – GAD and OCD are likely to impair functioning most of the time and in most situations, while SAD and phobias are usually evident in specific situations, and functioning at other times and in other settings is not impaired.

Phobias

Phobias are diagnosed when a specific stimulus or setting precipitates an anxiety reaction. Phobias are generally divided into those that involve social situations, and those where the fear is precipitated by a specific stimulus (commonly referred to as simple phobias, or specific phobias). Specific phobias are common and are considered to be the most frequently occurring psychological disorder during adulthood (APA, 2000). Specific phobias are usually categorized into those where the feared stimulus is an animal (for example, a spider or a snake), a natural phenomenon (a storm, or water), a stimulus associated with blood or injury (an injection, or the sight of blood), a specific situation (being in enclosed places, or flying in an airplane), or other stimuli (for example, fear of contracting an illness). Some of these are especially common during childhood, including fear of insects, storms, dark, germs, or costumed characters (like clowns). These specific phobias usually result in anxiety only while the feared situation or object is present, and functioning through other parts of the day is not usually impaired. For this reason, specific phobias are rarely treated pharmacologically, especially in children and adolescents, and are usually treated psychologically by administering a cognitive-behavioral treatment known as exposure with response prevention, which may be administered by gradually increasing the exposure (as in systematic desensitization).

Phobias involving social situation, however, may present with more debilitating symptoms. Individuals with social phobia experience anxiety whenever they are among other people (not members of family), and often avoid social situations. This impairs their ability to build friendships and develop appropriate social skills. Individuals with social anxiety disorder may present with significant isolation and may prefer solitary activities. This may especially impair the functioning of an adolescent, who will shy away from friends and seem very awkward while among peers. These teens are more likely to become victims of bullies, thus further exacerbating their social discomfort. One variant of social phobia that is especially common during childhood is school phobia. Children with this disorder avoid school and present with severe anxiety when taken to school and forced to separate from the parent. As with separation anxiety disorder, the anxiety reaction may take a form of severe tantrums. While school phobia commonly occurs in individuals who present with separation anxiety disorder, in some cases children do not seem anxious during other times of separation from parents or the home, except when they are required to go to school. Because social phobias usually impair daily functioning more so than simple phobias, they are sometimes treated pharmacologically.

Separation Anxiety Disorder

SAD may be thought of as a form of specific phobia that is relatively common in young children and more rare during adolescence. Children with SAD exhibit age-inappropriate and excessive anxiety about being separated from an attachment figure (usually, the parent who spends the most time with the child), or going out of the home. This usually occurs at times when the separation takes place (or is about to take place), but in some cases the children worry well in advance of the separation. In addition, children exhibit fear that either the child or the parent will become hurt or lost, or another harmful event may occur, like being kidnapped. When separation takes place, children may resort to temper tantrums, pleading, screaming, and other avoidance behaviors, and these symptoms tend to gradually intensify (Albano et al., 2003). When away from home or the parent, some children may require constant reassurance that the parent is OK (for example, by asking the parent to call them frequently). Children with SAD may refuse to attend school or daycare, may avoid extracurricular activities and social events, and often 'shadow' the parent, following him or her from room to room. Bedtime is also difficult, and children with SAD often insist on sleeping in parent's bed. During the night, nightmares may commonly occur and the content may be associated with the child or the parent getting hurt. While most cases seem idiopathic, in some cases SAD may occur after a stressful event.

Generalized Anxiety Disorder

At one time, the childhood version of this disorder was called overanxious disorder of childhood, but this disorder is now considered to be a childhood presentation of GAD. A child or adolescent with GAD must present excessive anxiety or worry for the majority of the time in a 6 month period of time. The individual cannot control their worry or seems to worry for little or no reason. Most of the time the worries are unrealistic or excessive (for example, worrying that a robber may break into the house), although the youngster may also exhibit worries about adult concerns, such as family finances and the safety of their home (Bell-Dolan & Brazeal, 1993). Sometimes, symptoms may present as notable restlessness. Sleep disturbance may also be evident, including difficulties falling asleep, problems staying asleep, or restlessness during sleep. Fatigue and difficulties with concentration are often reported, and may stem from the sleep disturbance of the cumulative effects of autonomic hyperarousal. Muscle tension is also common, and more likely to be reported by adolescents. Other physical symptoms may also accompany the anxiety, including heart palpitations, sweating, trembling, and dry mouth. Patients may also experience respiratory reactions and gastrointestinal symptoms, such as nausea or diarrhea.

Obsessive Compulsive Disorder

Like GAD, OCD is also likely to present impairing symptoms through most of the day, and the severity of symptoms usually is much more notable. While either obsessions or compulsions are minimally sufficient for the diagnosis, most patients present a combination of both groups of symptoms (APA, 2000). Obsessions are recurrent and persistent thoughts, impulses, or images that happen intrusively and occur at improper times, causing anxiety or distress. Compulsions are repetitive acts or behaviors that a child or adolescent feels he or she needs to carry out in response to the obsessions in order to reduce the anxiety. The compulsions temporarily reduce the distress, but the obsessions reoccur, precipitating more compulsions. Unlike adults, children with this disorder do not usually recognize that their behavior is excessive or unreasonable, but adolescents may begin to recognize that the obsessions and compulsions are not rational. However, recognition of the nonsensical nature of these components does not help increase the control over these symptoms, and individuals with OCD often feel even more distress when they recognize that the obsession and compulsions are unnecessary, but cannot stop them from occurring.

In children and adolescents, most common obsessions include fears of contamination; fears of harm to self or others; need for symmetry, exactness, or order; concerns with religious or moral conduct; or forbidden sexual or aggressive thoughts. Most common obsessions in children include decontamination rituals (like excessive hand washing), checking, ordering, and rearranging (Albano *et al.*, 2003), but counting, confessing, praying, reassurance seeking, touching, or tapping may also be evident (Keeley *et al.*, 2007). These obsessions and compulsions are very time consuming and interfere with most daily functioning at home, in school, and with peers.

Secondary Symptoms

Children or adolescents with anxiety disorders experience autonomic hyperarousal that may precipitate various physical symptoms, including headaches, stomachaches, nausea, vomiting, and heart palpitations. Over time, these may result in significant health problems, including gastrointestinal disorders and cardiovascular problems. When a child or adolescent has exhibited symptoms of anxiety for a long time, especially when these are accompanied by physical complaints, an in-depth medical examination is necessary.

Children and adolescents with anxiety disorders exhibit problems in many settings, especially including school. Those with GAD or OCD are likely to experience relentless, persistent fears and worry, and their ability to concentrate on learning usually is significantly impaired. The quality of work may suffer, they may forget to write down assignments, and may miss significant portions of lectures and class work, because their mind is preoccupied with the anxiety. Their grades are likely to drop, and they may also exhibit reluctance about (or downright refusal of) attending school. When anxiety about school is present, the child's or adolescent's morning routine is likely to be affected, and procrastination about getting ready in the morning is likely to be evident.

Many children and adolescents with anxiety disorders also present difficulties in social settings. If they have situational fears, they may exhibit symptoms when such a situation occurs. When others recognize the anxiety, the child or adolescent exhibiting it may get picked on or teased. Those who exhibit obsession and compulsions are likely to find it difficult to interact with peers, since the repetitive nature of the obsessions and compulsions will interfere with the ability to participate in play dates, sporting events, and other situations in which children and adolescents commonly are involved. Overall, when children and adolescents present significant symptoms of anxiety, they are likely to exhibit impairment in many aspects of their lives. Thus, treatment of these symptoms is needed to help them return to normal functioning and become able to participate in age-appropriate activities and pursuits.

RULE-OUTS AND COMORBID DISORDERS

Anxiety disorders commonly co-occur with other disorders, and some disorders not classified as anxiety disorders may include features of anxiety, complicating the diagnosis. It is imperative for mental health professionals to carefully examine all symptoms in order to perform a comprehensive differential diagnosis. In order to select an appropriate therapeutic compound, the diagnosis must be parsimonious, but at the same time it must account for all symptoms that are evident. To assist clinicians, this section reviews the disorders commonly associated with anxiety that need to be examined when rule-outs and comorbidities are considered.

Mood Disorders

Depression and anxiety frequently co-occur. In one study, 10–15 percent of children and adolescents with anxiety disorders also had clinical depression, and about 25–50 percent of youths with depression also had an anxiety disorder (Axelson & Birmaher, 2001). Anxiety disorders and depression are both considered 'internalizing' disorders where stress is experienced through internal discomfort (rather than behavioral disturbances commonly associated with 'externalizing' disorder, like ADHD). Hyperarousal is characteristic of anxiety disorders, but may also be a feature of depression (presenting as agitation, as discussed in Chapter 6), as well as mania (Chapter 7). In addition, those who experience chronic discomfort secondary to long-standing symptoms of anxiety may also develop depression. Consequently, when a patient presents with symptoms of anxiety, it is usually necessary to rule out the presence of a mood disorder.

Depression

A child or adolescent with an anxiety disorder may exhibit withdrawal, apathy, and limited motivation when facing anxiety-provoking situations. For example, a child with SAD may dread detachment from the parent and display symptoms of depression when away from home, but will usually exhibit relief when reunited with the attachment figure.

Adolescents with social phobia will exhibit flatness and social with-drawal when among peers, but these symptoms usually resolve at home. However, because symptoms of anxiety disorders often cause unpleas-ant outcomes in the youngsters' familial, social, and academic life, chil-dren and adolescents who live with chronic symptoms of anxiety may gradually develop symptoms of depression, fatigue, poor concentration, and sleep disturbance. In addition, some research findings suggest that youth who experience comorbid anxiety and depression exhibit higher levels of anxiety as compared to those without depression (Laurent & Potter, 1998). Thus, if symptoms of anxiety and depression are present, a compound should be selected that may address both groups of symp-toms, or an addition of another supplement may become necessary.

Mania or Agitation

Anxiety may precipitate agitation, and even more commonly, agitation and mania may include features of anxiety. For example, Harpold *et al.* (2005) reported that 51 percent of youth with bipolar disorder had at least one comorbid anxiety disorder. Because the overlap is so common, clinicians must determine whether comorbid presentation of mania and/ or agitation with symptoms of anxiety require multiple diagnosis and treatment strategies to address both sets of symptoms.

This distinction may be especially difficult when symptoms of a mixed episode are present. These commonly include agitation and may also involve a discomfort that may sometimes present as anxiety. However, the subjective experience usually is not one of fear, but more of apathy, anger, and restlessness. If such symptoms are also accompanied by significant anxiety, then both groups of symptoms must be captured with appropriate diagnosis. In such situations, it is likely that both disorders will need to be treated with specific compounds, although in some cases one supple-ment may have beneficial effects on both groups of symptoms. Clinicians should compare the discussion of compounds in this chapter with the compounds discussed in Chapter 7. Since some compounds are discussed in both chapters, these may be a good place to start when treating comor-bid mania/agitation and anxiety.

Disruptive Disorders

Although symptoms of anxiety are not commonly mistaken for dis-ruptive behaviors, and anxiety and disruptive behaviors may represent opposite ends of a conceptual spectrum of internalizing/externalizing disorders, anxiety symptoms can coexist with symptoms of some dis-ruptive disorders.

ADHD

As discussed in Chapter 5, ADHD is an externalizing disorder in which children and adolescents exhibit persistent patterns of inattention/disorganization and/or hyperactivity/impulsivity. Although very different from the internalizing symptoms of anxiety disorders, ADHD and anxiety disorders are sometimes comorbid, and studies report that 25–35 percent of individuals with ADHD also present symptoms of at least one anxiety disorder (Tannock, 2000). Symptoms of anxiety can usually be differentiated from symptoms of ADHD with little difficulty, but sometimes poor concentration, nervousness, and not following instructions may be mistaken for symptoms of ADHD while these may be secondary to anxiety disorders (Albano *et al.* 2003). However, when symptoms of both disorders co-occur, each may change the expression of the other (Barkley, 2006). For example, individuals with ADHD and anxiety tend to exhibit less impulsivity (Barkley), and comorbid ADHD and anxiety may result in more aggression (Tannock). In addition, when symptoms of OCD and ADHD are simultaneously present, the combination often results in significant impairment and high levels of aggression.

When symptoms of ADHD and anxiety disorders coexist, the selection of effective compounds may become more difficult. Generally, supplements that increase catecholaminergic activity, such as stimulants, are effective in reducing symptoms of ADHD, but the same compounds are also associated with increasing anxiety in those susceptible to these symptoms. Thus, stimulants and related compounds often are not a good choice for individuals with comorbid ADHD and anxiety. Instead, some compounds have been shown to be effective in management of both anxiety and ADHD, and readers should review this chapter and Chapter 5 to see which compounds seem supported for the management of both sets of symptoms (for example, inositol). When monotherapy is not sufficient, the use of compounds to separately manage symptoms of ADHD and anxiety may be necessary.

Tic Disorders

Of the three specific tic disorders recognized in the DSM system Tourette's disorder (TD) is the least common, but it is most likely to co-occur with an anxiety disorder – OCD. Normally, compulsions and tics can easily be differentiated – compulsions are accompanied, and preceded by, anxiety, and are performed to relieve it. The tics, however, are not associated with any fears and are performed impulsively, usually without much thought accompanying or preceding them. However, the compulsions and tics may coexist, and therefore all unusual behaviors performed by a patient should carefully be examined, especially when anxiety is also evident. In addition, DSM requires the presence of obsessions *or* compulsions for the diagnosis of OCD, and so it is possible that someone can be diagnosed with OCD based on obsessions only, and in such a case, compulsions will not be evident. Thus, comorbid TD and OCD may exist when tics (motor and vocal) and anxiety-driven obsessions (but not compulsions) are evident. As always, when a patient presents symptoms of two or more disorders simultaneously, all must be treated, although it is probably best to address the disorders one at a time, starting with the one that presents the most debilitating symptoms. As with other cases where symptoms of two or more disorders are simultaneously apparent, readers should check the compounds discussed in each relevant chapter to determine whether any one supplement is known to simultaneously address symptoms of both disorders. If so, administering that compound is the most logical place to start, but if sufficient response is not evident, use of multiple supplements may be necessary.

Adjustment and Trauma

As children and adolescents grow, they encounter many stressors that require adaptation, and may also experience traumatic events. In response, children and adolescents may develop symptoms of anxiety, including fears, nervousness, worry, or separation anxiety. These symptoms resemble the symptoms of many anxiety disorders, and so it is important to rule out an adjustment to stress or trauma before an anxiety disorder is diagnosed.

Adjustment Disorders

Children and adolescents who have been exposed to family conflicts, moves, or parental separation, or similarly stressful events may experience various symptoms of anxiety. Within the DSM system, these may meet the criteria for various forms of adjustment disorder (APA, 2000), and some specific subtypes of adjustment disorder include symptoms of anxiety. Youngsters who experience such emotional reactions commonly benefit from counseling and psychotherapy in order to help them cope with the stressors. If anxiety is apparent, adjunct use of an anxiolytic supplement may be beneficial. However, clinicians should administer treatment that comprehensively focuses on helping the child or adolescent cope with the stressful events.

Post-Traumatic Disorders

Children and adolescents who have been exposed to severe trauma, such as abuse, loss of a parent, severe injury, or exposure to a major catastrophe, may exhibit symptoms of acute stress disorder (ASD) or post-traumatic stress disorder (PTSD). Although these are classified within the DSM system as anxiety disorders, they are differentiated from the other disorders discussed in this chapter by the significant severity and wide range of symptoms. Children with ASD or PTSD usually exhibit substantial disturbance of overall functioning, including severe anxiety and hypervigilance, sleep disturbance and nightmares (which do not necessarily need to contain trauma-related content), reliving the event through play (or other forms of flashbacks), and avoidance of (and/or detachment from) trauma-related stimuli. Often, significant depression and behavioral disturbances also accompany these symptoms.

When clinicians encounter children or adolescents with ASD or PTSD, all symptom groups must be managed. Intensive psychotherapy and/or psychiatric treatment is likely to be necessary, and anxiety should not be treated in isolation. While using an anxiolytic supplement may be helpful, it is not likely to be effective unless the other symptoms are also being addressed. Unfortunately, this will usually mean that multiple supplements will need to be used, and such cases should be approached with extreme caution, since the use of multiple supplements has rarely been researched, especially in the pediatric population.

Medical Disorders

Many medical conditions may be accompanied by anxiety. Endocrine problems, in particular, are often associated with anxiety. Hyperthyroidism usually results in restlessness, irritability, and nervousness. Hyperglycemia and adrenal tumors (for example, pheochromocytoma) may also produce similar symptoms. These disorders should be ruled out, especially if the onset of symptoms is sudden and pronounced. Because such disorders need to be treated medically, it is necessary to carefully perform a differential diagnosis, including a medical check-up.

Immunological problems are also associated with anxiety, particularly when obsessions and compulsions are also evident. When symptoms begin, or are notably exacerbated, after a bacterial infection, such as strep throat or scarlet fever, it is possible that symptoms of anxiety are secondary to PANDAS.

PANDAS

Pediatric Autoimmune Neuropsychiatric Disorder Associated with Steptococcus (PANDAS), also discussed in Chapter 10, is a syndrome of various symptoms associated with strep infections, one of pediatric, infection-triggered autoimmune neuropsychiatric disorders (PITANDs).

Symptoms of PANDAS usually include anxiety and, in some cases, full-blown obsessions and compulsions are evident. While in some cases a child appears totally anxiety free before a strep infection, and develops symptoms afterwards, in other cases some prodromal symptoms are evident and PANDAS significantly exacerbates prior anxiety.

Although causal factors have not yet been sufficiently identified, it is presumed that some children are born with genetic vulnerabilities to anxiety and obsessions/compulsions, and when these children experience Group-A beta-hemolytic streptococcal infection, antibodies are produced that then affect cells in the basal ganglia, particularly in the caudate nucleus and putamen. Thus, the symptoms result from an interaction of these antibodies with neurons in those regions of the brain (Snider & Swedo, 2004), and neuroinflammatory factors may also be involved (Swedo, 2002).

Treatment of PANDAS is different than treatment of strep-unrelated anxiety. The presence of antibodies is usually verified by performing a blood test, although in some cases symptoms appear to be strongly correlated with strep infections but blood tests come out negative for strep antibodies. PANDAS is often treated with the administration of immunomodulatory therapies, usually intravenously, and plasma exchange treatment has also been utilized, with varying degrees of success (Allen et al., 1995; Swedo, 2002). Since symptomatic treatment of anxiety is often done concurrently with medical interventions to address the immunological problems, treatment of PANDAS is usually performed by medical, pediatric specialists (most frequently, pediatricians, pediatric neurologists, or pediatric psychiatrists).

ETIOLOGY

Although specific symptoms vary to some extent, all anxiety disorders share many common etiological features. All involve the overactivation of the limbic system and the release of stress hormones, and a subsequent cascade of physical reactions associated with the activation of the sympathetic nervous system. In fact, some believe that symptoms of different anxiety disorders are essentially various presentations of the same etiology, and are likely to progress and change by morphing into one another while maintaining common core features, or temporarily receding into subsyndromal levels and reappearing again in some form (Stahl, 2008). Indeed, there is some evidence that this conceptualization may be on target. For example, one study revealed that after 12 years, only 3 percent of patients previously diagnosed with GAD, and only 10 percent of patients previously diagnosed with panic disorder still met the diagnostic criteria for those diagnoses, while a much larger group 'morphed' into other syndromes and became diagnosed with a different anxiety disorder on follow up (Starcevic, 2006). In addition, the majority of research findings reveal that the same compounds seem to help reduce anxiety in its various presentation, regardless of the specific DSM diagnosis (Stahl).

The major monoamines (serotonin, norepinephrine, and dopamine) are involved in the symptoms of all anxiety disorders, as are additional neurotransmitters (GABA and glutamate) and a number of stress hormones. Structural and functional changes in some brain areas associated with the anxiety response have also been identified, especially involving the functioning of the locus coeruleus, a portion of the brain in the upper brain stem associated with the triggering of the activity of major catecholaminergic pathways (especially those for norepinephrine).

Phobias and Separation Anxiety Disorder

Phobias become apparent when a specific stimulus (object or a situation) trigger an activation of the limbic system, HPA axis, and other endocrine and neurological systems, resulting in a state of panic when a person confronts the feared stimulus. Chronic vulnerability to overactivation of the locus coeruleus and/or the amygdala seems to underlie these states, although in absence of the feared stimulus the patient usually appears symptoms free. When facing the object of fear, the amygdala, anterior cingulate cortex, and orbitofrontal cortex quickly become overactivated, beginning a rapid cascade of reactions that may lead to a full-blown panic attack, during which the limbic system activates the HPA axis and a release of stress hormones takes place that further activates peripheral portions of the sympathetic nervous system. As a result, the classic symptoms of panic become evident, including rapid heart beat, elevated blood pressure, rapid respiration, dilation of pupils, cardiovascular changes associated with redirection of blood flow into the muscles, immunosuppression, and other changes associated with the fight–flight reaction.

The feeling of anxiety is so uncomfortable that patients who experience it seek to avoid the situations that precipitate such reactions. Unfortunately, reduction of anxiety through avoidance behaviors reinforces the connection between the amygdala and the periaqueductal gray and teaches the brain that avoidance is an effective means of avoiding anxiety (Stahl, 2008). As avoidance behaviors continue, this learning strengthens and the avoidance becomes automatic, even in situations that bear limited resemblance to the feared stimulus, and the patient resorts to avoidance behaviors quickly and automatically. Along the way, the limbic system becomes further sensitized to any stimuli associated with the feared object, because all of them are avoided. To reverse this process, psychological treatments based on the principle of exposure with response prevention have proven very effective, and usually are performed *in vivo*, gradually exposing the patient to the feared stimulus and preventing the avoidance from taking place. Generally, these approaches are considered to be the treatment of choice for phobic behaviors, but if the behaviors approach is impractical or produces insufficient response, the use of an adjunct anxiolytic may be helpful.

Generalized Anxiety Disorder

GAD is characterized by a chronic worry, tension, and hyperarousal, as well as restlessness, irritability, fatigue, difficulties with concentration, and sleep disturbance (usually, any form of insomnia). These symptoms begin with the overactivation of the amygdala, perhaps by overactivity in the locus coeruleus, which in turn stimulate the remaining portions of the limbic system and the hypothalamic–pituitary–adrenal (HPA) axis. GAD, in particular, is associated with the activation of the cortico-striatal-thalamo-cortical (CSTC) loops associated with chronic states of tension (Stahl, 2008). In GAD, the malfunctioning of the amygdala and CSTC loops is 'persistent and unremitting yet not severe' (Stahl, 2008, p. 728). Thus, patients with GAD report chronic discomfort and a feeling of being 'on edge' while experiencing diffuse tension and worry. Because the patient usually does not fear specific stimuli, avoidance behaviors are not associated with this disorder, and behavioral approaches based on exposure with response prevention are not usually appropriate. While cognitive-behavioral approaches may be helpful, the use of an anxiolytic compound is often desirable to expedite patient's relief.

Obsessive Compulsive Disorder

Like GAD, OCD is characterized by chronic worry, tension, and hyperarousal. However, like phobias, OCD is also characterized by a persistent fear of an object or a situation (an obsession) that is relieved, at least temporarily, by performing a behavior connected with the fear (a compulsion). In this way, the compulsions are conceptually similar to behavioral activation associated with the fight–flight reaction, when the motor system is prepared to fight the stressor or flee the situation. In OCD, however, the activation of the motor system appears broader, and specifically includes the activation of the basal ganglia.

As with phobias, the compulsions result in a reduction of anxiety through avoidance behaviors, and therefore reinforces the connection between the amygdala and the periaqueductal gray and teaches the brain that compulsions are effective means of avoiding anxiety (Stahl, 2008). This learning strengthens and the avoidance becomes automatic, so that every situation that stimulates an obsession results in the performance of compulsions to quickly and automatically avoid the anxiety. As with phobias, the limbic system becomes further sensitized and the connection between obsessions and compulsions is reinforced. To reverse this process, psychological treatments based on the principle of exposure with response prevention have proven effective, but their success depends on the severity of the obsession and compulsions. Although the behavioral approach may be helpful, more severe cases usually require the use of an anxiolytic to reduce the anxiety to more manageable levels.

Summary of Research Findings

As mentioned above, the etiology of anxiety disorders is usually conceptualized as a group, and few studies have examined brain changes associated with specific anxiety disorders. Genetic studies reveal that anxiety disorders, as a group, are much more common in children of parents who have a history of any anxiety disorder, and genetic linkage is thought to account for one-third of the variability in the levels of fear and anxiety experienced by children (Albano *et al.*, 2003). Similarly, studies show that monozygotic twins are much more likely to exhibit symptoms of anxiety than dizygotic twins (Eley, 2001).

Neuroanatomical Abnormalities

Patients with history of anxiety have been found to exhibit changes in the size of the amygdala and regions of the temporal lobe in close proximity to the amygdala. In addition, those susceptible to anxiety have been found to exhibit smaller regional gray matter volume in the right hippocampus, as well as smaller regional brain volume in the left anterior prefrontal cortex, especially in females (Yamasue *et al.*, 2008). Some studies have shown that the left amygdala is smaller than the right amygdala in patients with anxiety disorders (Kim & Gorman, 2005), and a study of children with GAD confirmed this finding (De Bellis *et al.*, 2000).

Children with SAD have also been shown to exhibit brain differences. Kim and Gorman (2005) reported that children with SAD exhibited anatomical changes in the right hemisphere of the brain, and Pini *et al.* (2005) found that patients with SAD exhibited significantly lower densities of peripheral GABA receptor, suggesting that inhibitory circuits may be underactive in those individuals. Additionally, patients with OCD reveal changes in the orbitofrontal cortex, including increases in gray matter and a decrease in white matter, as well as increased blood flow in the region. Moreover, other studies reported more detailed results. For example, Menzies *et al.* (2008) found that patients with OCD demonstrated increases in white matter in a large region of right inferior parietal region, and a decrease in a right medial frontal region. These findings are especially exciting, because non-clinical first-degree relatives also revealed the same changes, possibly pointing to genetic brain changes that may be part of the inherited vulnerability for the disorder.

Neurophysiological Abnormalities

Consistent with hypotheses that implicate amygdala overreactivity in the pathophysiology of anxiety disorders, findings of several studies consistently reveal that individuals with high levels of trait anxiety exhibit high basolateral amygdala activity (Savitz & Drevets, in press). For example, patients with GAD exhibit hyperactive neurotransmitter circuits between the cortex, thalamus, amygdala, and hypothalamus, and overactivity of noradrenergic neurons arising from the locus coeruleus, while serotonergic function arising from the dorsal raphe nucleus seems hypoactive. In addition, overactivity of noradrenergic neurones arising from the locus coeruleus may produce excessive excitation in the brain areas implicated in GAD (Nutt, 2001). Although serotonin can inhibit the activation of the locus coeruleus, and therefore reduce norepinephrine activation of the amygdala, it seems that patients with GAD do not exhibit a proper balance of the two neurotransmitters (Kim and Gorman, 2005). Similarly, GABA may also inhibit norepinephrine activation of the amygdala, but patients with GAD have been shown to exhibit fewer GABA receptors, particularly in the amygdala, as well as a genetic mutation that reduced GABA receptor binding ability (Millan, 2003).

When patients exhibit symptoms of a phobia, activation of the amygdala and the locus coeruleusis evident. This causes anticipatory anxiety (strengthened by avoidance behaviors), and presence of the feared stimulus activates the hypothalamus, thalamus, and the sympathetic nervous system, precipitating a panic reaction (Gorman *et al.*, 2000). Similar findings have been also reported about children with SAD, who seem to exhibit higher levels of catecholamines and lower levels of serotonin, and therefore may exhibit hyperactivation of the limbic system because serotonin is not able to exert its inhibitory action (Masi *et al.*, 2001).

In addition to these changes, patients with OCD exhibit further problems with brain areas that control motor function. Increased metabolic activity in the cortico-basal ganglia network seems to combine with hyperactive neurotransmitter circuits between the cortex, basal ganglia, and thalamus, and hypofunctioning of serotonergic neurons arising from the rostral raphe nucleus may result in insufficient inhibitory effects on the hyperactive brain pathways. Furthermore, overactivity of dopaminergic neurons arising from the substantia nigra may further contribute to the excessive excitation of the relevant brain regions (Graybiel & Rauch, 2000).

SUPPLEMENTS WITH LIKELY EFFICACY

Like depression, anxiety is an area of psychopharmacology where many naturopathic compounds have been studied. While kava has established efficacy with adults and consistently has been shown to be effective in decreasing symptoms of anxiety, no studies thus far have been performed with children and adolescents, and some risk of hepatotoxicity may be present, and consequently the supplement is included in this section. In addition, some other compounds have also revealed at least some efficacy, but research has primarily been done with adult patients, and clinicians must use caution when applying results of these studies to pediatric patients.

Anxiolytic medications work by increasing the amount of activity in the serotonergic pathways, as well as altering the glutamate–GABA balance in favor of inhibitory effects. Supplements that accomplish similar changes in the brain have been shown to be effective in managing symptoms of anxiety.

Kava

Kava (*Piper methysticum*), alsto referred to as kava kava, is a tall bush indigenous to the South Pacific, especially Hawaii, Fiji, Samoa, Tonga, Tahiti, New Guinea, and New Zealand. Its root is typically ground, and indigenous cultures have also chewed it, prepared it as an infusion, or brewed it to use for celebratory and ceremonial occasions for thousands of years. In addition, it has been used as a gift to symbolize the resolution of a social conflict, and 'partaken as an after-work drink to relax' (Spinella, 2001, p. 212). It has peen prized because, unlike many herbal herbs that cause sleepiness, kava's relaxant effects seem to occur without significant drowsiness.

Kava has been used in the west at least since the eighteenth century, and is approved by Germany's Commission E as a treatment for nervous anxiety and stress (Medical Economics, 2007). In addition to its anxiolytic effects, kava is also known for its analgesic, antibacterial, antifungal, anti-inflammatory, antithrombotic, and muscle relaxant properties (Medical Economics, 2007). Kava supplements are generally available in capsules that range from 100–500 mg, a liquid, and tea bags for brewing. As with all supplements, capsules and tablets are preferred because the exact dosage is easier to control, although those who do not like to swallow pills may prefer to use the liquid.

Evidence of Efficacy

Although case reports of the benefits of kava as an anxiolytic date back some 200 years (Connor & Davidson, 2002), controlled research is more recent and seems to have started in the late 1980s. Controlled studies in Europe have revealed that clinical effects are usually evident after 4 weeks of treatment, but in some cases, treatment for 8 weeks was necessary before significant symptom reduction was noted (Kinzler *et al.*, 1991). Symptoms of various anxiety disorders seem to respond well to treatment with kava, including agoraphobia, specific phobia, generalized anxiety disorder, and adjustment disorder with anxiety (Connor & Davidson). By the end of the 1990s, some 14 randomized clinical trials were conducted around the world and results revealed that kava was far superior to placebo and safe when used at 60–240 mg/day for up to 25 weeks of treatment (Pittler & Ernst, 2000). An update reviewed 11 controlled trials with a total of 645 participants and revealed similar results (Pittler & Ernst, 2003).

Head-to-head studies comparing kava and prescription anti-anxiety medications have also been performed. Kava has been shown to be equally effective as oxazepam (a benzodiazepine anxiolytic) with fewer side effects (Lindenberg & Pitule-Schodel, 1990), and other studies similarly compared kava with other benzodiazepines and buspirone, and find comparable efficacy (Lee *et al.*, 2007). In the largest, multicenter, randomized, placebo-controlled trial, 129 patients were given kava, buspirone (a serotonergic anxiolytic) or opipramol (a tricyclic anxiolytic primarily used in Germany) and found that 70 percent of patients given kava responded well (at least a 50 percent reduction in symptoms), and 60 percent attained symptom remission (Boerner *et al.*, 2003). In another study, patients who were originally on a benzodiazepine were started on kava and gradually the dose of kava was increased while the benzodiazepines were tapered and eventually discontinued. Results revealed that after 3 weeks on kava as monotherapy, the anxiolytic effects were similar to that previously seen with the benzodiazepine, and far superior to placebo (Malsch & Kieser, 2001).

Very few studies have investigated the use of kava with children or adolescents, although case reports, primarily published on naturopathically oriented websites, suggest that kava is effective in adolescents. In addition, in rare cases, serious hepatotoxicity has been reported, but remains controversial (as further discussed below). Clinicians and parents should weigh these factors very carefully. If a trial of kava is undertaken, regular medical monitoring of liver function should be performed, and the American Botanical Council recommends that any use of kava for more than 1 month should be done under medical supervision (Blumenthal, 2003).

Pharmacodynamics

Kava contains dozens, if not hundreds, of constituents. Psychoactive ingredients are presumed to be the many kavapyrones and kavalactones, including kavain, dihydrokavain, yangonin, methysticin, and dihydromethysticin (Spinella, 2001). Kavain and dihydrokavain are presumed to be the most permeable to the blood–brain barrier.

Kavalactones facilitate the functioning of GABA A receptors, in a manner that is similar to benzodiazepines, but kavalactones do not appear to bind to benzodiazepine receptors. The overall effect involves positive allosteric modulation of chloride channels, increasing the influx of chloride and hyperpolarizing the cell. The increase in GABA activity may also be secondary to kavain's suppression of thromboxane, which further enhances GABA activity. In addition, kavalactones inhibit calcium channels, and various kavalactones may do so additively, producing a reduction of calcium influx by as much as 70 percent. Thus, the psychoactive effect involves broad inhibition of neuronal firing. Several kavalactones have also been found to inhibit sodium channels, further contributing to the inhibitory effect (Spinella, 2001).

Kavalactones may have other psychoactive properties. Kavain and methysticin weakly block the reuptake of norepinephrine, but seem to have no effect on serotonin. The effect on dopamine is inconsistent, with levels rising in some parts of the brain and dropping in others (Spinella, 2001). Kavalactones may also reversibly block platelet MAO B enzymes, and this effect does not seem evident until at least 3 or 4 weeks of treatment (Uebelhack et al., 1998). This may be responsible for some of the latency of clinical response observed in research trials.

Pharmacokinetics

Kava lactones are rapidly absorbed in the small intestine and transported to the liver, where they undergo metabolism via the CYP 450 system of enzymes. Although the specific pathways have not yet been identified, 2D6 may be the primary pathway (see further discussion of adverse effects). Importantly, however, kava constituents seem to inhibit 1A2, 2C9, 2C19, 2D6, 3A4, and 4A9/11 enzymes, thus making the use of kava problematic with most prescription medications (Medical Economics, 2007). After the first pass effect, kava enters systemic circulation and is absorbed by various tissues in the body. Several kavalactones cross the blood–brain barrier, but may do so competitively, making it difficult to predict which ones are most psychoactive. Peak levels of kavalactones in the plasma occur about 2 hours after oral administration, and metabolites of kava are excreted in the urine, while unabsorbed portions are excreted in the feces (Anke & Ramzan, 2004).

Dosing

In research, typical dose for adults is 70–240 mg/day (0.8–2.8 mg/kg/day) of kava, or 60–120 mg/day (0.7–1.4 mg/kg/day) of a standardized preparation of 30 percent kavalactones (Lee *et al*., 2007). Dose with children and adolescents should start at the low end of the range and gradually titrate upwards, and clinicians should keep in mind that 4 weeks or more may be necessary before therapeutic effect is evident, and therefore a few weeks at each dose level may be needed before it will be apparent whether the dose is effective. The supplement may be administered in divided doses, although it is usually given in the evening.

Adverse Effects

Most regard kava to be safe and effective, especially in low doses, and that fears of adverse effects have caused many to use kava at doses that are unnecessarily low (Connor & Davidson, 2002). Mild reactions include gastrointestinal upset, dizziness, headache, and dermatological reactions, including 'kava dermopathy' after prolonged heavy use, a yellowing of the skin. Changes in vision, mydriasis, and disturbances in eye tracking have also been reported, as well as impaired motor reflexes and rare difficulties in motor coordination, including choreoathetosis, all of which reversed upon discontinuation (Medical Economics, 2007; Lee *et al*., 2007).

The greatest concern surrounds the risk of liver damage. Over 60 cases of hepatotoxicity have been reported around the world, and many of these required liver transplants (Currie & Clough, 2003), including a 14-year-old girl who had been taking kava supplements (at unspecified dose) for 3 months (Campo *et al*., 2002). Concern over hepatotoxicity has caused some countries to restrict the use of kava and require a prescription. In some cases, it is apparent that adulterants added to kava may have been responsible for the liver damage, and methods of extraction may also be involved. In addition, some of those with liver damage have been found to exhibit low levels of endogenous CYP 2D6 enzyme (Currie & Clough), which may be responsible for most of kava's metabolism. This is further confirmed by data that suggests that in many cultures, heavy use of kava (at doses hundreds of times greater than doses used during supplementation) reveal no history of hepatic damage (Currie & Clough). Waller (2002) performed a high-level review of all available data and concluded that serious adverse hepatic effects that can be traced to kava use are extremely rare, and involve very few individuals who may be hypersensitive to it or reveal an idiosyncratic reaction. Another published report estimated that of approximately 250 million daily doses of kava administered in the 1990s, only two individuals revealed hepatotoxicity secondary to kava, and in both cases the supplement was used far above the recommended dose (Schmidt & Nahrstedt, 2002). Consequently, most regard kava as safe when used at the doses recommended above, although patients who take kava should have their liver function monitored regularly, especially if the supplement will be used for more than 1 month.

The use of alcohol is contraindicated when kava supplementation is utilized. Kava and alcohol may have additive, if not synergistic, effects because they both increase GABA transmission and exert similar inhibitory effects. Even more importantly, both kava and alcohol induce liver enzymes, and the combination of the two may further predispose patients for liver damage. This is very important to consider in adolescents, since many teenagers tend to experiment with alcohol, especially if they also have a history of symptoms of anxiety (Albano et al., 2003).

Additional factors should also be considered. In some cases, patients who used kava started to exhibit symptoms of depression, especially with long-term use (Blumenthal, 2003). Generally, patients with a history of depression should avoid using kava. Because depression and anxiety often coexist, the supplement may not be appropriate for that group of patients.

Because of kava's extensive inhibition of liver enzymes, the use of kava should be avoided with the vast majority of medications, including anticoagulants, antiplatelet medications, heparins, thrombotic agents, amantidine, muscle relaxants, and most psychoactive agents (antidepressants, anxiolytics, mood stabilizers, etc.). Patients need to remember that even over-the-counter medications should be avoided with kava. For example, acetaminophen (sold in the US as Tylenol), poses some risk of hepatotoxicity, especially when used regularly, and using kava with Tylenol may increase the risk of liver damage. Parents of patients who take kava must be advised against using any medications concurrently with the supplement unless the combination is cleared (and monitored) by a medical professional.

Use of kava is contraindicated during pregnancy. Female adolescents who take kava and are suspected of being sexually active must be advised of this risk, and should use contraception to prevent pregnancy. If oral contraceptives are used, since they are metabolized by a CYP 3A4 pathway that is inhibited by kava, their plasma levels may increase, potentially causing unpredictable results. Once again, medical professionals prescribing the contraceptives must be aware that kava will be used concurrently and must approve (and monitor) the combination.

Inositol

Inositol is an isomer of glucose and is present in high concentrations in the brain. It was once classified as part of the B vitamin group and was designated vitamin B8, but was then found to be synthesized by the human body and was declassified as a vitamin. Inositol is found in many foods, including high-bran cereals, fruit, nuts, and beans. Inositol is available in several forms, and only some of these are appropriate for psychiatric use. These include inositol and myo-inositol. Other forms, such as inositol hexaphosphate, inositol nicotinae, and D-chiro-inositol have not been shown to have mental health effects and are used to treat cancer, vascular diseases, and insulin resistance. Supplemental inositol is available in capsules of various strengths, generally ranging from 500–1000 mg. Inositol powder is also available.

Evidence of Efficacy

As discussed in Chapter 6, supplementation with inositol may offer some benefits in treating depression. In addition, a number of small studies reported that inositol has been found effective in reducing symptoms of anxiety. In a double-blind, placebo-controlled, cross-over study, 25 patients with panic disorder exhibited decreases in anxiety that were significantly greater than responses to placebo, even though the placebo effect in the study was reported to be quite large (Benjamin *et al.*, 1995). In addition, Fux *et al.* (1996) investigated the use of inositol to treat symptoms of OCD and found that a dose of 18 g/day was effective in reducing symptoms of OCD over a 3 month trial. Although a head-to-head comparison with prescription medications was not performed, the authors noted that the degree of improvement was comparable to that seen with SSRIs. Another study also found inositol to be effective in OCD-spectrum disorders, including trichotillomania (Seedat *et al.*, 2001). After reviewing several studies as well as the pharmacology of the nutrient, Levine (1997) concluded that inositol appears effective for the same conditions commonly treated by SSRIs, including depression, anxiety, and OCD. At this time, although results of research studies are still preliminary, reference resources on child and adolescent psychopharmacology (for example, Bezchlibnyk-Butler & Virani, 2007) list inositol as a safe and potentially effective 'natural' treatment alternative.

Pharmacodynamics

The mechanism of action of inositol is not fully understood. Inositol may be involved in neurotransmitter synthesis and is a precursor to the phosphatidylinositol (PI) cycle, an important intracellular second messenger system. By changing the PI cycle, inositol may exert intracellular changes that are similar to those seen when a post-synaptic receptor is activated, but without the need to activate that receptor. Thus, it may 'fool' the cell into thinking that it is activated (Belmaker *et al.*, 2002). Consequently, it may be involved in regulating the activity of monoamines (especially serotonin, with possible action on dopamine and norepinephrine) as well as other neurotransmitters. This serotonergic activity may be involved in inositol's anxiolytic properties.

Pharmacokinetics

Inositol is absorbed from the small intestine. It is hypothesized that inositol is metabolized to phosphatidylinositol and then converted to phosphatylinositol-4,5-bisphosphate, which is a precursor to second-messenger molecules. Unfortunately, little else is known about the pharmacokinetics of inositol, and time to peak and elimination half-life have not been established. Thus far, no effect on liver metabolism has been identified.

Dosing

Although there is no recommended daily intake for inositol, the average daily dietary intake is estimated to be about 1g/day (Medical Economics, 2008a). Inositol is dosed at much higher levels than other supplements. Therapeutic doses usually range from 12–18g/day, taken in divided doses (usually two to three times per day). Inositol is also available as a powder that dissolves easily in water or juice. This may be a good option for those who have difficulties swallowing pills. Dosing usually starts at 2g twice per day, increasing to up to 6g three times per day (Settle, 2007). Inositol can be taken with or without food. Onset of clinical effect is usually observed in 2–4 weeks.

Adverse Reactions

Inositol is generally well tolerated at doses of up to 20 g/day (Settle, 2007). In children, the studied dose (for ADHD, as discussed in Chapter 5) was 50 mg/kg/day (Alvarado *et al.*, 2004). Common adverse effects are mild and may include gastrointestinal upset, such as nausea, diarrhea, and flatulence. Rarely, an increase in blood glucose levels has been observed (Belmaker *et al.*, 2002). At high doses, there are rare reports of decreased peripheral nerve conduction (Settle). The supplement is considered safe to use with other medications, but few studies have investigated such combinations.

Inositol is contraindicated during pregnancy because it may induce uterine contractions (Settle, 2007). Female adolescents who take inositol and are suspected of being sexually active must be advised of this risk, and should use contraception to prevent pregnancy.

Because of its antidepressant effects, inositol may be associated with a small increase in suicidal tendencies in those patients who present with symptoms of depression. Clinicians should carefully monitor patient response and intervene if an increase in suicidal thoughts or plans becomes evident. In addition, inositol is also associated with a small risk of inducing hypomanic or manic symptoms, and case reports exist of patients 'switching' from depressive to manic symptoms (Potter *et al.*, 2009). Careful monitoring of dose/response and adverse effects is necessary.

SUPPLEMENTS WITH POSSIBLE EFFICACY

In addition to supplements discussed above, a few other compounds may also have some efficacy in treating symptoms of anxiety. However, since the data that supports the use of the following supplements is extremely limited, clinicians should proceed with caution, and consider the use of the compounds discussed in this section as experimental.

St. John's Wort

As described in Chapter 6, St. John's Wort (*Hypericum perforatum*) is an herb that exists in many species throughout the world, and it is widely used as an antidepressant. It is available in a variety of preparations, including capsules, liquid, oils, and raw herb to be brewed as tea. St. John's Wort contains a plethora of active ingredients, including flavonoids, naphthodianthrones, phloroglucinols, phenolic acids, terpenes, and xanthones (Spinella, 2001). These exert a variety of psychoactive effects, and several of these are described below.

Of all herbal supplements, St. John's Wort is the one that has been researched most extensively and there is strong support for its efficacy in reducing depressive symptoms. The use of St. John's Wort as an anxiolytic is more recent, but a few studies suggest that is may be effective. Davidson and Connor (2001) reported case studies of patients with generalized anxiety disorder who responded well to St. John's Wort at doses of 900 mg twice daily (BID), and tolerated it with minimal side effects. Improvement was seen in about 4 weeks and after using the compound for a year, patients continued to exhibit clinical improvement without adverse effects or relapse. A similar study was performed with patients with OCD and found that after 3 months of treatment, patients exhibited significant clinical improvement (Taylor & Kobak, 2000). Thus far, there appear to be no studies that investigated the use of St. John's Wort with children or adolescents with anxiety disorders.

Because of the plethora of active ingredients, the mechanism of action of St. John's Wort is very complex. Its antidepressant effects are likely secondary to weak monoamine oxidase inhibition (MAOI), as well as catechol-O-methyl transferase (COMT) inhibition, and collectively these effects may contribute to higher levels of monoamines in the brain. Its anxiolytic effects may be related to agonist activity at GABA benzodiazepine receptors, serotonin reuptake inhibition, and activation of mu and kappa opioid receptors (Spinella, 2001). All in all, it is likely that various ingredients are responsible for the anxiolytic effects of St. John's Wort, and utilizing the whole plant with its multiple constituents may have a synergistic effect (Butterweck, 2003).

St. John's Wort is absorbed from the gastrointestinal tract and the most active ingredients are lipophyllic, aiding its absorption. Hyperforin reaches maximum plasma levels in about 3 hours, and hypericin reaches these levels in about 4 hours. Half-life for hyperforin is about 9 hours, but the half-life for hypericin is much longer and may reach 24 hours (Spinella, 2001). Long-term dosing of 300 mg three times per day (TID) revealed that steady state was reached after 4 days of treatment (Spinella, 2001).

St. John's Wort utilizes the CYP450 enzyme system for metabolism, but the exact pathways have not been identified thus far (Medical Economics, 2007; Chatterjee *et al.*, 1998; Stahl, 2008). However, the herb exerts significant effects on liver metabolism. While the ingestion of the herb appears to induce liver metabolism, perhaps by inducing P-glycoprotein, hyperforin has also been found to significantly induce CYP 3A4 enzyme (Lee *et al.*, 2007). Because this enzyme is responsible for the metabolism of many medications, the use of St. John's Wort with prescription medications should generally be avoided.

For adults, the standard dose is 300 mg, and because of hyperforin's short half-life, the herb must be taken three times per day (TID). Usually, it is recommended that standardized extracts with 0.3 percent hypericin should be used (Medical Economics, 2007). In children, the usual starting dose in 150 mg TID, and the dose is gradually increased until about 900 mg/day in teenagers, although lower doses in younger children, and higher doses in mature teens may be needed.

St John's Wort is generally well tolerated and minimal side effects are reported. Sometimes, gastrointestinal irritation, nausea, constipation, and feeling of uncomfortable fullness has been reported (Medical Economics, 2007). Usually, taking the compound with food may reduce these difficulties. Fatigue and/or restlessness has also been reported in some cases (Spinella, 2001). Frequent urination has also been reported.

Photosensitivity has been reported with the use of this compound. This means that some individuals who take the herb become more sensitive to sunlight and may easily experience sunburns. The mechanism of this problem is attributed to increased sensitivity to ultraviolet waves (UVA and UVB). Patients who take St. John's Wort should be monitored for this reaction and, if one is observed, use of sun blocking sunscreens will be necessary. For children and adolescents who spend a lot of time outside, this problem must especially be monitored.

St. John's Wort is contraindicated during pregnancy due to evidence of damage to reproductive cells (Medical Economics, 2007). Female adolescents who take St. John's Wort and are suspected of being sexually active must be advised of this risk, and should use contraception to prevent pregnancy. However, oral contraceptives are metabolized by the same CYP 3A4 pathway that is induced by St. John's Wort, and breakthrough bleeding and pregnancy have been reported as a result of the increased metabolism of oral contraceptives (Lee *et al.*, 2007). Sexually active females must be aware of this risk and utilize other forms of birth control.

Cardiovascular effects have been reported in a minority of patients, and these may include swelling and an increase in heart rate. Even more importantly, a small risk of hypertension appears to be present in some patients. Although MAOI activity appears to be a minor component of this herb's pharmacodynamics, it may pose some risk that is similar to prescription MAOI medications. Patients who take MAOIs must avoid products that contain tyramine, because decreased regulation of the MAO enzymes may lead to excess levels of noradrenaline, causing unsafe levels of blood pressure. Foods rich in tyramine include most aged food products, including cheese and aged meats, and tyramine-rich food products are plentiful in the typical American and European diet.

The exact degree of this risk is not yet known, and thus far only one case has been reported that presented with a hypertensive crisis potentially due to St. John's Wort (Medical Economics, 2007). However, clinicians should use caution and monitor the blood pressure of patients who take St. John's Wort (especially after meals), at least in the initial phases of treatment.

Perhaps the greatest risk associated with the use of St. John's Wort is its effect on the liver, and the resultant potential for significant drug interactions. Generally, St. John's Wort should not be utilized whenever patients take prescription medications. Of particular concern are protease inhibitors, anticoagulants, anticonvulsants, antiretrovirals, immunosuppressants, cardiovascular drugs, and anticancer drugs (Lee *et al.*, 2007; Medical Economics, 2007). This list is by no means exhaustive. Usually, a 14 day washout period is often recommended when stopping or starting St. John's Wort.

Although a specific 'black box' warning that applies to all antidepressants is not issued for St. John's Wort, because of its antidepressant action, St. John's Wort may be associated with a small increase in suicidal tendencies in those patients who present with symptoms of depression. Clinicians should carefully monitor patient response and intervene if an increase in suicidal thoughts or plans becomes evident. In addition, St. John's Wort is also associated with a small risk of inducing hypomanic or manic symptoms (Bezchlibnyk-Butler & Jeffries, 2007), and some patients who have tendencies toward symptoms of bipolar disorder may exhibit 'switching' from depressive to manic symptoms. Once again, careful monitoring of dose/response and adverse effects is necessary.

Tryptophan and 5-Hydrohytryptophan

Tryptophan, also referred to as L-tryptophan, is an essential amino acid. Of all essential amino acids, it is the one that is least abundant. It is a protein with many functions in the body, and it is a building block for many endogenous substances. It is also a precursor for serotonin. Consequently, it has been researched as a hypnotic and an antidepressant.

Supplementation with tryptophan has been attempted for many years, and studies report inconsistent results. Because it competes to cross the blood–brain barrier, levels of tryptophan seem to be unpredictable and the response does not appear to be uniform. However, a modified version of tryptophan, 5-hydroxytryptophan (5-HTP) appears to cross the blood–brain barrier less competitively and seems to show more promise in results of research studies.

Some open and controlled trials reveal that tryptophan and 5-HTP may offer some benefits to treat symptoms of anxiety. Kahn and Westenberg (1985) performed a small, open trial and found that 10 patients with anxiety disorders treated for 12 weeks with 300 mg/day of 5-HTP (with 50 mg of carbidopa TID) exhibited significant reductions in anxiety. The authors then performed a double-blind study with 45 patients and found that the group taking 5-HTP exhibited similar reduction in anxiety to the group taking clomipramine, a tricyclic anxiolytic (Kahn *et al.*, 1987). Other research also reveals that supplementation with tryptophan and/or 5-HTP is effective in patients who are described as 'low serotonin producers' (Settle, 2007). Consequently, it is reasonable to expect that supplementation with tryptophan or 5-HTP may offer some benefits in reducing symptoms of anxiety.

In neurons, tryptophan is converted into 5-HTP, which is then further converted to serotonin (5-hydroxytryptamine, or 5-HT). Theoretically, supplementation with either should increase levels of serotonin in the brain, but because of the blood–brain barrier competition mentioned above, supplementation with 5-HPT seems to increase synaptic levels of serotonin more effectively (Settle, 2007). Increase in serotonergic activity is associated with the anxiolytic effects of medications such as SSRIs and some TCAs, and consequently the pharmacodynamics of the anxiolytic mechanism of 5-HTP may involve similar effects of serotonergic activity agonism, although 5-HTP seems to accomplish this by increasing the availability of the precursor, rather than the reuptake inhibition mechanism utilized by prescription anxiolytics (SSRIs and TCAs).

Following ingestion, tryptophan is absorbed from the small intestine and metabolized in the liver. However, 5-HTP is more easily transformed into serotonin in the small intestine, and therefore to prevent this effect, carbidopa is sometimes taken with 5-HTP to delay its demabolism. The portions not synthesized during first pass effect enter systemic circulation and become distributed to the brain and other tissues. The half-life of tryptophan and 5-HTP is presumed to be very short due to its rapid conversion into serotonin, and appears unrelated to the duration of the clinical effect, since anxiolytic action is likely due to the increase in serotonin.

Tryptophan tablets are generally available in tablets and capsules with dosages ranging from 50–1000 mg, and 5-HTP is dosed similarly. Because research studies identified a very wide range of effective dose, trial and error is likely to be necessary to determine the appropriate dose for a specific patient. Children and adolescents should begin with a dosage of 50–100 mg and the dose should gradually be titrated until clinical response is evident. Doses above 1000 mg/day should only be used under medical supervision.

Tryptophan and 5-HTP are usually well tolerated, although some patients may exhibit daytime drowsiness, dizziness, and dry mouth. At higher doses, additional problems with nausea, lack of appetite, and headaches may become evident (Medical Economics, 2007). Because tryptophan and 5-HTP may exert sedative effects, concurrent use of other compounds that exert similar effects (for example, alcohol) should be avoided.

Tryptophan and 5-HTP are associated with a small risk of cardiac dysfunctions. Because tryptophan is converted into serotonin in the brain as well as peripherally, increases in serotonin may become evident in tissues and muscles, including the heart. When taken with carbidopa, these effects are not seen (Xu et al., 2002).

Tryptophan and 5-HTP need to be used cautiously with patients who have been diagnosed with diabetes or exhibit family history of diabetes. One of tryptophan's metabolites, xanthurenic acid, has been found to have a diabetogenic effect in animals. Although no cases in humans have been reported, caution should be exercised.

Valerian

Valerian (*Valeriana officinalis*) is a medicinal plant endogenous to Europe and Asia and widely introduced in North America. Various portions of the plant are consumed for medicinal reasons, including the flowers, fruit, and leaves. However, it is valerian root that is considered to be most psychoactive and its extracts are used as hypnotics and anxiolytics. Although its use as a hypnotic is well supported (as discussed in Chapter 9), there is some research that also confirms its usefulness as an anxiolytic.

In one German study, 49 patients with anxiety responded to valerian and found it efficacious at a level similar to diazepam (a prescription benzodiazepine anxiolytic, sold in the US as Valium), and valerian was perceived to be superior when considering the risk–benefit ratio (Panijel, 1985). Similarly, Leuschner et al. (1993) found valerian approximately equal in efficacy to diazepam or chlorpromazine (an anxiolytic neuroleptic). A more recent trial also revealed that valerian was effective in reducing symptoms of anxiety in patients with adjustment disorder with anxious mood (Bourin et al., 1997). These findings are preliminary, but suggest that valerian may offer some benefits in treating symptoms of anxiety.

Like most herbal compounds, valerian may have as many as 150 individual compounds (Morin et al., 2007). Consequently, its action is likely to be very broad. Although the effects of the specific constituents have not been identified, the overall effect of supplementation with valerian is the depression of central nervous activity that may be due to changes in the affinity of cortical membrane receptors, including hyperpolarization (Andreatini & Leite, 1994). This is probably the result of changes in the activity of GABA, the major inhibitory neurotransmitter in the brain. As GABA levels increase, chloride channels on cell membranes open and the cells become hyperpolarized. Valerian increases activity of GABA in a variety of ways. Valerian may block, and perhaps reverse, the reuptake of GABA, thus increasing synaptic concentrations of GABA. In addition, valerian may also inhibit the metabolism of GABA, and may even act as a precursor for GABA synthesis (Spinella, 2001). Just as is evident in the action of benzodiazepines, as GABA activity increases, anxiolytic effects become apparent.

Valerian is supplied in capsules, tablets, and liquid preparations, as an extract to be taken as drops (in a base, as in apple sauce) or dissolved in a tincture. Liquid preparations are absorbed more quickly, and tablets and capsules may take about 30–60 minutes longer to be absorbed. Pharmacokinetics are not well established, but onset of effect is generally seen in less than 1 hour. Various compounds present in valerian are metabolized through different mechanisms and at different rates, further complicating its use. However, it is apparent that clinical effects generally wear off after about 4–6 hours. Moreover, some have suggested that continued use of valerian, at the effective dose, does not result in tolerance to the effect (Spinella, 2001).

When used with adults as a hypnotic, daily doses range from 100–1800 mg, depending on the method of ingestion and the amount of the active compounds present in preparations available from different manufacturers. Studied dosages range from 1.5–3 g of actual herb or root, or 400–900 mg of an extract, taken up to 1 hour before bedtime. Bezchlibnyk-Butler and Jeffries (2007) recommend a dose of 200–1200 mg/day (with adults). With children and adolescents, about 20 mg/kg is used for hypnotic effect (Francis & Dempster, 2002). Usually, when used as an anxiolytic, lower doses are utilized to prevent sedation. Thus, it is apparent that the lowest possible dose should be started and dosage should gradually be titrated. Doses above to 20 mg/kg/day ratio should only be used under medical supervision.

Valerian is usually well tolerated, although a minority of patients may exhibit some adverse effects. Some patients may report some gastrointestinal discomfort and headaches, as well as feeling of restlessness and heart dysrhythmias. These are generally more common with higher doses or when the compound is used for extended periods of time, but individual patient response should carefully be monitored. At higher doses, additional problems may become evident, including severe headaches, nausea and vomiting, dizziness, stupor, and cardiac dysfunction.

Valerian is associated with a small risk of hepatic damage. This risk is significantly increased when patients already take medications or other supplements that carry a similar risk. For this reason, use of valerian with other supplements should generally be avoided, unless the other supplement has no documented risk of hepatotoxicity. Use of valerian with medications should only be done under careful medical supervision. Even when valerian is used in monotherapy, some recommend periodic liver function tests to monitor the health of the liver (Bezchlibnyk-Butler & Jeffries, 2007).

Because valerian is a sedative, concurrent use of other compounds that exert similar effects (for example, alcohol) should be avoided. Because alcohol also exerts liver effects, it is especially important to make sure that patients who take valerian do not drink alcohol. While this is not usually a risk for children, this needs to be stressed when valerian is used with adolescents.

Valerian may interfere with the absorption of iron. For this reason, those who require iron supplementation should not take the two compounds together, and should take iron at other times of day (Medical Economics, 2007).

Theanine

Theanine, also known as L-theanine, is a non-protein amino acid mainly found naturally in green tea (*Camellia sinensis*) and some mushrooms (*Boletus badius*). Theanine is related to glutamine, is speculated to increase levels of GABA, serotonin, and dopamine. Theanine may also interact with Kainate and NMDA receptors for glutamate. Theanine has been available in Japan as a nutritional supplement marketed to reduce stress, produce feelings of relaxation, and improve mood (Kimura *et al.*, 2007). Recently, theanine has also been marketed in the US.

Anxiolytic effects are presumed but not well documented. In animal studies, theanine has been shown to stimulate GABA (A) receptors (Egashira *et al.*, 2007), and oppose caffeine stimulation (Kakuda *et al.*, 2000). Studies in humans are more rare. In one study, Lu *et al.* (2004) found theanine to be as effective as alprazolam (a benzodiazepine anxiolytic, sold in the US as Xanax) in improving a sense of relaxation. A subsequent study confirmed these effects and found theanine to be effective in reducing the physiological effects of the stress response and the psychological experience of anxiety (Kimura, 2007). Although theanine is generally well tolerated, use of theanine in the pediatric population is considered experimental and clinicians must proceed with much caution.

Theanine supplements are generally available as tablets and capsules in doses between 50 and 200 mg. Although theanine is present in most green teas, the amount is unpredictable. Generally, two to three cups of green tea may contain between 30 and 50 mg of theanine (Medical Economics, 2008a), but this depends on the specific leaves being used and the brewing method. For this reason, it is best to avoid using theanine in tea when clinical effects are desired. Anxiolytic effects in adults are usually seen with doses of 200 mg/day (2.3 mg/kg/day). Pharmacokinetics are not well established, but theanine appears to be absorbed from the small intestine. Peak blood levels are reached between 0.5 and 2.0 hours after consumption (Nathan *et al.*, 2006). Theanine crosses the blood–brain barrier and may be taken up by the cells via a sodium-coupled active transport process. No guidelines about effective dosage ranges have been established.

Theanine supplements are usually well tolerated and no adverse effects have been reported thus far. However, pregnant and nursing mothers should avoid using the supplement. Female adolescents who take theanine and are suspected of being sexually active must be advised to use contraception to prevent pregnancy.

Ginger

Ginger (*Zingiber officinale*) is a tropical perennial that grows in Asia, west Africa, and the Caribbean. Ginger is well known as a spice, but its medicinal uses date back thousands of years. Ancient Greeks and Romans imported ginger from Asia, and it was known in China in the fourteenth century bc (Spinella, 2001). It is even mentioned in the Koran as a divine drink. More recently, it is recognized in the world for a variety of medicinal properties, including antiemetic, anti-inflammatory, antimicrobial, antioxidant, antithrombotic, cardiotonic and antimigraine effects, and it is approved by Germany's Commission E as a treatment for loss of appetite, travel sickness, and dyspepsia (Medical Economics, 2007).

Ginger has several active constituents, including aromatic ketones and terpenoids, and some of these may have anxiolytic properties. These psychoactive effects may be secondary to the inhibition of 5HT 3 receptors, as well as eicosanoid inhibition, which results in greater GABA activity. GABA conductance may further be increased by inhibition of arachnoid acid metabolites (Spinella, 2001). In addition, abnormally higher levels of cortisol are usually released during stress reactions, and studies have shown that levels of cortisol reduce after ginger supplementation (Piccirillo *et al.*, 1994). Results of animal studies confirm ginger's anxiolytic properties (Vishwakarma *et al.*, 2002), and ginger is often used in Ayurvedic medicine to treat symptoms of anxiety (for example, see Huebscher & Schuler, 2003). Because ginger is well tolerated and poses very few risks, careful supplementation in children and adolescents may be warranted.

Ginger supplements are available in tablets and capsules ranging from 100–1000 mg. Chewable tablets are also available, and liquid and tea bags preparations may be obtained. Generally, the use of tablets and capsules is recommended because it is easier to control the dosage. In some studies, higher doses of ginger taken on an empty stomach were associated with the development of ulcers, and therefore it is recommended to take ginger supplements with a meal. Very little is known about pharmacokinetics of ginger, but animal studies suggest that following absorption and systemic distribution, it is rapidly cleared. However, serum binding was equally rapid, especially for one of the gingerol ketones (Spinella, 2001). At least some of the constituents of ginger are metabolized by the liver, and cross-metabolism of some of the constituents into others also seems evident (Spinella).

When used to treat nausea, dyspepsia, motion sickness, or arthritis, dosage generally range from 0.5–4 g/day. This can be converted to approximately 5.8–46.5 mg/kg/day. Children and adolescents should be dosed toward the lower end of this ratio, and gradually titrated while monitoring response and adverse effects. According to available data, ginger has a very wide therapeutic window and lethal doses have been reported to range from 250–680 mg/kg (Medical Economics, 2007). It is clear that the clinical range is a tiny fraction of this dose.

In doses listed above, ginger is generally well tolerated and adverse effects are rare. Some patients experience mild gastrointestinal distress, flatulence, bloating, and heartburn. In higher doses, some patients have experienced dermatitis, cardiac arrhythmias, and central nervous system depression.

According to Germany's Commission E, ginger is contraindicated during pregnancy. However, research studies failed to reveal any difficulties of malformations in the fetus, and ginger is sometimes used as an effective remedy for morning sickness (Medical Economics, 2007).

The use of ginger with some medications should be avoided. Concurrent use with anticoagulants may increase the risk of bleeding, and therefore the use of the supplement with any medications that decrease platelet aggregation should only be done under monitoring by medical professionals.

Taurine

Taurine is a non-protein organic amino sulfonic acid mainly found naturally in meat, fish, eggs, and milk. Humans also produce it from cysteine, but infants and children do so in much lower amounts, and some children lack the enzyme necessary for its metabolism. For this reason, taurine is added to most baby foods, as it is presumed to be necessary for normal retinal and brain development. Taurine has membrane stabilizing effects and consequently, as discussed in Chapter 7, it has been presumed to be involved in regulating neurotransmission and may have some efficacy in reducing symptoms of mania. It has also been suggested that it may have anxiolytic properties by altering the activity of the inhibitory glycine receptors, and animal studies confirmed this effect (Zhang & Kim, 2007). Taurine also seems to have an agonist effects on GABA A receptors (Jia *et al.*, 2008). Case studies in women support anxiolytic effects when taurine is used at a dose of about at 1000 mg/day (Bronson, 2001), and findings of controlled studies in humans reveal that taurine inhibits the release of norepinephrine, which may have antihypertensive as well as anxiolytic effects (Fujita *et al.*, 1987). Although these findings are preliminary, taurine supplementation has been shown to be safe over a wide dosage, and therefore a cautious trial in the pediatric population may be indicated.

Taurine is absorbed from the small intestine and enters the brain through sodium and chloride dependent transport systems. In the cell, taurine may keep potassium and magnesium inside the cell while keeping sodium out. Thus, it may affect neuronal firing. Remaining taurine is conjugated to form the bile salts and is excreted into bile, where it is transported to the duodenum to take part in the metabolism of various lipids. Excess taurine is excreted by the kidneys.

Taurine supplements are generally available as tablets and capsules and clinical doses range from 500 mg/day to 3 g/day in adults (Medica Economics, 2008a). Balch (2006) recommends a dosage of 500 mg three times per day (TID) to treat symptoms of bipolar disorder. Taurine supplements are usually well tolerated and no adverse effects have been reported thus far. However, pregnant and nursing mothers should only use the supplement under medical supervision.

Passion Flower

Passion flower (*Passiflora incarnata*) is indigenous to many parts of the world, except Europe and Africa, although various species of passion flower have now been naturalized in those regions. Various species of passion flower are native to the US, especially the middle and southeastern regions of the country. Only a few species have psychotropic properties, including *Passiflora incarnata*, and perhaps *P. coerulea* and *P. edulis* (Spinella, 2001). Passion flower has long been used by Native American Indians for its sedative and anxiolytic effects (Kowalchick & Hylon, 1987). It is also recognized in other parts of the world for these properties. Passion flower is approved by Germany's Commission E to treat nervousness and insomnia but, as discussed in Chapter 9, its hypnotic effects are not widely supported. As a supplement, passion flower is available in liquid and capsules.

Passion flower has many constituents, including flavonoids, maltol, and indole alkaloids. Active ingredients include chrysin, vitexin, coumerin, and umbelliferone (Spinella, 2001). Chrysin is the most studied component. Along with other flavonoids, chrysin has been shown to bind to benzodiazepine receptors sites and acts as an agonist for GABA activity, especially at A type GABA receptors. This has an inhibitory effect on the brain, accounting for passion flower's anxiolytic properties. In animal studies, psychoactive effects of passion flower were reversed by benzodiazepine antagonists, and the overall effect in the brain has been compared to that of diazepam (Valium) (Wolfman *et al.*, 1994).

Some studies began to confirm passion flower's effectiveness as an anxiolytic in humans. Bourin *et al.* (1997) found that the herb was effective in reducing symptoms in patients with adjustment disorder with anxiety. Akhondzadeh *et al.* (2001) performed a small, double-blind, randomized study in which the effects of passion flower were compared with anxiolytic properties of oxazepam (a benzodiazepine). Results revealed similar efficacy and less adverse effects with the use of passion flower. Larzelere and Wiseman (2002) found similar efficacy when they reviewed a number of small studies, and a recent review in the Cochrane system revealed that studies are beginning to emerge that support its efficacy (Miyasaka et al., 2007). Although no studies have thus far been performed with children or adolescents, supplementation with passion flower is regarded as safe and adverse effects are quite rare. Consequently, clinicians and parents may want to consider a cautious trial of passion flower to treat symptoms of anxiety.

Little is known about passion flower's pharmacokinetics, but its half-life may be short because the supplement is generally taken two to three times per day. When brewed as tea, about 150 ml (1 cup) of boiling water is poured over about 1 teaspoon. of dried herb are brewed for about 10 minutes, and drunk two to three times per day (Medical Economics, 2007). When used in capsules, children and adolescents should start with a low dose (200 mg capsules seem to be the lowest available) and used twice to three times per day. Dosage may slowly be adjusted upward while monitoring response and adverse effects.

Passion flower is usually well tolerated and side effects are rare. When initiated, treatment with passion flower may exert sedative effects, so monitoring of response is necessary. Passion flower may contribute to blood thinning, so those who take anticoagulant medications should avoid using passion flower. This may include over-the-counter medications, such as aspirin and ibuprofen. Use of passion flower is contraindicated during pregnancy. Female adolescents who take passion flower and are suspected of being sexually active must be advised of this risk, and should use contraception to prevent pregnancy.

Chamomile

Chamomile, (*Matricaria recutita*) sometimes also referred to as German chamomile, is an herb that is native to Europe, Africa, and Asia, and is now also grown in North America. Chamomile has been used medicinally for thousands of years and was known by ancient Greek, Roman, and Egyptian cultures. It is now approved by Germany's Commission E to treat cough and bronchitis, fevers, cold, inflammation, infection, wounds, and burns. It is available as a supplement in capsules, as well as tea bags and liquid extract.

Chamomile contains terpenoids, flavonoids, and lactones, including matricin and apigenin. Chamomile may have sedative effects because apigenin binds to benzodiazepine receptors and potentiates the activity at GABA A receptors (Viola *et al.*, 1995). Apigenin also stimulates uptake of tyrosine, resulting in increased monoamine production (Morita *et al.*, 1990). Apigenin may also inhibit the MAO enzyme, further increasing the availability of monoamines (Spinella, 2001). Increase in serotonin may especially be related to its anxiolytic effects.

Animal models confirm that chamomile has anxiolytic effects, and a small number of case studies in humans also supports its sedative properties (Medical Economics, 2007), although its use as a hypnotic has been discredited (as discussed in Chapter 9). Because few risks are associated with its use, and the herb is usually well tolerated, a cautious trial in children and adolescents may be warranted.

Very little is known about the pharmacokinetics of chamomile. Doses in adults vary widely and range from 25 mg to 2000 mg per day. Half-life may be short because it is often recommended to take chamomile three times per day. Usually, chamomile is ingested when brewed as a tea and tablets are more difficult to locate, but may offer better dosage control. Liquid extract is generally dosed at 1–4 ml three times per day (TID), and tincture is dosed at 15 ml three to four times per day (TID or QUID). Children and adolescents should start at low doses TID and gradually titrate upwards while response and adverse effects are carefully monitored.

Chamomile is usually well tolerated and side effects are rare. Patients with allergies to plants in the daisy family (including ragweed) should avoid chamomile because an allergic reaction may be triggered. When initiated, treatment with chamomile exerts sedative effects, so monitoring of response is necessary. Chamomile may contribute to blood thinning, so those who take anticoagulant medications should avoid using chamomile. This may include over-the-counter medications, such as aspirin and ibuprofen.

Use of chamomile is contraindicated during pregnancy because it may stimulate uterine contractions. Female adolescents who take chamomile and are suspected of being sexually active must be advised of this risk, and should use contraception to prevent pregnancy.

SUPPLEMENTS NOT LIKELY TO BE EFFECTIVE

It is not possible to review all compounds that, at one time or another, have been tried to treat symptoms of anxiety and have not shown to be effective, or lack sufficient rationale about how they may affect brain action to promote sleep. However, some of these compounds are sometimes marketed as anxiolytics, despite the lack of evidence of efficacy. Clinicians who seek to practice in the area of naturopathic psychopharmacology should be aware of compounds that continue to be propagated despite evidence to the contrary.

GABA

As discussed in Chapter 4, GABA is a major neurotransmitter in the central nervous system that is ubiquitous and affects the firing of all neurons by increasing membrane polarization. Most GABA receptors are ionotropic and regulate the influx of chloride into the cell. As chloride levels increase in the cell, the negative charge also increases, and the cell becomes more and more difficult to stimulate.

A number of medications target GABA neurotransmission and have been shown to be effective in treating mood disturbance (especially mania and agitation), anxiety, and tics. Consequently, naturopaths sometimes recommend GABA supplementation, and various forms of GABA tablets and capsules are available on the market.

Unfortunately, these are of very limited value. GABA does not easily cross the blood–brain barrier (Foster & Kemp, 2006), and the majority of GABA becomes metabolized and/or excreted before it can enter the brain. Although some peripheral effects have been observed, like muscle relaxation, few psychogenic effects seem evident. When administered at high doses (at 1000 mg or higher), supplemental GABA does, in fact, appear to begin to cross the blood–brain barrier, but surprisingly, the effects are not the inhibition that is expected, and a mix of sedation as well as increased anxiety becomes evident (Abdou *et al.*, 2006). Thus, GABA supplements appear to show no benefits in treating symptoms of anxiety.

Ginkgo

Ginkgo (*Ginkgo biloba*), sometimes also spelled ginko, and also known as the maidenhair tree or kew, is an ancient tree primarily endogenous to China but now widely grown in various parts of the world, usually under controlled conditions. Ginkgo has been used for thousands of years and was known in ancient China for its benefit in treating memory loss and breathing ailments (Spinella, 2001). It is widely used in Europe, and ginkgo prescriptions account for up to 4 percent of all medication prescriptions in some countries (Spinella). Over the past few decades, its use has been becoming more popular in the US. When used as a supplement, it is ingested in capsules or liquid extracts.

Ginko has many active ingredients, including various flavonoid glycosides, biflavones, and terpene lactones. Its psychoactive mechanisms primarily include an increase in acetylcholine activity, which it appears to accomplish by increasing the uptake of choline into the cells, and increasing the release of acetylcholine into the synapse (Spinella, 2001). This action is probably responsible for ginkgo's well-documented benefits in improving memory. However, some of ginkgo's constituents may also inhibit MAO enzymes (both A and B types), as well as increases in serotonergic neurotransmission and elevating levels of GABA (Spinella). Consequently, it has been presumed to have some anxiolytic properties.

Results of research studies, however, have not confirmed these effects. In animal models, some studies reported preliminary results, but these have never been replicated in humans. In addition, use of ginkgo may pose some risks. It potently inhibits platelets and cases of spontaneous bleeding have been reported with its use, including hemorrhaging and hematomas (Medical Economics, 2007). Use of ginkgo has also been associated with a decrease in seizure threshold (Gregory, 2001). Even more importantly, use of ginkgo is associated with a risk of developing Stevens Johnson syndrome (Davydov & Stirling, 2001), a potentially fatal condition in which death of skin cells causes the epidermis to separate from the dermis, and children and adolescents are especially at risk for this disorder. All in all, weighing the lack of evidence of anxiolytic properties and the potential risks of using ginkgo, it seems clear ginkgo supplements should not be used in the pediatric population.

Serine

Serine is non-essential amino acid supplied from food or synthesized by the body from a number of metabolites, including glycine. Serine is found in soybeans, nuts (especially peanuts, almonds, and walnuts), eggs, chickpeas, lentils, meat, and fish (especially shellfish). Serine is produced by the body when insufficient amounts are ingested. It is metabolized from ketones and glycine, and retroconversion with glycine also occurs.

As with most amino acids, when food is ingested that contains serine, the molecule is extracted in the small intestine and absorbed into circulation. There, it travels through the body, crosses the blood–brain barrier, and enters neurons, where it gets metabolized into glycine and many other molecules. Thus, the amount of serine in cells is regulated through these metabolic processes. If too little is ingested, more serine is converted from various sources. When too much is ingested, only a portion is converted to glycine, and the remainder is metabolized into folate and many other proteins.

As with all precursors, only a limited amount of serine is converted to glycine, and supplementation seems to be of limited value. Although non-peer reviewed sources list it as effective in treatment of a variety of symptoms of psychological disorders (especially, depression and anxiety), there is no empirical research to support these claims. Thus, although supplementation with serine is not associated with significant adverse effects, benefits are unlikely, and therefore clinicians are advised to avoid using serine supplements.

SUMMARY

In order to help clinicians select the compounds that are most likely to be effective, an algorithm was developed and is presented in Figure 8.1. Patients with no history of depression may start with a cautious trial of

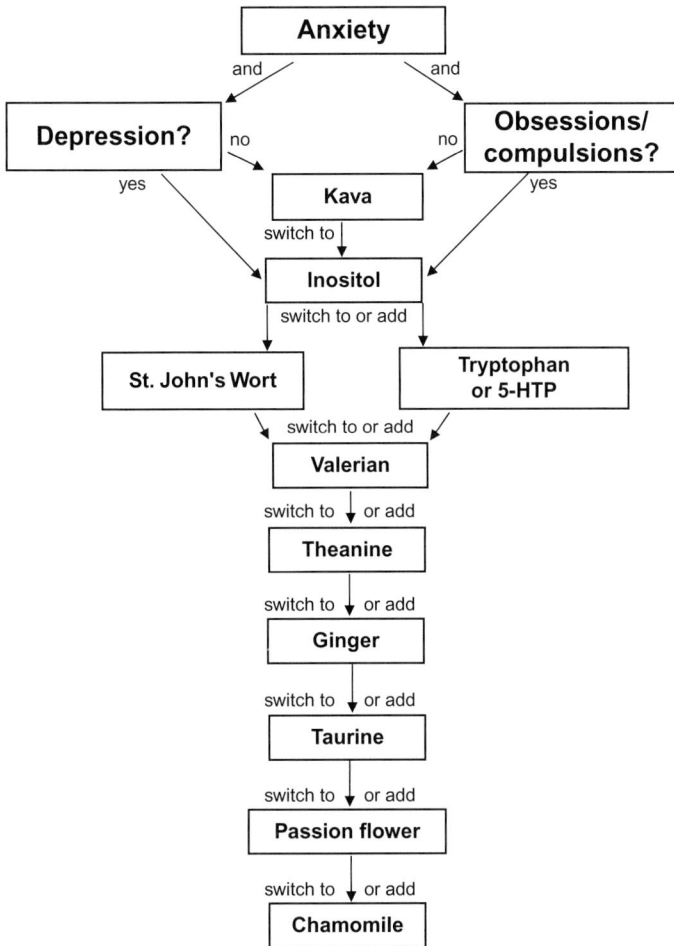

FIGURE 8.1   Algorithm for treatment of anxiety with naturopathic supplements.
© Elsevier 2009.

kava, and if insufficient response is evident, patient should switch to inositol. If needed, St. John's Wort or tryptophan/5-HT may be added or switched to as monotherapy, but because of similarities in their action, the two should not be used together. Valerian may also be added to this combination, or used as monotherapy. In descending order, theanine, ginger, taurine, passion flower, and chamomile may also be attempted, and no more than two of these should be combined with each other.

Instead of starting with kava, patients with obsession and/or compulsions should start with inositol, and then switch to or add St. John's Wort, since these two compounds appear to reveal at least some efficacy in clinical trials for treatment of symptoms of OCD. If these are not sufficiently effective, valerian may be added or used as monotherapy. If needed, theanine, ginger, taurine, passion flower, and chamomile may also be attempted, and no more than two of these should be combined with each other.

If multiple supplements are being administered, extreme caution must be exercised and, ideally, medical monitoring should be utilized.

Chapter 9

Sleep

Sleep disturbances are among the most frustrating problems that parents of children and adolescents encounter. Traditionally, sleep problems have been associated with adults or the elderly. However, it is now widely recognized that children and adolescents also present various symptoms of sleep disturbance that need proper treatment. However, symptoms of sleep disturbance may be hard to identify. Children often complain that they do not like to go to sleep and try to delay bedtime. Most parents see this behavior as an attempt to act more grown up and a way to seek privileges associated with being older. However, children may exhibit legitimate difficulties with sleep, and delaying bedtime may be a way for the child to try to avoid the problem. Parents and clinicians need to carefully consider whether problems at bedtime are a sign of sleep disturbances.

These problems are compounded in adolescents. Most teenagers enjoy staying up at night, and view that portion of the evening as a time during which they have privacy and freedom to do things they enjoy. It is also a way to assert their independence and perceived maturity. However, teenagers may exhibit problems with sleep that are related to the irregularity in schedules that is commonplace among many adolescents. If they are involved in sports, it is likely that sporting events and practices may take place at different times of day and evening. The same may be true of other activities, like clubs and youth groups. While these pursuits are beneficial to teens in many ways, they often prevent them from keeping a consistent daily schedule. Thus, the daily rhythm of waking, going to school, doing homework, relaxing, and going to bed is disrupted, and the sequencing may be different day to day. In addition, many school districts begin their school days very early, sometimes at 7:00 a.m. If the teens are bussed, they may need to leave the house 30–60 minutes earlier. Adding the time it takes a teenager (especially, a teenage girl) to get ready for school, this means that the teen may need to wake up as early as 5:00 a.m. In order to get at least 8 hours of sleep, the teen needs to go to bed at 9:00 p.m. However, most teens consider this to be much too early, and therefore those teens who start school early in the morning usually miss a significant amount of sleep each school day. Over time, this contributes to sleep dysregulation and may become a factor leading to a sleep disorder.

SYMPTOMS OF SLEEP DISORDERS

DSM-IV-TR (APA, 2000), divides sleep disorders into two broad categories. Dyssomnias are disturbances in the amount or timing of sleep. The most common dyssomnia is insomnia, a disturbance that causes the person to get an insufficient amount of sleep at night. Various types of insomnias are currently identified, based on the time of night during which the disturbance occurs. In addition to insomnia, some may experience hypersomnia. However, hypersomnia is much more rare than insomnia, and some of the variants (like Klein-Levin Syndrome) are poorly understood. Hypersomnia does not lend itself well to naturopathic treatment, and therefore it will not be included in this chapter. The category of dyssomnias also includes disturbances in sleep timing. While this topic is relevant to teenagers and may sometimes be caused by irregularities in the teenagers' schedules (as discussed above), the treatment usually involved restoring sleep during proper times, and therefore the strategies are similar to those used to treat symptoms of insomnia. For this reason, disorders characterized by disturbances in sleep timing will not be discussed separately in this chapter.

In addition to dyssomnias, the DSM system also includes parasomnias, disorders characterized by abnormal behaviors that occur during sleep. These may or may not interfere with the patient's quality of sleep, although they may interfere with the quality of sleep of the parents. For example, sleepwalking, or night terrors, are relatively common among children, and the vast majority of patients grow out of these problems on their own. However, hearing their child scream while in the middle of sleep is usually difficult for parents to ignore, and therefore most will come into the child's room and try to comfort their child (assuming that the child experienced a nightmare), even though the child usually does not lose sleep because of this episode, and the best course of action is to leave the child alone and let him or her continue sleep. Once again, parasomnias do not lend themselves well to naturopathic treatment, and therefore they are not covered in this chapter.

Before symptoms of sleep disturbance can be outlined, it is necessary to develop an understanding of normal sleep and the patterns of changes that our brain and body routinely goes through during a typical night. With this as a model, it will become easier to identify the deviations that may occur from this normal pattern, and the effects of these deviations on the overall health of the patient. Thus, this chapter will discuss normal sleep and insomnia, helping the readers to recognize how various forms of insomnia affects different portions of the normal sleep pattern.

Normal Sleep

In order to discuss normal sleep, two aspects must be discussed – the stages of sleep that the child's or adolescent's body must go through during a typical night, and how much sleep is normally needed in order for sleep to serve its restorative functions.

Stages of Sleep

During a normal night's sleep, children and adolescents typically experience two different types of sleep – dream states, usually referred to as REM sleep, and non-REM sleep. When dreaming, we experience a rapid movement of our eyes (REM), which is not seen during non-dreaming sleep (non-REM). Both serve different functions and must occur in a precise sequence.

When we lie down to fall asleep, we initially drift off into light sleep during which our consciousness is not yet altered. In other words, if we awake from this stage, we think we were not yet asleep. During this stage, our brain waves, as evident on the electroencephalogram (EEG), are similar to those characterized by states of wakefulness – fairly rapid, with limited amplitude. Sometimes this type of sleep is referred to as Stage 1 sleep or alpha sleep. The function of this stage is to begin to prepare the brain for the changes that will come in the following stages.

After about 15–20 minutes, we typically progress on to the next stage, one that is a little 'deeper' – the brain waves slow down a little, and the amplitude increases. On the EEG, these are referred to as beta waves, and this stage of sleep is sometimes referred to as Stage 2 sleep or beta sleep. As with Stage 1, this is a transitional stage that further prepares the brain for the next stages. Stages 1 and 2 are sometimes collectively referred to as fast-wave sleep, since the brain waves evident during those stages are not very different from the brain waves evident during wakefulness.

After another half-hour or so, the brain waves slow down again and we enter Stage 3 sleep. By now, theta brain waves become apparent – these are much slower, and have much greater amplitude than waking brain waves. The purpose of this stage is to prepare the brain for the next stage, which serves many important physical functions. This stage, which may last from a few minutes to a half-hour or more, is the first of the slow-wave sleep stages.

An hour or so after falling asleep we typically enter Stage 4 sleep, the deepest sleep. Delta brain waves are evident on the EEG – the amplitude is very high, and the frequency is low (around 1 Hz). This is the stage of sleep during which important restorative functions take place. Immune cells are synthesized from bone marrow. Growth hormone is released into the blood stream. Wound healing is accelerated. It seems that this is the stage of sleep that is indispensable, especially for children and adolescents. If sleep disturbance prevents the body from entering delta sleep, growth, immune, and other basic bodily functions will be interfered with. The amount of time spent in this stage differs based on age. Children spend half their night sleep in delta sleep, while the elderly rarely enter delta sleep at all. In addition, being ill is also associated with increased duration of Stage 4 sleep – perhaps to give the body a change to produce more white blood cells.

Next, the brain waves accelerate again, and we enter REM sleep. The brain waves again exhibit a fast pattern, and movement of eyeballs becomes evident. This is the stage of sleep during which we dream. REM sleep is among the least understood, and its functions are not clear. People who are depressed tend to spend more time in REM sleep, but it is hard to determine whether this is a contributing factor to depressive symptom, or just the result of them. There are many hypotheses about the reasons we need REM sleep, mostly derived from sleep-deprivation studies where subjects were awaken during the onset of REM sleep (thus, interfering with the proper sequence of sleep stages). Participants in those studies revealed difficulties with memory, concentration, and emotional control. In fact, studies of extreme REM sleep deprivation were halted after some participants later committed suicide. Today, it is believed that REM sleep is necessary for consolidation of long-term memory, and contributes to the brain's ability to process emotions.

Through the night, the body cycles between non-REM and REM sleep. At first, the body goes through Stages 1, 2, 3, and enters Stage 4 sleep. This first delta sleep episode is the longest. When it is over, the body enters REM sleep, and the first episode is the shortest. For the remainder of the night, the body transitions back and forth between delta and REM sleep, each time decreasing the time in delta sleep and increasing the time in REM sleep. By the end of a typical 8 hour sleep, we have spent the last hour or so in REM sleep.

Amount of Sleep

As mentioned before, children and adolescents spend more time in Stage 4 sleep than adults. However, studies have not yet identified changes in the amount of REM sleep between children, adolescents, and adults. Thus it is apparent that the amount of time needed in delta sleep determines the minimum length of sleep necessary for persons of different ages. Infants and toddlers spend most of their time sleeping. Gradually, as children enter school age, it seems that about 10 hours of sleep is necessary, and by adolescence the amount of time decreases, but only by a little, and teenagers still need about 9 hours of sleep. It is likely that they still need to spend a significant amount of time in Stage 4 sleep because they are still growing. Adults typically need 8 hours of sleep, and the amount of time spent in Stage 4 decreases with age, while the amount of time spent in REM sleep increases. It is unknown whether this increase in REM serves a specific function, or whether this is just a replacement for the time no longer needed in Stage 4 sleep.

Another factor must also be considered. In addition to the amount of sleep, it is necessary for the body to obtain the proper amount of sleep in one continuous block. The transition from wakefulness to Stage 4 sleep is a drastic one and changes in brain waves are very significant. Thus, in order for the brain to get to Stage 4 sleep, the preceding stages must take place in order, and in the proper amount of time. Once Stage 4 sleep completed its cycle, the remaining REM sleep may occur on and off – for example, many individuals may wake for a bathroom break when going into this stage. However, waking during the sequence preceding Stage 4 will interrupt the cycle and reset the need to proceed through it in order, thus potentially interfering with the proper amount of time needed for some of the sleep stages.

Whether or not to nap is a topic that is closely related and often debated. Usually, a nap is not a substitute for a proper night's sleep, but the relationship between napping and night-time sleep is a complex one. The danger in napping is that it will interfere with the onset of sleep during the normal night-time sleep period. In other words, napping during the day will make a person less tired when it is normally time to go to sleep. As a result, the person may stay up longer, thus interfering with the proper amount of night-time sleep, resulting in being tired the next day, then napping, and then again interfering with sleep onset at night. This cycle must be avoided.

On the other hand, napping can sometimes be helpful, but keeping in mind the need for delta sleep is paramount. When sleep disturbance is severe enough to interfere with delta sleep, napping is not likely to restore it, since the brain needs a long time to prepare to enter Stage 4 sleep, and naps usually do not last several hours. On the other hand, if the night-time sleep was long enough to satisfy the need for delta sleep, it is possible that a short nap may be somewhat helpful. Interestingly, however, napping does not seem to restore the REM deficit associated with sleeping shorter than necessary at night, so the real benefit of napping is still unknown.

Insomnia

Insomnia is a general term for a condition where the person does not get a sufficient amount of sleep. The term 'sufficient' is relative. When diagnosing sleep problems, clinicians should consider not only the amount of sleep commonly needed by people of similar age, but also whether the amount of sleep typically obtained by the patient seems to be right for him or her. For example, teenagers generally need about 9 hours of sleep. If a teenager wants to get a proper amount of sleep and sets aside the sufficient amount of time (i.e., goes to bed at an hour that allows for a 9 hour sleep before waking), but is not able to sleep during a sufficient portion of that time, insomnia may be evident. Conversely, if a teenager seems to sleep 9–10 hours per night, and still wakes up tired and feels groggy for a long time afterward, hypersomnia may be evident.

Insomnia is commonly divided into subtypes by the time of night when the sleeplessness occurs. Early-onset insomnia, also referred to as sleep-onset insomnia, is evident when a person lies down to fall asleep and cannot do so for an unusually long period of time. Usually, people fall asleep in about 15–20 minutes. People with early insomnia sometimes report lying in bed for hours without being able to go to sleep. In extreme cases, when the insomnia lasts through the night, the lack of sleep may cause significant physical problems. When the insomnia is severe enough to result in a deprivation of Stage 4 sleep, functions associated with this stage of sleep will likely be adversely affected. Most of the time, however, the insomnia may last for an hour or two, and eventually the person falls asleep. Thus, sufficient amount of sleep will occur to complete the delta sleep cycle, although REM deprivation is likely to be evident.

Sleep-maintenance insomnia occurs when awakening takes place during the night, after sleep onset took place. Middle-onset insomnia occurs when a person wakes in the middle of the night and cannot fall back asleep for a long time. This may occur spontaneously, or when the person wakes up to go to the bathroom. During normal sleep, it is not unusual to wake up to urinate, or because of a noise nearby, but people normally are able to fall back asleep without difficulties. However, when an individual exhibits symptoms of middle insomnia, he or she cannot fall back asleep after those normal awakenings. Middle insomnia does not affect Stage 4 sleep quite as much – since delta sleep occurs early in the night, much of its cycle may have completed. However, REM deprivation and its sequelae are commonly apparent with middle insomnia.

Sleep-maintenance insomnia may also occur in the early morning hours. Late-onset insomnia is evident when a person is able to fall asleep without difficulty and sleeps through much of the night, but wakes much earlier than expected and cannot get back to sleep, even though he or she feels tired. As with middle-onset insomnia, the delta sleep cycle probably completed, but REM deprivation will be apparent.

When children and adolescents experience insomnia, they commonly report feeling groggy and tired in the morning. They have difficulties attending in school and, in extreme cases, may fall asleep in school. They are forgetful and have difficulties keeping track of their responsibilities and chores. During homework, they report that they cannot concentrate and they forget assignments, complete work with many errors, etc. In addition, they are likely to be irritable and may exhibit an increase in tantrums. Because they feel tired, they may also withdraw from activities and friends. It is clear that symptoms of insomnia significantly affects functioning at home, in school, and with peers.

RULE-OUTS AND COMORBID DISORDERS

Insomnia is a common symptom of many psychological disorders. In those cases, treating insomnia without addressing the other symptoms of the underlying disorder is not likely to result in much improvement. On the other hand, insomnia may also lead to the development of additional symptoms, and, in those cases, treating the insomnia first and foremost is necessary. Clinicians need to perform a careful differential diagnosis when they encounter children and adolescents with insomnia.

Mood Disorders

Insomnia is a core symptom of mood disorders (APA, 2000). Sleep disturbance is part of the biological features of both depression and bipolar-spectrum disorders, and the specific way in which sleep becomes disturbed in these conditions varies from patient to patient.

Depression

A small percentage of individuals with symptoms of depression present a so-called atypical variant of symptoms, including hypersomnia. However, insomnia is much more common (Birmaher *et al.*, 1996), and it is considered one of the biologically based vegetative symptoms of depression. Insomnia may present differently in children and adolescents.

Children are more likely to present with early insomnia, that is, difficulties falling asleep. This may become evident in various ways. While some children may be able to directly disclose that they have problems falling asleep after they lie in bed, many children may not report sleep disturbance in this way. Instead, children may exhibit reluctance with going to bed and may state that they are not tired at bedtime. Once parents attempt to put the child to bed, he or she may frequently leave the room to ask questions, use the bathroom, etc. Since it is common for children to do so simply because they do not want to go to bed, the presence of such behaviors does not necessarily signal sleep problems. However, when these behaviors are present, and in addition the child seems sad, affectively flat, withdrawn, and/or easily agitated, it is possible that the sleep disturbance accompanies symptoms of depression. In this situation, instead of treating the insomnia, it is important to first and foremost treat the symptoms of depression. While a hypnotic supplement may be used as an adjunct, the initial focus of treatment needs to be on the depressive symptoms.

Teenagers may present similar sleep problems in various parts of the night. At bedtime, adolescents may stay up late watching television, playing with video games, or spending time on the computer. In addition, adolescents may also present insomnia at other times of the night, including awakenings in the middle of the night or waking up too early in the morning. As with children, it is important to be vigilant about other symptoms of depression, including withdrawal, flatness of affect, sadness, loss of appetite, and/or agitation, and when these symptoms accompany sleep disturbance, the treatment needs to focus on addressing all of the symptoms of depression, not just sleep disturbance.

Bipolar Disorder

As discussed in Chapter 7, a small number of children or adolescents may present with symptoms of bipolar-spectrum mood disturbance. While symptoms of 'classic' mania – excessive pursuit of pleasure, grandiosity, severe flight of ideas, and rapid/pressured speech – are rare in this population, hypomanic or mixed episodes are more likely, where patients present with significant agitation, restlessness, and difficulties with concentration. Such symptoms are likely to be accompanied by sleep disturbance, including insomnia and nightmares. Children and adolescents may express sleep difficulties by exhibiting difficulties settling down when it is time for bed, frequently waking up in the middle of the night (and, sometimes, engaging in activities when they awake), or waking early in the morning with a high amount of energy. In some cases, children and adolescents may seem to require less sleep than most children, although this is not necessarily a reliable sign of bipolar symptoms. However, when times of reduced need for sleep seem to coincide with agitation and/or significant energy, and if such periods seem to occur cyclically, it is possible that the change in sleep patterns may be a sign of mood disturbance.

If clinicians identify symptoms of manic, mixed or hypomanic episodes, it is important to aim treatment strategies at managing all of those symptoms, rather than focusing on sleep disturbance in isolation. While a supplement to aid sleep may be used as an adjunct, treatment strategies should aim to address all of the symptoms of mood disturbance.

Anxiety Disorders

Children and adolescents may express symptoms of anxiety in a variety of ways, and anxiety disorders that commonly occur in this population are discussed in detail in Chapter 8. Insomnia is a common feature of many of these disorders. In addition, some research indicates that, in many cases, sleep disturbance is a prodromal sign of a developing anxiety disorder (Neckelmann, 2007). Some anxiety disorders are especially likely to be accompanied by sleep disturbance.

Separation Anxiety Disorder

Children who experience significant anxiety when separated from their primary parents and caretakers are likely to present these symptoms not only at times when the separation involves out-of-home settings (for example, going to school), but also when the child is separated from the parent in other circumstances – for example, when the parent is about to leave to go shopping, or when the child is put to sleep in his or her own room. When going to sleep, children with separation anxiety disorder often cry, protest, and become very upset. When the parent tries to force the issue, the child often continues to carry on for a long time and sleep onset is greatly delayed. If the child wakes in the middle of the night, he or she is likely to seek out the parents again and the cycle of crying and becoming upset may start over.

When children present symptoms of separation anxiety during the day and at night, it may be helpful to try to use a hypnotic agent to help the child relax and go to sleep, but significant anxiety and emotional distress are likely to interfere with sleep even if a sleep-promoting supplement is used. Clinicians need to address all symptoms of separation anxiety disorder in order for improvement to become apparent.

Social Phobia

Children and adolescents with social anxiety disorder (also known as social phobia) feel most anxious when around others, especially in situations outside the home that involve a larger group of individuals (for example, school, the playground, or other settings where a larger number of peers is likely to be present). Consequently, it may seem that individuals with social phobia should be relatively anxiety free at home. However, children and adolescents are likely to exhibit apprehension about situations when social situations are forthcoming. Since school is one social situation many children and adolescents with social phobia find anxiety provoking, those youngsters are likely to start thinking about next day's school attendance while going to sleep, and they often become anxious while they ruminate about what may happen the next day, what their friends may say to them, etc. As they become more anxious, they are less likely to be able to fall asleep.

When mental health professionals encounter children and teens who exhibit difficulties falling asleep, they should inquire about the thought process that takes place while the children or adolescents lie in bed. When symptoms of anxiety are identified, a comprehensive treatment approach will be needed to address this problem. While using a sleep-promoting agent may be helpful, the treatment should address other symptoms of anxiety as well.

Generalized Anxiety Disorder

Generalized anxiety disorder (GAD) is conceptually similar to social phobia, except that anxiety-provoking situations do not necessarily involve social situations, and the anxiety is more free flowing and not clearly connected to specific settings or situations. Consequently, the anxiety is likely to be evident throughout the day, as well as at night. Not surprisingly, children or adolescents who seem anxious much of the time will likely exhibit similar tendencies at night, and their ability to go to sleep will be affected. Those children and teens are likely to lie in bed worrying or ruminating about some anxiety-provoking situations or settings, and they may attempt to delay bedtime.

As with social phobia, when mental health professionals encounter children and teens who exhibit chronic tendencies toward significant worry and anxiety, these should be addressed with interventions that comprehensively target all symptoms. While using a sleep-promoting agent may be helpful, the treatment should address other symptoms of anxiety as well.

Adjustment and Trauma

Children and adolescents who have undergone traumatic experiences are likely to exhibit a variety of difficulties. Some may display changes in mood, agitation, depression, and related symptoms. Others may display much anxiety and withdrawal. In addition to emotional changes, many children and teenagers may exhibit changes in behaviors, including acting out and difficulties with being managed. All of those problems are likely to be accompanied by sleep difficulties, and the severity of sleep problems will usually correlate with the severity of other symptoms that are evident.

Post-Traumatic Disorders

Acute stress disorder (ASD) and post-traumatic stress disorder (PTSD) are two disorders that may develop in children and adolescents who have been exposed to severe trauma, such as abuse, loss of a parent, severe injury, or exposure to a major catastrophe. Children with ASD or PTSD will usually exhibit substantial disturbance of overall functioning, including anxiety and hypervigilance, nightmares (which do not necessarily need to contain trauma-related content), reliving the event through play (or other forms of flashbacks), and avoidance of (and/or detachment from) trauma-related stimuli. Significant sleep disturbance often accompanies these symptoms, and children and teens with these disorders may avoid going to sleep because they fear the onset of nightmares, or because they feel more vulnerable when they are asleep.

When clinicians encounter children or adolescents with ASD or PTSD, all symptom groups must be managed. Intensive psychotherapy and/or psychiatric treatment is likely to be necessary, and sleep disturbance should not be addressed in isolation. While using a hypnotic may be helpful, it is not likely to be effective unless the other symptoms are also being addressed.

Adjustment Disorders

Children and adolescents who have been exposed to less severe stressful events, like family conflicts, moves, or parental separation, may

experience less severe variants of emotional and behavioral disturbances. Within the DSM system, these may meet the criteria for various forms of adjustment disorder (APA, 2000). While sleep disturbance
is not a core symptom of these reactions, it is nevertheless commonly
seen in children and teens who are under stress and have experienced
an upsetting event. Youngsters who experience such emotional reactions commonly benefit from counseling and psychotherapy in order to
help them cope with the stressors. If insomnia is apparent, an adjunct
use of a hypnotic agent may be beneficial. However, clinicians should
administer treatment that comprehensively focuses on helping the child
or adolescent cope with the stressful events.

ETIOLOGY

As discussed previously, insomnia may occur at various points of the
night, including the onset of sleep, the middle of the night, or the final
phase of sleep early in the morning. To understand the regulation of
sleep, it must be recognized that different mechanisms are involved in
the onset of sleep and the maintenance of sleep through the night. Both
are reviewed below.

Onset of Sleep

Sleep is regulated by several parts of the brain. The reticular formation, a portion of the brain stem, is involved in regulating alertness.
During waking hours, various regions of the reticular formation release
dopamine, norepinephrine, and serotonin, and activate the pathways for
these neurotransmitters that in turn regulate many psychological functions, including attention and focusing, cognitive processes involved in
problem solving and decision making, and emotional functioning. When
individuals exhibit difficulties falling asleep, it is apparent that these portions of the brain remain too active and do not begin to decrease activity (Nofzinger et al., 2005). Consequently, the brain continues to exhibit
levels of activity associated with wakefulness and sleep onset is delayed.

The hypothalamic–pituitary–adrenal axis has especially been implicated in this hyperarousal (Richardson et al., 2005). The hypothalamus
regulates the functioning of the pituitary, which in turn regulates most hormone release. Since the reticular formation activates the hypothalamus, it
is possible that overactivation of the brain stem leads to overactivation of
the hypothalamus, which in turn does not send the necessary signals to the
pituitary to begin to slow down brain activation in preparation for sleep.

Melatonin seems to play a major role in preparing the brain for sleep. It is a neurotransmitter and a hormone, synthesized from serotonin in some areas of the brain, especially including the pineal gland and the retina. The retina begins to release melatonin when light patterns change and more darkness is evident (as is the case at night, the time when most people sleep). The pineal gland releases melatonin in response to circadian rhythms that signal that it is time to go to sleep. The paraventricular nucleus of the hypothalamus responds by signaling the brain stem to lower the release of various stimulatory neurotransmitters, including norepinephrine, acetylcholine, serotonin, and histamine. The ventrolateral preoptic area also contributes to this process by increasing the release of GABA, especially in nerve pathways that lead to the brain stem. As the brain stem begins to slow the release of excitatory neurotransmitters, drowsiness is experienced and sleep onset is promoted.

Maintenance of Sleep

As sleep is initiated, the brain gradually slows neuronal activity and brain waves evident on the EEG become increasingly slower. At the same time, the amplitude of these waves is magnified. This appears to be regulated by thalamic neurons that connect with various portions of the cortex and gradually begin to be hyperpolarized and fire in slow bursts. Along with these changes, blood flow and glucose metabolism decrease by more than 40 percent (Hobson, 1999). This change in firing stimulates the pituitary to activate the endocrine system and the immune system. Greater releases of hormones are evident, and production of white blood cells is increased. While the exact mechanisms that propel these processes are not known, adenosine seems to play a role. During states of wakefulness, adenosine is gradually released and becomes accumulated, eventually contributing to the feeling of fatigue and drowsiness. During sleep, levels of adenosine seem to regulate the amount of time the body spends in non-REM sleep – the more adenosine was accumulated during waking hours, the more time the body will spend in non-REM sleep. This process may especially be relevant to children and adolescents, since they spend a greater amount of time in non-REM sleep than adults.

REM sleep seems to be regulated by different mechanisms. Since REM sleep involves brain waves that are closer in speed and amplitude to those seen during wakefulness, excitatory neurotransmitters seem to be involved in promoting and maintaining REM episodes. Acetylcholine activity, in particular, has been shown to regulate REM episodes, and people exposed to acetylcholine antagonists spend less time in REM sleep, while those who take acetylcholine agonists exhibit longer REM episodes and shorter intervals between REM sleep portions (Sitaram *et al.*, 1978). Acetylcholine nuclei in the peribrachial area of the brain stem seem to especially be involved in this regulation.

Although acetylcholine neurons seem to directly trigger REM episodes, the length of each REM stage is probably regulated by other neurotransmitters, especially norepinephrine and serotonin. As these neurons 'awake' and begin firing, they inhibit the firing of the acetylcholine neurons and REM episodes come to a close. The thermostat that regulates the length of these episodes is not known, but circadian rhythms regulated by the suprachiasmatic nucleus are thought to be responsible for the regulation of REM stages. The cycle of neuronal firing in the suprachiasmatic nucleus normally runs about 24 hours, but disturbances are common, and these are referred to as 'free wheeling cycles.' In some cases, the circadian cycles may run less than 24 hours (for example, 20 hours), and therefore when sleep is not initiated each time the cycle is completed, REM episodes may occur more frequently, since after falling asleep, the suprachiasmatic nucleus may suppress non-REM sleep and enter REM episodes prematurely. In other cases, free wheeling cycles may run longer than 24 hours (for example, 25 hours). When this occurs, problems falling asleep may become evident and time spent in REM may be decreased. When the cycle of REM/non-REM sleep is disturbed, night-time awakenings can occur.

SUPPLEMENTS WITH ESTABLISHED EFFICACY

Strategies that aim to address insomnia generally target the specific portion of the night during which sleep problems occur – falling asleep at the beginning of the night, awakening in the middle of the night, or waking up too early in the morning. This is accomplished by administering sleep-promoting agents with various half-lives. Those with short half-life are used to address early insomnia, and those with longer half-lives are used to address sleep problems in the middle of the night and in the early morning. Naturopathic agents, however, are only used to promote sleep at the beginning of the night, and most have short half-life. Only one has sufficiently been researched to establish its efficacy in empirical trials.

Melatonin

Melatonin is a neurotransmitter and a hormone that is involved in triggering the 'sleep switch.' When melatonin is released, brain stem reduces the activation of catecholamine, acetylcholine, and histamine pathways, and a feeling of sleepiness is experienced. It is possible that insomnia results from the insufficient activation of the 'sleep switch' and as a result the brain continues to remain in a state of full wakefulness when it is time to go to sleep. This may be due to an insufficient amount of melatonin being converted from serotonin. To remedy this problem, supplemental melatonin can be taken at about the time when the patient should begin to get ready for bed.

Many neurotransmitter and hormones are not effective when taken exogenously. Sometimes, these chemicals become completely metabolized before entering systemic circulation, and in other cases the compound may survive metabolism but does not cross the blood–brain barrier. For this reason, the vast majority of neurotransmitters are useless when taken as supplements. However, melatonin does not become fully metabolized on first pass effect and crosses the blood–brain barrier, and therefore supplementation with melatonin has been shown to be useful.

Evidence of Efficacy

Results of numerous studies have found that melatonin is effective as a treatment for initial insomnia (Medical Economics, 2008a). The presumption in this line of research is that raising melatonin levels to those that should be evident during normal states of sleepiness restores normal sleep patterns. Unfortunately, the specific dose required to exert this effect has not been established, and various research studies utilized dosages of 0.3–5 mg, although the median dose in these studies fell between 2 and 3 mg (Medical Economics). In a more recent double-blind study, a two-stage design was utilized to compare the use of melatonin to benzodiazepine and placebo in adults with initial insomnia. Results revealed that melatonin was not only more effective than placebo, it also exerted more beneficial effects than the benzodiazepine and eventually patients on benzodiazepine switched to the melatonin with good results (Bursztajn, 1999). In a similar study, Garfinkel et al. (1999) obtained similar results, and melatonin was also found to be effective in addressing sleep disturbance associated with major depression ((Dolberg et al., 1998). Although melatonin has been shown in several studies to decrease the time to sleep onset and increase sleep duration, it has not been shown to improve sleep quality (Almeida Montes et al., 2003). Consequently, it is considered to be a better treatment for initial insomnia rather than sleep problems that occur during the middle of the night or in the early morning.

In children, similar results have been obtained. For example, in a double-blind, placebo-controlled study with 62 children, melatonin has been shown to promote sleep onset in children ages 6–12 without significant adverse effects (Smits *et al.*, 2003). Another study found similar results with children previously diagnosed with Asperger's disorder (Paavonen *et al.*, 2003). Weiss *et al.* (2006) also obtained positive effects using a combination of sleep hygiene and melatonin to treat children and adolescents with ADHD who exhibited initial insomnia. These studies seem to have obtained positive results with a median dose of 5 mg, but lower doses have also sometimes found to be effective (Brzezinski *et al.*, 2005). In addition, adverse events have been reported to be minimal and no rebound insomnia upon discontinuation was evident.

Some, however, have cautioned that melatonin may not be safe for everyone. In a small study of children and adolescents with neurologic disorders, six individuals, aged 6 months to 18 years, were given 5 mg of melatonin at bedtime. Although sleep latency improved in all subjects, four of the six participants (all of whom had prior history of seizures) exhibited increased frequency of seizures (Medical Economics, 2008a). Consequently, it is apparent that melatonin should not be utilized with individuals with neurological problems and seizures.

Pharmacodynamics

The main effect of melatonin is derived from its binding to its own endogenous receptors. Three types have been identified. One of which, the MT3 receptor, is not involved in sleep mediation and may play a role in immune function and anti-oxidant activity. However, the MT1 and MT2 receptors mediate sleep, and melatonin binds to these post-synaptic receptors directly (Stahl, 2008). More specifically, the MT1a subtype of the MT1 receptor seems to be prevalent in the suprachiasmatic nucleus of the hypothalamus, and stimulation of this receptor activates the 'sleep switch.' It is a g-protein coupled metabotropic receptor that alters the activity of catecholamines, acetylcholine, and histamine by decreasing its release in the brain stem. Thus, the primary hypnotic effect of melatonin comes from direct stimulation of the MT1a postsynaptic receptor.

Pharmacokinetics

Melatonin is absorbed from the small intestine and is then partially metabolized in the liver into 6-hydroxymelatonin, an inactive metabolite that is excreted by the kidneys. The remaining portion enters systemic circulation and travels to the brain and other tissues. The onset of effect varies widely, and peak concentrations are reported to occur about

60 minutes after ingestion. The half-life is short, generally ranging from about 20–50 minutes (Bezchlibnyk-Butler & Jeffries, 2007). The onset of effect usually occurs in about 30 minutes, but some studies reported more significant latency. For this reason, some recommend taking melatonin in the evening, a few hours before bedtime. When used regularly in this manner, it seems that the release of endogenous melatonin may be advanced by as much as 3 hours, and sleep onset may become more regular. In addition, with chronic dosing, some lipid storage of melatonin may occur, further increasing the availability of melatonin at bedtime (Medical Economics, 2008a).

Dosing

In research studies, melatonin is generally dosed anywhere from less than 1 mg to about 5 mg, although some research studies used doses as high as 10 mg. Most researchers, however, recommend doses up to 5 mg and doses above 5 mg may not contribute additional beneficial effect (Bezchlibnyk-Butler & Jeffries, 2007), and doses above 3 mg for longer periods of time may require medical supervision (Medical Economics, 2008a). Melatonin supplements derived from animals should be avoided.

Doses less than 1 mg are considered to be 'physiological doses' – that is, minimal doses exerting some physiological effects within the body. Clinical doses are usually higher. Melatonin in generally available in capsules of 3, 5, or 10 mg, although lower doses may sometimes be found on the Internet. It seems prudent to begin the administration of melatonin at a dose of 2 or 3 mg, and a trial of 2 weeks should be performed before the dose is increased. With minimal response, the dose may be increased to 5 mg. If partial response is evident, cautious trials of higher doses may be attempted, but medical supervision should be sought.

Although melatonin has a quick onset of effect and a short half-life, it seems that its effects do not become fully evident for at least 1 hour. In fact, some suggest that melatonin is most effective when administered about 2 hours before bedtime (Bezchlibnyk-Butler & Jeffries, 2007). For this reason, it seems appropriate to recommend that melatonin be taken about 1–2 hours before bedtime.

Adverse Effects

Melatonin is usually well tolerated, although a minority of patients may exhibit some adverse effects. A minority of patients may report some gastrointestinal discomfort and headaches. Although melatonin has short half-life, a minority of patients report a morning 'hangover' effect, including grogginess, lethargy, and difficulties with concentration.

These are generally more common with higher doses, but individual patient response should carefully be monitored.

Patients who take medications or naturopathic supplements that alter the action of monoamines (especially, serotonin) should generally avoid the use of melatonin, and psychotic reactions with concomitant use have been reported (Medical Economics, 2008a). However, melatonin has also been shown to be effective in improving sleep of patients with schizophrenia (Bezchlibnyk-Butler & Jeffries, 2007), so the presence of a psychotic disorder is not necessarily an automatic contraindication.

Although research findings indicate that melatonin may help reduce insomnia associated with depression, in other cases, melatonin may exacerbate depression (Medical Economics, 2008a). Thus, those patients who are depressed need to carefully be monitored when they are treated with melatonin.

At higher doses (usually, above 5 mg), additional problems may become evident, including disorientation, amnesia, suppression of sexual drive, hypothermia, and retinal damage. For this reason, doses above 5 mg should only be used under careful monitoring by a medical prescriber. In addition, one study reported a correlation between decreased gonadal development and use of melatonin in children (Commentz et al., 1997). A decade old, the study thus far has not been replicated. However, parents concerned about this potential risk should consult their medical professional to discuss this possible risk.

SUPPLEMENTS WITH LIKELY EFFICACY

Some nutritional and herbal compounds have been investigated and results of research studies show promising results. In some cases, these compounds have been established to be effective in adults but have not been extensively researched with children. Compounds that may be effective, but do not yet show adequate efficacy in research studies, are reviewed in this section.

Valerian

Valerian (*Valeriana officinalis*) is a medicinal plant endogenous to Europe and Asia and widely introduced in North America. Various portions of the plant are consumed for medicinal reasons, including the flowers, fruit, and leaves. However, it is valerian root that is considered to be most psychoactive and its extracts are used as hypnotics and anxiolytics.

As discussed in Chapter 8, the use of valerian as an anxiolytic is experimental, but its use as a hypnotic is better supported. In Germany, Commission E has approved valerian as a naturopathic supplement to treat sleep disorders, and research evidence from numerous studies with adults supports its effectiveness. However, very few studies have been done with children or adolescents.

Evidence of Efficacy

A systematic review of randomized clinical trials, some of which were placebo controlled, revealed that valerian is an effective treatment for insomnia, and its repeated, short-term use reduced sleep latency, improved quality of sleep, and promoted sleep maintenance (Stevenson & Ernst, 2000). Another meta-analysis examined 16 studies that researched the use of valerian with a total of 1093 patients, and found similar results, although a wide range of dosages were evident, making it difficult to form recommendations about effective doses (Bent et al., 2006). Other studies have reported similar results. In a multicenter, placebo-controlled study of 121 patients, Vorbach et al. (1996) found that about two-thirds of the patients reported significant improvement on valerian, while less than one-third improved on placebo. Positive effects of using valerian have also been reported to be related to a change in sleep architecture, including decreased time in Stages 1 and 2 of sleep, and increased duration of REM sleep (Schulz et al., 1994).

The use of valerian with children or adolescents has rarely been researched. In one small study, five children and adolescents (aged 5–14 years) were given doses of 20 mg/kg of valerian in a double-blind, cross-over, placebo-controlled trial. Results revealed that valerian was helpful in decreasing sleep latency, increasing sleep quality, and improving ratings of sleep quality (Francis & Dempster, 2002). Other, small studies, reported similar findings (Bezchlibnyk-Butler & Jeffries, 2007). It is apparent, therefore, that evidence is beginning to emerge about the effectiveness of valerian with this population, but further studies are needed to confirm these findings.

Pharmacodynamics

Like most herbal compounds, valerian has many active ingredients. By one count, valerian may have 150 individual compounds (Morin et al., 2007). Consequently, its action is likely to be very broad, and its hypnotic effects may be one of many other effects that this herb may precipitate.

Although the effects of the specific constituents have not been identified, the overall effect of supplementation with valerian is the depression of central nervous activity, including drowsiness, muscle relaxation, sedation, and a decrease in anxiety. Some data suggests that these effects may be primarily caused by valerenic acid, but other ingredients in valerian extracts may magnify this effect (Medical Economics, 2007).

This sedative effect may be due to changes in the affinity of cortical membrane receptors, including hyperpolarization (Andreatini & Leite, 1994). This is probably the result of changes in the activity of GABA, the major inhibitory neurotransmitter in the brain. As GABA levels increase, chloride channels on cell membranes open and the cells become hyperpolarized. Valerian increases activity of GABA in a variety of ways. Valerian may block, and perhaps reverse, the reuptake of GABA, thus increasing synaptic concentrations of GABA. In addition, valerian may also inhibit the metabolism of GABA, and may even act as a precursor for GABA synthesis (Spinella, 2001). As GABA activity increases, sedation becomes apparent and sleep onset is promoted.

Pharmacokinetics

Valerian is supplied in capsules, tablets, and liquid preparations, as an extract to be taken as drops (in a base, as in apple sauce) or dissolved in a tincture. Liquid preparations are absorbed more quickly, and tablets and capsules may take about 30–60 minutes longer to be absorbed. Pharmacokinetics are not well established, but onset of effect is generally seen in less than 1 hour. Various compounds present in valerian are metabolized through different mechanisms and at different rates, further complicating its use. However, it is apparent that clinical effects generally wear off after about 4–6 hours. Moreover, some have suggested that continued use of valerian, at the effective dose, does not result in tolerance to the effect (Spinella, 2001).

Dosing

To prepare an infusion, 2–3 g of the compound are added to a cup, or 1 teaspoon of the extract is added to about 150 ml of hot water (to brew, like a tea). Plant juice is also available for direct administration with a teaspoon or tablespoon. Capsules and tablets are ingested in the usual manner, and standardized preparations should be sought.

The daily dosage varies widely and exact recommendations are not established. Daily dose may range from 100–1800 mg, depending on the method of ingestion and the amount of the active compounds present in preparations available from different manufacturers. Studied dosages range from 1.5–3 g of actual herb or root, or 400–900 mg of an extract, taken up to 1 hour before bedtime. Bezchlibnyk-Butler and Jeffries (2007) recommend a dose of 200–1200 mg/day (with adults).

With children and adolescents, only one study established dosage guidelines, reporting effectiveness as a dose of 20 mg/kg (Francis & Dempster, 2002). Thus, it is apparent that the lowest possible dose should be started with children or adolescents, and dosage should gradually be titrated, every few days, until the 20 mg/kg ratio is evident. Doses above this ratio should only be used under medical supervision.

Adverse Effects

Valerian is usually well tolerated, although a minority of patients may exhibit some adverse effects. Some patients may report some gastrointestinal discomfort and headaches, as well as feeling of restlessness and heart dysrhythmias. These are generally more common with higher doses or when the compound is used for extended periods of time, but individual patient response should carefully be monitored.

Valerian is associated with a small risk of hepatic damage. This risk is significantly increased when patients already take medications or other supplements that carry a similar risk. For this reason, use of valerian with other supplements should generally be avoided, unless the other supplement has no documented risk of hepatotoxicity. Use of valerian with medications should only be done under careful medical supervision. Even when valerian is used in monotherapy, some recommend periodic liver function tests to monitor the health of the liver (Bezchlibnyk-Butler & Jeffries, 2007).

Because valerian is a sedative, concurrent use of other compounds that exert similar effects (for example, alcohol) should be avoided. Because alcohol also exerts liver effects, it is especially important to make sure that patients who take valerian do not drink alcohol. While this is not usually a risk for children, this needs to be stressed when valerian is used with adolescents.

Valerian may interfere with the absorption of iron. For this reason, those who require iron supplementation should not take the two compounds together, and should take iron at other times of day (Medical Economics, 2007).

At higher doses, additional problems may become evident, including severe headaches, nausea and vomiting, dizziness, stupor, and cardiac dysfunction. Doses above the 20 mg/kg ratio should only be used under careful monitoring by a medical prescriber.

Tryptophan

Tryptophan, also referred to as L-tryptophan, is an essential amino acid. Of all essential amino acids, it is the one that is least abundant.

It is a protein with many functions in the body, and it is a building block for many endogenous substances. It is also a precursor for serotonin, and as such, it is a precursor for melatonin. Consequently, it has been researched as a hypnotic, and some studies support its efficacy. However, research with children and adolescents is very limited.

Tryptophan is also a precursor for Vitamin B3 as well as several important enzymes. Since tryptophan must be ingested in food, the WHO has set a typical recommended daily intake for tryptophan at 4 mg/kg of body weight (WHO, 2007). Tryptophan is found in a wide variety of protein-containing foods, including eggs, cheese, meat (especially turkey), fish, wheat, rice, potatoes, and bananas.

Supplementation with tryptophan has been attempted for over 40 years. However, in the late 1980s, 1500 cases of eosinophilia-myalgia syndrome, including 30 deaths, were caused by contaminated batches of tryptophan. In 1989, sale of tryptophan supplements was banned in the United States, but recently it was revealed that problems in manufacture were responsible for these deaths and the supplement is potentially safe. Consequently, sales of tryptophan as a supplement were allowed to resume in 2001, and the FDA ban on tryptophan supplement importation was lifted in 2005. However, all along, prescription tryptophan has been available for sale. At this time, Monarch Pharmaceuticals continue to manufacture a prescription capsule of tryptophan at a strength of 500 mg (Medical Economics, 2008b).

Evidence of Efficacy

Tryptophan has been researched for over four decades. Although much of the research focused on supplementation with tryptophan to augment the action of antidepressants (see Chapter 6), some studies were performed that investigated its efficacy as a hypnotic. Because tryptophan was withdrawn from market for over a decade, and was only reintroduced recently, most of the research is dated. Several small studies exist that suggest that improvement in sleep is seen with the use of tryptophan supplements. The data supports claims that sleep latency is reduced, and some studies also suggested that overall length of sleep also improved. A recent study that examined age-related sleep effects confirmed tryptophan's efficacy in improving sleep onset. In research studies, dosages have ranged from 1–15 g (1000–15,000 mg), and because of this wide margin, it is difficult to estimate the dosage at which clinical effects are expected (Medical Economics, 2007). In addition, thus far the use of tryptophan has not been researched with children or adolescents.

Pharmacodynamics

Tryptophan is a precursor for serotonin, and, consequently, it also acts as an indirect precursor for melatonin. When administered as a supplement, tryptophan crosses the blood–brain barrier and is thought to exert its clinical effect by acting in the suprachiasmatic nucleus of the hypothalamus to increase the synthesis of melatonin. Melatonin then binds to post-synaptic receptors, especially the MT1a. When higher levels of melatonin are evident, the 'sleep switch' is activated and brain stem functions decrease the activation of monoaminergic pathways, promoting sedation and sleep.

Pharmacokinetics

Following ingestion, tryptophan is absorbed from the small intestine and metabolized in the liver. In the liver, tryptophan undergoes several chemical reactions, including protein synthesis and oxidative catabolic reactions. The portion not synthesized during first pass effect enters systemic circulation and becomes distributed to the brain and other tissues.

Tryptophan is converted by the enzyme tryptophan hydroxylase into 5-hydroxytryptophan, which is then converted into serotonin with the assistance of B6-dependent aromatic amino acid decarboxylase. Serotonin is then converted to N-acetylserotonin, and finally to melatonin by the enzyme hydroxyindole-O-methyltransferase (Medical Economics, 2007).

When ingested, tryptophan supplements take about 30–60 minutes to be absorbed. Pharmacokinetics are not well established, but onset of effect is generally seen in less than 1 hour. The half-life of tryptophan is presumed to be very short due to its rapid conversion into serotonin and melatonin. However, the duration of clinical effects vary and generally last several hours. This is likely due to the increase in monoamines that is precipitated by the administration of tryptophan.

Dosing

Tryptophan tablets are generally available in tablets and capsules with dosages ranging from 50–1000 mg. Because research studies identified a very wide range of effective dose, trial and error is likely to be necessary to determine the appropriate dose for a specific patient. Children and adolescents should begin with a dosage of 50–100 mg about 1 hour before bedtime, and the dose should gradually be titrated, every few days, until clinical response is evident. Doses above 1000 mg/day should only be used under medical supervision.

Adverse Effects

Tryptophan is usually well tolerated, although some patients may exhibit daytime drowsiness, dizziness, and dry mouth. At higher doses, additional problems with nausea, lack of appetite, and headaches may become evident (Medical Economics, 2007). Because tryptophan is a sedative, concurrent use of other compounds that exert similar effects (for example, alcohol) should be avoided.

Tryptophan is associated with a small risk of cardiac dysfunctions. Because tryptophan is converted into serotonin in the brain as well as peripherally, increases in serotonin may become evident in tissues and muscles, including the heart. For this reason, some recommend that tryptophan supplements should only be taken with carbidopa, which blocks the conversion of tryptophan into serotonin until it crosses the blood–brain barrier (Xu *et al.*, 2002).

Tryptophan needs to be used cautiously with patients who have been diagnosed with diabetes or exhibit family history of diabetes. One of tryptophan's metabolites, xanthurenic acid, has been found to have a diabetogenic effect in animals. Although no cases in humans have been reported, caution should be exercised.

SUPPLEMENTS WITH POSSIBLE EFFICACY

In addition to the supplements discussed above, there is some data available that suggests that other compounds may also have some efficacy in treating insomnia. However, since the data that supports the use of the following supplements is extremely limited, clinicians should proceed with caution, and consider the use of the compounds discussed in this section as experimental.

Phenibut

Phenibut, also known as fenibut, phenigamma, and beta-phenyl-gamma-aminobutyric acid, is a derivative of the neurotransmitter GABA. It was developed in Russia, and there it has been used clinically since the 1960s to treat anxiety and related conditions, including insomnia (Lapin, 2001). Phenibut has anxiolytic properties and is commonly compared to benzodiazepines and baclofen. Structurally, phenibut is similar to GABA, with the addition of the phenyl ring. This allows the compound to more easily cross the blood–brain barrier, but also changes its activity profile (Shulgina, 1986). Like baclofen, phenibut extensively binds to GABA B receptors, but its psychoactive effects are similar to those of benzodiazepines.

Although phenibut primarily binds to GABA B receptors, it also increases release of GABA and has some effect on GABA A receptors. GABA B receptors may be involved in inhibition of the release of some neurotransmitters (for example, monoamines), and GABA A receptors regulate the activity of chloride channels. When open, the influx of chloride hyperpolarizes the membrane and cell firing decreases. By affecting both GABA A and B receptors, phenibut may exert sedative, hypnotic, and muscle relaxant properties. Phenibut may also exert serotonergic effects (Nurmand *et al.*, 1980), but these hypothesized effects have not been confirmed.

When administered as a hypnotic, usual doses range from 250–500 mg. Since most of the drug is excreted unchanged (Lapin, 2001), it is apparent that the compound is not metabolized by the liver and enters systemic circulation unchanged. Onset of effect is generally within an hour, and plasma half-life has been reported to be about 5 hours (Shulgina, 1986).

Adverse effects of phenibut may include a morning hangover effect, including grogginess, lethargy, and difficulties with concentration. In higher doses, and when used for longer periods, discontinuation may result in withdrawal effects similar to those seen with benzodiazepines, including acute anxiety, insomnia, agitation, and, in some cases, seizures. Tolerance to phenibut can develop quite rapidly, and when the compound is used for long periods of time, it is usually discontinued for a day or 2 every 5 days or so (Chojnacka-Wójcik *et al.*, 1975).

Phenibut may inhibit some liver enzymes, and, consequently, there is a potential for drug interactions. While the specific liver enzymes have not be identified, phenibut is not recommended with opiate analgesics. In addition, other compounds that affect GABA, including benzodiazepines, hypnotics, and alcohol, should be avoided.

Hops

Hops is the flower cones of the hop plant (*Humulus lupulus*). It is an ingredient of beer, but is also consumed as a tea. As a supplement, it is sold as liquid, powder, or in tablets and capsules. Some research evidence has suggested that hops may promote sedation, and in folklore hops flowers have been placed on the pillow with the belief that the smell helps induce sleep (Spinella, 2001). Results of some research studies suggested that hops may exert anxiolytic and sedative effects

(Kowalchik & Hylon, 1987), and hops has been shown to improve sleep in some male subjects (Widy-Tyszkiewicz & Schminda, 1997), particularly when added to 170 mg of valerian. It is approved as a sleep aid by Commission E. The use of hops in children and adolescents has not been researched.

The pharmacology of hops has not been established. Its sedative effect is deemed to be secondary to the action of one of its constituents, dimethylvinyl carbinol, a volatile alcoholic compound that may exert an effect within the GABA system of neurotransmission. This hypothesis, however, has not been confirmed, and some admit that the basis of the sedative effect is not fully known, although it is considered to be well established (Bradley, 1992).

When used as a sedative hypnotic, it is usually given in a single dose of 1–2 g before bedtime. If a liquid extract is used, 0.5–2 ml should be given, or 1–2 ml should be dissolved in a tincture. An infusion may also be prepared, where boiling water is poured over 1–2 g of ground hop cones (where 1 teaspoon of the powder equals about 0.4 g of the active compound).

Hops is usually well tolerated and adverse effects are not common. As with other sedative hypnotics, morning hangover may be evident characterized by sleepiness, lethargy, and problems with concentration. With the exception of valerian, hops should not be used with other sedatives, including alcohol, and it is contraindicated in pregnancy. When used with female teens who may be sexually active, the need for consistent use of contraception must be stressed. In rare cases, blood disorders (hemolysis), severe allergic reactions (anaphylaxis), and jaundice have been reported (Medical Economics, 2007). The fresh plant also exacerbates respiratory allergies in some patients. In addition, some sources recommend against the use of hops with patients who present a history of depression (Medical Economics), although exacerbation of depression with hops is not well documented.

Rauwolfia

Rauwolfia (*Rauwolfia serpentina*), also spelled ravolphia, is a medicinal shrub in the milkweed family. Its root is ground into a powder and packaged in this form or sold in tablets or capsules. It is a compound commonly used in Asian medicine, including traditional Ayurveda medicine native to India. Its active components are alkaloids and about 50 have been identified, although the primary psychoactive components appear to be reserpine, rescinnamine, and deserpidine (Spinella, 2001). The primary effect of these alkaloids is the blockage of vesicular storage of monoamines, ultimately leading to greater degradation of these neurotransmitters by the MAO enzyme and an overall decrease in neuronal activity in monoamine pathways. Thus, the overall effect is inhibitory and sedative.

Rauwolfia is best supported as an antipsychotic (see Chapter 11), and in eastern medicine it also continues to be used as a tranquilizer. The compound is approved by Commission E for the treatment of hypertension and insomnia. However, its utility is limited by its wide-ranging effects. When administered, rauwolfia reduces blood pressure and may result in dizziness. In addition, rauwolfia exerts a significant antagonistic effect on dopamine. Although this may promote sedation and sleep, it may also cause unpleasant side effects commonly associated with antipsychotic medications, including problems with coordination and stereotypic movements. If utilized, rauwolfia should carefully be monitored for adverse effects, and it seems most prudent to recommend its occasional use only with adolescents, not children. The typical dose is 600 mg/day, taken about 1 hour before bedtime. Since the use of rauwolfia results in a decrease of monoamine activity, those who take this compound should be monitored for the possible onset of depressive symptoms. In addition, rauwolfia is contraindicated during pregnancy, so if it is used with adolescent females, they need to be counseled about the need to use contraception (Medical Economics, 2007).

SUPPLEMENTS NOT LIKELY TO BE EFFECTIVE

It is not possible to review all compounds that, at one time or another, have been tried to treat symptoms of insomnia and have not shown to be effective, or lack sufficient rationale about how they may affect brain action to promote sleep. However, some of these compounds are sometimes marketed to improve sleep, despite the lack of evidence of efficacy. Clinicians who seek to practice in the area of naturopathic psychopharmacology should be aware of compounds that continue to be propagated despite evidence to the contrary.

Kava

Kava (*Piper methysticum*), sometimes referred to as kava is an herb that is approved by Commission E for the treatment of anxiety, stress, restlessness, tension, and agitation. It contains a plethora of active ingredients, including many kava lactones. Because of its efficacy in treating symptoms of anxiety, some have assumed that it is also effective as a hypnotic. Indeed, one small, open-label study found that 24 adults improved their sleep habits on the compound (Wheatley, 2001). However, the results of this study have been questioned by many because of significant methodological flaws (Medical Economics, 2007). In addition, other researchers have obtained results that suggested that kava is not effective as a sleep aid (Morin *et al.*, 2007).

Kava is widely used as an anxiolytic and adverse effects are rare. However, in some cases, use of kava has been associated with potential risks of severe liver injury (FDA, 2002), and the sale of kava is regulated in many countries, where kava is only dispensed with a medical prescription. Milder adverse effects are more common, including changes in vision, mydriasis, and disturbances in eye tracking, as well as impaired motor reflexes and rare difficulties in motor coordination, including choreoathetosis. In addition, because of kava's extensive inhibition of liver enzymes, the use of kava should be avoided with the vast majority of medications. All in all, given the possible danger and the minimal evidence of efficacy, use of kava as a hypnotic is not recommended.

Chamomile

Chamomile (*Matricaria Recutita*), also referred to sometimes as German chamomile, is an herb that it approved by Commission E to treat cough and bronchitis, fevers, cold, inflammation, infection, wounds, and burns. It is believed by some to have sedative and anticonvulsant effects, and a small amount of research supports these effects (Medical Economics, 2007). As discussed in Chapter 8, it may offer some benefits as an anxiolytic, and consequently some have argued that it may have some hypnotic effects, but many researchers disagree and maintain that chamomile is not effective as a sleep aid (Morin *et al.*, 2007). Indeed, there is no empirical evidence supporting its use as a hypnotic (Medical Economics). While no significant dangers are associated with the use of chamomile and the herb is usually well tolerated, its use as a sleep aid is not likely to produce any beneficial effects and parents and clinicians are encouraged to try more effective alternatives.

Passion Flower

Passion flower (*Passiflora incarnata*) is an herb that is approved by Commission E to treat nervousness and insomnia, but its hypnotic effects are not widely supported. As discussed in Chapter 8, passion flower may offer some limited benefits as an anxiolytic, but the use of the herb as a sleep aid needs further investigation. Currently, its use as a hypnotic falls into the category of 'unproven uses' (Medical Economics, 2007, p. 634). Indeed, another review of literature concluded that passion flower is not effective as a sleep aid (Morin *et al.*, 2007). While no significant dangers are associated with the use of passion flower and the herb is usually well tolerated, its use as a sleep aid is not likely to produce any beneficial effects and parents and clinicians are encouraged to try more effective alternatives.

Scullcap

Scullcap (*Scutellaria lateriflora*), sometimes also spelled skullcap, is an herb that has sometimes been presumed to be effective for hysteria, nervous tension, epilepsy, chorea, and other psychological disorders. A review of literature concluded that its psychogenic effects are not proven and the use of the herb as an anxiolytic or a sleep aid needs further investigation, and its use for these reasons falls into the category of 'unproven uses' (Medical Economics, 2007, p. 739). Indeed, another review of literature concluded that scullcap is not effective as a sleep aid (Morin *et al.*, 2007). While no significant dangers are associated with the use of scullcap and the herb is usually well tolerated, its use as a sleep aid is not likely to produce any beneficial effects and parents and clinicians are encouraged to try more effective alternatives.

Lemon Balm

Lemon balm (*Melissa officinalis*) is a plant that is sometimes used in its dried form (or by extracting its oil) as an antibacterial, antiviral, and anti-oxidative agent. It is also approved by Commission E as a treatment for nervousness and insomnia, and it is commonly used in folk medicine to treat anxiety, gastric complaints (especially associated with stress), hysteria, melancholia, nervous palpitations, migraine, headaches, and high blood pressure. Homeopathically it is sometimes also used for menstrual irregularities. However, a review of literature concluded that its psychogenic effects are not proven and the use of the herb as an anxiolytic or a sleep aid falls into the category of 'unproven uses' (Medical Economics, 2007, p. 515). Indeed, another review of literature concluded that lemon balm is not effective as a sleep aid (Morin *et al.*, 2007). While no significant dangers are associated with the use of lemon balm and the herb is usually well tolerated, its use as a sleep aid is not likely to produce any beneficial effects and parents and clinicians are encouraged to try more effective alternatives.

Coenzyme Q10

Coenzyme Q10 is a vitamin-like substance that is sold as a nutritional supplement. It was discovered in 1957, and has since been used to treat a variety of disorders, including cardiac difficulties (especially, congestive heart failure), hypertension, high blood cholesterol, and some neurodegenerative diseases. Because it seems to drop blood pressure, some have also hypothesized that it may exert sedative and hypnotic properties. However, a review of literature revealed no data that support any psychogenic effects (Medical Economics, 2007), and another review of literature concluded that coenzyme Q10 is not effective as a sleep aid (Morin *et al.*, 2007). Since administration of coenzyme Q10 seems to lower blood pressure and alters cardiac function, and since its use as a sleep aid is not likely to produce any beneficial effects, parents and clinicians are discouraged from using coenzyme Q10 as a hypnotic.

SUMMARY

In order to help clinicians select the compounds that are appropriate given the specific cluster of symptoms evident in each patient, an algorithm was developed and is presented in Figure 9.1. This diagram takes into account the amount of research support available for each compound, as well as the specific mechanism of action of each supplement and its applicability to the treatment of various types of insomnia.

Patients with symptoms of sleep-onset insomnia should initially be tried on melatonin. If insufficient response is obtained, the patient should be switched to valerian, and hops may be tried as an adjunct. If insufficient response is again evident, valerian and hops should be discontinued, and tryptophan supplements may be attempted. If insufficient response is still evident, tryptophan should be discontinued and phenibut may be attempted, although it should not be used every day. As a last resort, phenibut can be discontinued and rauwolfia can be tried, with careful monitoring of physical and psychological effects.

Patients with symptoms of sleep-maintenance problems should essentially follow the same algorithm, but a trial of melatonin may be skipped, since it is not likely to be useful in middle-onset or late-onset insomnia.

With the exception of a simultaneous trial of valerian and hops, use of multiple supplements should be avoided.

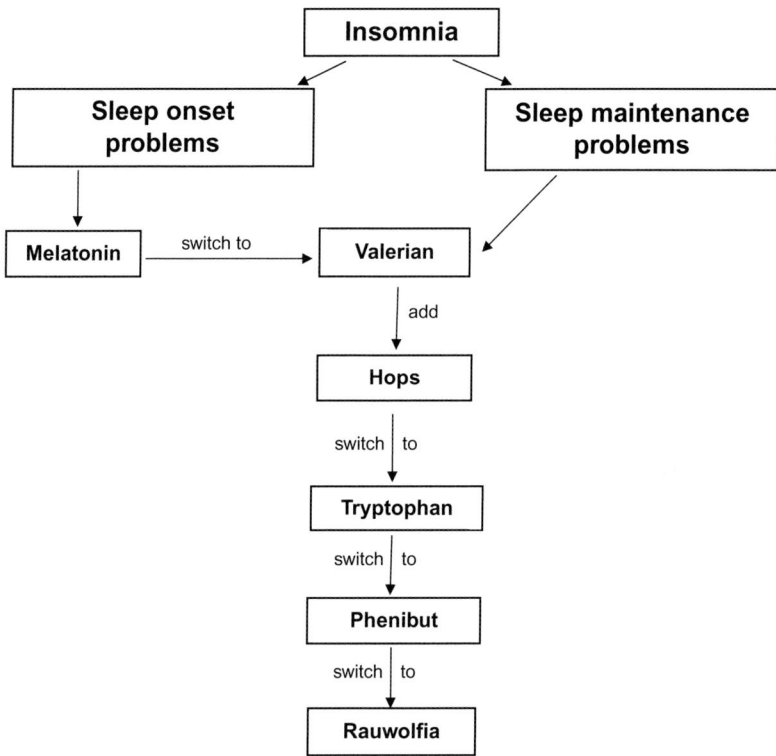

FIGURE 9.1   Algorithm for treatment of insomnia with naturopathic supplements.
© Elsevier 2009.

Chapter 10

Tic Disorders

With contributions from Debra Costanza and Nicholas Costanza

In 1885, Gilles de la Tourette was a 28-year old, practicing neurologist at the Salpetriere Hospital in Paris, France. Based on a description of nine patients he reviewed earlier with a condition characterized by multiple muscle tics, vocal noises, compulsive swearing, and other related behaviors, he began the journey of the discovery of the disorder that today bears his name.

A tic is a sudden, rapid, recurrent, non-rhythmic, stereotyped motor movement or vocalization. These occur spontaneously, although certain triggers (like stress) may be associated with increases in tic behaviors. The amount of control over these behaviors is very limited, and they are performed subconsciously, although awareness sometimes accompanies the tics. In some cases these may come and go, while others exhibit tics regularly and consistently. These differences must be examined when considering diagnostic and treatment options. DSM-IV-TR (APA, 2000) recognizes three specific tic disorders, and Tourette's is considered to be the most severe.

Tics are relatively common in children, less common in adolescents, and rare in adults. One review of research revealed that between 4 and 18 percent of children exhibit some form of tics during their development, and in the vast majority these disappear by adolescence (Peterson *et al.*, 2001a). Tourette's disorder, however, is rather rare and only occurs in about 0.05–0.3 percent of children, although some have placed the prevalence at about 10 times those rates (Robertson, 2003). Again, the vast majority of children with Tourette's eventually 'grow out' of the disorder, and the prevalence of Tourette's in adults is estimated to be about 0.01–0.02 percent (APA, 2000).

SYMPTOMS OF TIC DISORDERS

Children and adolescents with tic disorders exhibit repetitive sounds or motor behaviors, and in some cases both sets of symptoms are present.

Nutritional and Herbal Therapies for Children and Adolescents

These interfere with the youngster's ability to focus in school, hold a conversation, remain still when doing work, or attend places where it is necessary to remain still and quiet (for example, school, or a house of worship). Because these behaviors bring attention to the child or adolescent, patients with tic disorders often exhibit secondary social and emotional difficulties because they often encounter ridicule from their peers and frustration from adults around them.

Core Symptoms

Tics are generally divided into motor and vocal, and may further be divided into simple and complex. Simple motor tics are characterized by rapid, meaningless muscle contractions, such as eye blinking, and simple vocal tics include individual sounds, like grunting, or throat clearing. Complex motor tics are composite movements that involve the coordination of various muscle groups to perform a complex movement, such as touching, flexing, jerking, or stiffening of the head or neck, or striking oneself, and complex vocal tics include words or short phrases. The duration of the behavior generally separates the three tic disorders listed in the DSM.

Transient Tic Disorder

When a child or adolescent exhibits vocal and/or motor tics that occur many times per day, consistently (nearly every day) for a period of at least 1 month but less than 1 year, transient tic disorder (TTD) can be diagnosed. This is the most common of all tic disorders and may be evident in as many as 19 percent of all children (Bezchlibnyk-Butler & Virani, 2004). Generally, TTD is not diagnosed if the patient has a history of another tic disorder. Usually, tics come and go, and motor tics are more common than vocal tics. It is possible for children or adolescents to exhibit intermittent periods of tic episodes over many years, and the usual pattern is that the frequency of these tic episodes diminishes with age and eventually disappears.

TTD is rarely treated, and usually a wait-and-see approach is recommended. Because the tics come and go, there usually is no need for medical treatment, and therefore it is not likely that any naturopathic supplement will need to be used to treat symptoms of this disorder. If any treatment is needed, psychological approaches are generally utilized to help identify specific settings (like school or home) where the tics are more likely, and psychological states (like feeling anxious or stressed, sleepy and tired, or hungry) that may trigger the tic episodes.

Chronic Tic Disorder

Transient tics may progress to chronic tics. When a child or adolescent exhibits vocal *or* motor tics (but not both) that occur many times per day, consistently (nearly every day) for a period of at least 1 year, and the patient has not exhibited a tic-free period that lasted more than 3 consecutive months, chronic tic disorder (CTD) can be diagnosed. This disorder occurs in about 2–5 percent of all children (Bezchlibnyk-Butler & Virani, 2004). Only motor CTD or vocal CTD may be diagnosed, and both cannot coexist. Generally, CTD is not diagnosed if the patient has a history of Tourette's. Usually, tics are more consistent than those evident in TTD, and motor tics are more common than vocal tics. It is possible for children or adolescents to exhibit tics for many years, and the usual pattern is that the frequency and severity of tic episodes diminishes with age and eventually disappears.

CTD is not usually treated with medications, and therefore it is not likely that any naturopathic supplement will need to be used to treat symptoms of this disorder. As before, if treatment is needed, psychological approaches are generally utilized to help identify specific settings (like school or home) where the tics are more likely, and psychological states (like feeling anxious or stressed, sleepy and tired, or hungry) that may trigger the tic episodes. However, when the tics are very bothersome and/or embarrassing (for example, striking of oneself), or if vocal tics interfere with functioning in some settings (like in school), a trial of supplements may be utilized. In those cases, clinicians should try those compounds that have been shown to be effective in treating symptoms of Tourette's disorder (as described later in this chapter).

Tourette's Disorder

Either TTD or CTD may progress to Tourette's disorder (TD). When a child or adolescent exhibits vocal *and* motor tics that occur many times per day, consistently (nearly every day) for a period of at least 1 year, and the patient has not exhibited a tic-free period that lasted more than 3 consecutive months, TD can be diagnosed. Usually, tics are consistent (although active episodes usually wax and wane) and, along with vocal tics, complex motor tics are more common. Although symptoms of this disorder usually diminish with age and eventually disappear, a small portion of patients continues to exhibit symptoms into adulthood. TD is much more common in males, and some estimate the ratio to be as much as 10 : 1 (Bezchlibnyk-Butler & Virani, 2004).

The severity, number, location, frequency, and complexity of tics may change over time. Motor tics may include self-striking, or other extreme behaviors (including falling to the floor, jerking, twitching, flexing, etc.). Vocal tics may include barking, whistling, grunting, throat clearing, or other sounds. Complex vocal tics may include a variety of words, and rarely coprolalia (uttering of obscenities) may be evident, but it is neither common – less than 10 percent of patients with TD exhibit this symptom (APA, 2000) – nor necessary for diagnosis.

However, other unusual features may be present. Echolalia-like symptoms may be evident in a tendency to mirror the speech of others. Youngsters with TD may find themselves repeating, along with a body jerk, the last word or words of a sentence that they just heard. Echolalia may also occur when children read a word or even think of a word or of the object that the word represents (Comings, 1990). Palilalia (repeating one's own words) and echopraxia (mimicking of other people's actions) may also be evident. These can appear quite bizarre to others.

Symptoms of TD are usually more consistent and more evident than symptoms of TTD or CTD, and patients with TD usually present with greater impairment. For this reason, symptoms of TD are usually treated with medications. Those who wish to avoid using prescription drugs may try some of the naturopathic compounds reviewed later in this chapter.

Secondary Symptoms

Individuals with TTD usually have some control over their tics, and may be able to largely control them in social settings. They may be able to suppress them in school or when playing with peers, and then 'tic-out' when they get home. Thus, other than the frustration these may cause their parents and caretakers, symptoms of TTD usually do not result in major social impairment.

Symptoms of CTD may be more debilitating. Because the severity of the tics is usually more pronounced in CTD than TTD, the tics are more likely to be noticeable. Motor tics may be harder to suppress, and therefore they may be evident in a variety of social settings, including the classroom, the playground, or when visiting friends. Those young-sters who exhibit vocal tics may be especially likely to bring attention to themselves in school and with peers, and this may cause them much embarrassment. They may get reprimanded by adults and made fun of by peers. Consequently, children and adolescents with CTD may with-draw and appear socially awkward.

Individuals with symptoms of full-blown TD are most likely to exhibit additional impairment. Because the complex motor and vocal tics are difficult to hide, adults and peers usually recognize these symptoms, although they may not understand why the youngster is behaving in this way. Teachers may reprimand the child for being too disruptive, especially when vocal sounds are evident. Peers may make fun of the behaviors because they appear strange and unusual. The child usually feels different and exhibits social discomfort. Commonly, stress significantly exacerbates the tics, and therefore academic tasks that are harder for the child (for example, a classroom test) are more likely to by accompanied by tics. Unfortunately, during those times the tics become even more noticeable, and the social stigma and rejection is likely to increase.

Although parents and family members may be more understanding, the tics may also cause more stress at home. Usually children try to exert at least some control over the tics in social settings (like in school) and then 'tic-out' when they get home, releasing the pressure they felt to hold these in. Thus, tics at home are likely to be much more severe, pronounced, and disruptive to the family members. Even when adults express support and understanding, the children still feel bad because they know that the behavior is annoying, and they feel powerless to control it. Siblings may especially react by teasing. All of this is likely to cause the children with TD to exhibit low self-esteem, withdrawal, anger, and frustration.

RULE-OUTS AND COMORBID DISORDERS

Because living with pervasive tics is stressful, it is expected that anxiety and mood changes may accompany severe tic disorders, especially TD. However, it is apparent that TD frequently co-occurs with other disorders, perhaps because TD may share similar etiological factors with some other disorders.

Attention Deficit Hyperactivity Disorder

It is well established that some children with ADHD, when placed on stimulant medications, begin to exhibit tics. In the vast majority of cases, these are minor and disappear when the medication is discontinued. Indeed, children with ADHD present with no greater risk of having Tourette's than the general, non-clinical population, and is estimated at about 0.4 percent (Peterson *et al.*, 2001a). By contrast, between 25 and 85 percent of those with TD also have ADHD (Comings, 2000). It is clear, therefore, that those who exhibit symptoms of TD present a much higher likelihood of exhibiting symptoms of ADHD, and children and teens with TD should be evaluated for comorbid ADHD.

Symptoms of ADHD occur along the dimensions of hyperactivity/impulsivity and distractibility/disorganization. When children and teens exhibit significant motor and/or vocal tics, these are likely to impair their ability to pay attention. Because they may try hard to suppress these urges, their mental energy will be diverted away from the task at hand. Consequently, they will likely appear very distractible. However, since tics usually come and go, there may be periods during which the urges to tic are not evident. When possible, clinicians should assess patients to determine whether during these tic-free periods distractibility is also evident. If so, symptoms of comorbid ADHD may be present. If not, a diagnosis of TD may sufficiently account for all of the symptoms.

Symptoms of hyperactivity may be assessed similarly – if motor restlessness is present exclusively during tic episodes, TD likely accounts for all of the symptoms. If the hyperactivity and restlessness is present even without tics, comorbid ADHD may be apparent.

Symptoms of impulsivity, however, may be more difficult to distinguish. Tics take place when an urge to move or make a sound is not suppressed and the behavior takes place with little self-control over its production. Thus, a tic is an impulsive behavior. Children with TD tend to exhibit impulsivity in many ways, only one of which is exemplified by the tics. In addition, they may act impulsively in many situations, and may fail to properly exercise self-control whenever they experience a variety of urges. This difficulty in impulse control may be responsible for the high overlap between TD and ADHD reported in epidemiological studies. On the other hand, current diagnostic criteria for TD only focus on the presence of tics (APA, 2000). Consequently, those children and adolescents who exhibit significant history of tics (meeting the criteria for TD) and impulsivity in a variety of decision-making situations should be diagnosed with comorbid ADHD.

When symptoms of comorbid ADHD and TD are apparent, it is best to initially try to treat the symptoms of ADHD. Although common wisdom dictates that patients with tics should avoid stimulants, extensive reviews of research studies do not support this conclusion. True, if a patient is treated with a stimulant and begins to exhibit tics, the stimulant should be discontinued. However, as reviewed later in the chapter, results of many studies revealed that treatment of comorbid ADHD and TD with stimulants is often effective in reducing both sets of symptoms. Thus, clinicians who encounter such a diagnostic comorbidity should not be afraid to attempt stimulant treatment and carefully monitor the response.

Anxiety Disorders

Many youngsters who exhibit symptoms of TD have learned that others around them find them strange and bizarre, and may have reacted to social rejection by withdrawing from social situations. Consequently, symptoms of anxiety, especially social anxiety and shyness, are common among children and adolescents with TD (Coffey *et al.*, 1992). However, another mechanism may also be responsible for the overlap with symptoms of anxiety. As conceptualized by many, the impulse to produce a tic is not unlike a compulsion, and the overlap between obsessive compulsive disorder (OCD) and TD is significant. Thus, the symptoms of these two disorders need to be properly examined and differentiated.

Obsessive Compulsive Disorder

Compulsions are complex behaviors, usually resembling normal actions, which are performed in response to obsessions. Obsessions, the thoughts that drive the compulsions, are irrational fears that are relieved, at least for a moment, by performing the compulsive behavior. Because the relief is brief and the obsession usually reoccurs within moments, the pattern repeats itself, sometimes dozens of times. On the other hand, tics are behaviors that are usually less complex, briefer, and more discrete. Most importantly, tics are not driven by obsessions. While patients with TD often report a sense of mental pressure or physical tension before the tic, and a relief when the tic is performed, these sensations are not usually reminiscent of fear or anxiety. Thus, when the clinician is able to perform an in-depth interview with the patient, and the thought processes that accompany the behaviors are ascertained, a differentiation between the symptoms of the two disorders should be relatively straightforward.

Unfortunately, the matter is complicated because TD and OCD may co-occur (APA, 2000) although, because TD is so rare, reliable estimates of this comorbidity have not been established. If both disorders coexist, there should be qualitative difference between the tics and the compulsions. The compulsions should be accompanied, and preceded, by anxiety, and should be performed to relieve it. The tics, however, will likely have a different quality and will not be associated with any fears. In addition, since the DSM requires the presence of obsessions *or* compulsions for the diagnosis of OCD, it is possible that someone can be diagnosed with OCD based on obsessions only and, in such a case, compulsions will not be evident. Thus, comorbid TD and OCD may exist when tics (motor and vocal) and anxiety-driven obsessions are evident. As always, when a patient presents symptoms of two or more disorders simultaneously, all must be treated, although it is probably best to address the disorders one at a time, starting with the one that presents the most debilitating symptoms.

Mood Disorders

Symptoms of mood disorders usually do not mimic tics, and therefore differentiating mood symptoms from tics should not be difficult in most cases. The one exception may exist when symptoms of mania are evident. In those cases, especially when significant psychomotor agitation is present, motor hyperactivity may sometimes take on a repetitive, aimless quality characterized by behaviors that simply seem to be performed in response to an inner drive to move. However, in such situations, these behaviors will be evident only when other symptoms of mania or mixed-mania are evident, and will dissipate when mood symptoms resolve. Thus performing a differential diagnosis should not be difficult.

On the other hand, symptoms of TD may frequently coexist with a mood disorder, especially depression. Repetitive tics embarrass the patient and often result in negative reactions from peers and adults. In addition, because control over these behaviors is limited, the patient feels powerless to stop them. As a result, patients with TD commonly express distress and may exhibit symptoms of depression. Again, because TD is rare, rates of such comorbidities have not been established, but clinicians should be watchful for signs of depression among patients with TD. If these are evident, symptoms of both disorders must be treated. Since the depression is likely to be reactive in nature, counseling may be the preferred method, although serious symptoms of depression may require a pharmacological approach.

Neurological Disorders

Many medical conditions may be accompanied by abnormal movements. These may be secondary to neurodevelopmental delays, brain damage, immune problems, and a variety of other etiologies. Because these need to be treated medically, it is necessary to carefully perform a differential diagnosis and rule out these disorders.

Movement Disorders

Chorea, evident in disorders such as Huntington's, is 'a simple, random, irregular, and nonstereotyped movement that has no premonitory component and increases when the person is distracted' (APA, 2000, p. 110). Chorea may resemble fragments of normal movement, and the involuntary movements may be incorporated into voluntary movements (Mink, 2003). In many cases, these can usually be differentiated from tics because they are less repetitive and seem to be able to be incorporated into normal movements more easily.

Dystonias are movements that are slow and protracted, and often including twisting of the body accompanied by prolonged states of muscular tension. These appear different than tics, which are briefer, more rapid, and usually more repetitive. Athetoid movements are slow, irregular, usually writhing in character, and most frequently occur in the neck, fingers, and toes. By contrast, tics are more rapid and are not limited to these muscle groups.

Spasms are stereotypic, repetitive movements involving the same groups of muscles. Unlike tics, however, these are more prolonged and the movements are usually slower. Myoclonic movements, however, may be similar in character to simple motor tics and may include 'brief, simple, shock-like muscle contractions that may affect parts of muscles or muscle groups' (APA, 2000, p. 110). Unlike tics, however, myoclonic movements are usually also evident during sleep.

When any of the above abnormal movements are evident, a physician should be contacted to perform a careful medical examination and determine whether these are caused by underlying medical conditions. In addition, if the child or adolescent is on any medications, those should be evaluated to determine whether the movements might be caused by the medications' adverse effects.

PANDAS

Pediatric Autoimmune Neuropsychiatric Disorder Associated with Steptococcus (PANDAS), also discussed in Chapter 8, is a syndrome of various symptoms associated with strep infections, one of pediatric, infection-triggered autoimmune neuropsychiatric disorders (PITANDs). Commonly, symptoms of PANDAS include anxiety (in some cases, full-blown obsessions and compulsions are evident) and/or tics. In the 'classic' cases, a child appears totally symptom free (with regard to anxiety or tics) before a strep infection, and develops obsession, compulsions, and/or tics afterwards, although in some cases some prodromal symptoms are evident, so PANDAS may sometimes be a significant exacerbation of prior symptoms, rather than the onset of new symptoms.

The working hypothesis about the pathophysiology assumes that some children are born with genetic vulnerabilities to these problems. When these children experience Group-A beta-hemolytic streptococcal infection, antibodies are produced that then affect cells in the basal ganglia, particularly in the caudate nucleus and putamen. The symptoms result from an interaction of these antibodies with neurons in those regions of the brain (Snider & Swedo, 2004), and may include neuroinflammatory factors (Swedo, 2002).

Treatment of PANDAS is usually different than treatment of strep-unrelated tics. Initially, it is usually necessary to verify the presence of antibodies by performing a blood test, although in some cases symptoms appear to be strongly correlated with strep infections but blood tests come out negative for strep antibodies. Treatment of PANDAS generally involves the administration of immunomodulatory therapies, usually intravenously, and plasma exchange treatment has also been utilized, with varying degrees of success (Allen *et al.*, 1995; Swedo, 2002). While symptomatic treatment of tics is often done concurrently, it is necessary to try to address the immunological problems, and for this reason, PANDAS is usually treated by medical, pediatric specialists (most frequently, pediatricians, pediatric neurologists, or pediatric psychiatrists).

ETIOLOGY

For nearly 200 years, neurologists and psychiatrists have tried to understand the causes of TD. Some insisted that ticking behavior was analogous to seizures and constituted a florid form of hysteria. Then, medicine attempted to associate rheumatic fever, bacterial infections, and even syphilis with tics (Comings, 1990). Eventually, it was discovered that dopamine-blocking medication reduces symptoms of TD, and consequently the dopaminergic brain pathways have been implicated in producing the symptoms.

Since tics, both motor and vocal, are produced by the motor system, anomalies in the control and/or coordination of motor functions may be involved in producing the symptoms of TD. The major brain areas involved in the motor system are portions of the frontal lobes, the basal ganglia, and the cerebellum. The basal ganglia, in particular, are involved in coordinating and controlling motor activity, and are considered to be the most major relay station for motor impulses. Other motor disorders, including Parkinson's and ADHD, have been shown to result, at least in part, from functional changes in these ganglia, and symptoms of TD may similarly be caused by problems in this brain area. The basal ganglia are primarily regulated through dopaminergic nerve pathways, with additional contributions from other monoamines, including norepinephrine and serotonin. Consequently, problems in these pathways have been presumed to underlie symptoms of TD.

The etiology of TD seems to be closely related to genetics and familial patterns, and some genes involved in transmitting the dopaminergic deficits have been identified. Generally, polymorphisms of dopamine transporter (DAT) genes are presumed to be responsible for the functional differences in the brain. Yoon *et al.* (2007) studied over 200 individuals with TD, matched with normal controls, and identified genetic abnormalities in D4 and DAT dopaminergic receptors, as well as in dopamine β-hydroxylase enzyme, and the acid phosphatase locus 1 (ACP1) gene. Genotyping of 27 informative SNP markers from all subjects identified three subgroups, TD with ADHD, TD without ADHD, and normal controls, and was able to reliably predict these categories. Similar studies have also revealed that abnormalities in D2 receptors is similarly linked to both disorders (Barkley, 2006). Thus, as is the case with ADHD, it is apparent that TD may be caused by a variety of factors, including several different, heritable, dopaminergic receptor abnormalities.

Interestingly, some have observed that physical activity, including strenuous exercise, has a calming effect on symptoms of TD (Khalsa, 1997). Because exercise induces the release of endorphins, opioids may have some role in regulating symptoms of TD. Unfortunately, these suggestions, while compelling, have not been empirically verified.

Summary of Research Findings

Available results of research studies convincingly suggest that anomalies in the brain motor system are responsible for symptoms of TD. Brain scans have consistently revealed anatomical differences in areas responsible for motor coordination and planning. The findings of functional studies have been contradictory, but results of recent research are beginning to reconcile prior inconsistencies. It is becoming clear that the pathophysiology of TD is more complex than previously thought.

Neuroanatomical Abnormalities

Anatomical disturbances in patients with TD have been identified by MRI, CAT, and other brain imaging studies. Generally, smaller volumes in cortical, striatal, and thalamic circuits have been observed. For example, Gerard and Peterson (2003) found volume reductions in the putamen, caudate nucleus, and globus pallidus, as well as an absence or reversal of the volumetric asymmetry normally found in portions of the basal ganglia (for example, the caudate nucleus). Other studies have also reported volumetric abnormalities of the dorsal prefrontal area (Peterson *et al.*, 2001b), frontal white matter (Fredericksen *et al.*, 2002), and frontal gray matter (Hong *et al.*, 2002).

In one study, ferritin levels were correlated with caudate volume and were found to be inversely related in healthy comparison subjects but not in the subjects with TD, suggesting that a normal association of ferritin with caudate volume is disrupted in persons with the disorder. In contrast, ferritin level did not correlate with putamen volume in the comparison subjects, but correlated positively with putamen volume in the TD group. In addition, the caudate and putamen were smaller in the TD subjects who had lower ferritin levels than in normal controls who had lower ferritin levels (Gorman *et al.*, 2006). Although the mechanisms by which iron and ferritin may be involved in producing these results is not known, these studies again confirm that subjects with TD exhibit lower brain volumes in portions of the basal ganglia.

In addition, MRI scans of corpus callosum revealed that mean callosal curvature in patients with TD was less rounded than normal control subjects, suggesting that structural interhemispheric connectivity may be aberrant in the brains of patients with TD (Plessen *et al.*, 2006). Again, abnormalities were especially evident in portions related to frontal and striatal functions. These findings further contribute to the evidence that abnormal features of the basal ganglia and related brain regions seem to be evident in individuals with symptoms of TD.

Neurophysiological Abnormalities

Traditionally, it has been presumed that overactivity in dopaminergic brain pathways underlies symptoms of TD. This evidence comes from a variety of sources. It has long been observed that some children with ADHD treated with stimulants develop tics that usually dissipate when the medication is discontinued. Because psychostimulants essentially are dopamine reuptake inhibitors, they indeed increase dopaminergic activity in the brain, and therefore tic behaviors in some children appear to be correlated with this effect.

Further evidence for dopaminergic hyperactivity in TS comes from reviewing the mechanism of action of medications found to be effective in managing symptoms of TD. Traditionally, typical antipsychotics (for example, haloperidol) have been used and reveal good efficacy (Bezchlibnyk-Butler & Virani, 2004) providing they can be tolerated with minimal adverse effects. Typical antipsychotics are dopamine blockers, significantly reducing dopaminergic activity in the entire brain. Thus, it seems that reducing the stimulation of dopaminergic pathways improves symptoms of TD.

Similar results have been obtained in medications that reduce brain levels of a closely related catecholamine. Alpha-2 adrenergic agonists clonidine (Catapress) and guanfacine (Tenex) stimulate pre-synaptic autoreceptors for norepinephrine thus decreasing norepinephrine release.

This mechanism of actions has been shown to be effective in reducing tics. Additionally, other medications effective in reducing symptoms of TD similarly aim to reduce the overall stimulation of the brain by changing the balance between glutamate and GABA. For example, anticonvulsants reduce the action of glutamate and/or increase the activity of GABA, thus reducing brain stimulations. Some of these anticonvulsants, like topiramate (Topamax), have also shown efficacy in reducing tics.

However, the relationship between brain stimulation, levels of dopamine, and tics is more complex than it was initially expected. Although early prospective studies reported association between the use of stimulants and the exacerbation of tics, more recent review of many placebo-controlled studies revealed that patients with comorbid ADHD and TD, treated with stimulants, usually showed an improvement in *both* sets of symptoms (Palumbo, 2004). Thus, the relationship between dopaminergic stimulation and symptoms of TD seems to be much more complex.

There is increasing evidence that the basal ganglia are involved in the pathophysiology of TD. Children with TD are likely to reveal abnormal EEGs (Dedmon, 1990), and a review of research revealed that in some studies, changes in EEG patterns were identified in ancillary motor areas of the basal ganglia in the brains of patients with TD at the time they experienced the urge to tic, and these changes were able to predict whether a tic took place (Ernst & Rumsey, 2000). Positron emission tomography (PET) studies of patients with TD have shown increased glucose metabolic rates in the prefrontal striatal system, including the caudate nuclei and the orbital gyri of the frontal lobes (Jadresic, 1993). However, these findings are not consistently obtained. In some studies, reduced glucose metabolism seems evident in the frontal, cingular, and insular cortices, and other studies also identified blood hypoperfusion of basal ganglia and the thalamus in patients with TD (Ernst & Rumsey). Some studies also revealed that temporolimbic pathways may be involved, suggesting that a hyperactivity of the amygdala may contribute to tic behaviors (Ernst & Rumsey). This may explain why stress seems to precipitate tic episodes for some patients with TD.

More recent studies provide evidence that allows us to understand the pathophysiology involved in symptoms of TD in more detail. It is now apparent that the dysregulation of the basal ganglia involves underactivation of some areas, and overactivation of others. The most sophisticated studies performed to date reveal that the right middle and superior temporal gyrus, caudate nucleus, anterior cingulate cortex, and anterior frontal lobe are more active in patients with TD than in controls, while the right posterior cingulate cortex, and bilateral putamen, globus pallidus, and thalamus are less active in patients with TD (Ernst & Rumsey, 2000). Since these portions of the basal ganglia are extensively innervated with dopaminergic pathways, it is apparent that dopaminergic activity may be overabundant in some of these areas, while deficient in others. In addition, person-to-person variations in these patterns were evident. This complicates treatment approaches, and necessitates open-mindedness when treatments are sought for symptoms of TD.

SUPPLEMENTS WITH LIKELY EFFICACY

Unfortunately, at this time it is apparent that no naturopathic supplements have consistently revealed efficacy in reducing tics, and therefore no compounds at this time should be considered to have established efficacy in treating symptoms of TD or CTD. However, the action of medications proven to reduce tics provide some guidance about which supplements may be associated with decrease in tic symptoms. To date, medications that reduce dopaminergic activity in the brain show the most consistent efficacy in reducing tics. Thus, the natural compound that exerts similar effects in the brain is most likely to be effective.

Rauwolfia

Rauwolfia (*Rauwolfia serpentina*), also spelled ravolphia, is a medicinal shrub in the milkweed family. Its root is ground into a powder and packaged in this form or sold in tablets or capsules. It is a compound commonly used in Asian medicine, including traditional Ayurveda medicine native to India. Its active components are alkaloids and about 50 have been identified, although the primary psychoactive components appear to be reserpine, rescinnamine, and deserpidine (Spinella, 2001).

Supplementation with rauwolfia has been performed in western medicine since the 1950s (Spinella, 2001), primarily for the purpose of treating psychosis (as discussed in Chapter 11). This use has mostly been replaced with the availability of atypical antipsychotic medications, because they are able to successfully treat symptoms of psychosis with fewer risks of motor side effects. However, rauwolfia supplements (especially those that contain reserpine) are still sometimes used as adjuncts to a prescription antipsychotic (Spinella).

Evidence of Efficacy

Although rauwolfia has long been used to treat various motor abnormalities including tics, in Ayurvedic and Chinese medicine (for example, Becker, 2003), it seems that no empirical studies of its benefits in reducing tics have been performed. However, studies have been per-formed that revealed that the efficacy of rauwolfia, especially reserpine, is similar to that of typical antipsychotics (Spinella, 2001), with simi-lar psychoactive effects. Thus, it is reasonable to expect that rauwolfia, especially those supplements that contain reserpine, will be effective in reducing tics in at least some patients.

Pharmacodynamics

Reserpine has been shown to block vesicular storage of monoamines (including dopamine). Consequently, these neurotransmitters remain longer in the cytoplasm, and are more likely to be destroyed by monoamine oxidase, the enzyme that destroys all monoamine neuro-transmitters. As a result, depletion of monoamines becomes evident in central and peripheral neurons, and levels of monoamine neurotrans-mitters released with each neuronal action are significantly decreased. In addition, the effects of this action seem evident a few days to a few weeks after discontinuation of the supplement (Spinella, 2001).

Pharmacokinetics

Little is known about the pharmacokinetics of rauwolfia or reserpine. Following administration, the compound is absorbed and enters systemic circulation, where it crosses the blood–brain barrier and is absorbed into cell bodies of monoaminergic neurons. Rates of metabolism or excretion have not been established, but effects have been known to last for days or weeks after discontinuation of the compound. Although some have hypothesized that this continued effect is evident because this is how long it takes neurons to synthesize new vesicles to store the monoamines (Spinella, 2001), it is also possible that reserpine may have active metabolites that continue to affect the neuron and take much longer to be eliminated from the body.

Dosing

Rauwolfia supplements are generally available in tablets and capsules. Whole and crude forms are also available, but because dosing is more difficult to establish and monitor, the use of these forms is not recom-mended. Adult daily dose is usually 600 mg of rauwolfia or 6 mg of reserpine (Medical Economics, 2007). Thus, the daily dose may be about 7 mg/kg of rauwolfia supplement, or 0.07 mg/kg of reserpine. While this dose may be appropriate for adolescents, children should start much lower. It is preferable to purchase the tablet preparations for use with children, since these can be scored to begin with a low dose. Because rauwolfia is sedating, it may be better to take the compound at night.

Adverse Effects

Use of rauwolfia carries a risk of significant side effects. To begin with, patients who take rauwolfia (or reserpine) are at a significant risk of developing symptoms of depression, and this effect is presumed to be directly caused by the pharmacodynamic properties of the compound – the depletion of monoamine neurotransmitters. Consequently, youngsters who take rauwolfia or reserpine supplements must carefully be monitored for the onset of depressive symptoms.

In addition, rauwolfia exerts a significant antagonistic effect on monoamines, including dopamine. In some patients, this effect may decrease tics, but in others it may cause unpleasant motor side effects associated with antipsychotic medications, including problems with coordination and stereotypic movements. In extreme cases, and if the compound is used for long periods of time, it is possible that it may carry a risk of tardive dyskinesia (TD) that is similar to other conventional antipsychotics, although the link between TD and use of rauwolfia (or reserpine) has not been established. However, because TD is irreversible, it is prudent to exercise extreme caution when using this compound.

In eastern medicine rauwolfia continues to be used as a tranquilizer, and the compound is approved by Commission E for the treatment of hypertension and insomnia. Rauwolfia is sedating. When administered, it reduces blood pressure and may result in dizziness. Although in low doses patients may develop tolerance to these effects, blood pressure of patients who take rauwolfia should regularly be monitored.

In addition, rauwolfia is contraindicated during pregnancy, so if it is used with adolescent females, they need to be counseled about the need to use contraception (Medical Economics, 2007).

SUPPLEMENTS WITH POSSIBLE EFFICACY

In addition to rauwolfia, a few other compounds may also have some efficacy in treating tics. However, since the data that supports the use of the following supplements is extremely limited, clinicians should proceed with caution, and consider the use of the compounds discussed in this section as experimental.

Lecithin and Choline

Lecithin is a naturally occurring fatty substance referred to as phospholipid. Although the term lecithin is sometimes used generically to refer to a wide variety of lipids (including choline and glycine), it is most commonly associated with phosphatidylcholine, a precursor for choline. It is naturally found in several foods, including egg yolks, soybeans, nuts, and whole grains, as well as in organ meats. Because lecithin is not considered an essential nutrient, no recommended daily allowance (RDA) has been established. Generally, dietary intake of lecithin ranges from 1–5 g/d, but some have proposed that current trends toward low-fat diets may be producing lecithin deficits (Potter *et al.*, 2009).

Choline is a partly essential nutrient that is usually grouped within the Vitamin B complex. Although not a standard amino acid, it is a natural amine found in the lipids that make up cell membranes. It is a co-factor required for the synthesis of acetylcholine. Although small amounts are produced by the body, most choline must be ingested in food. Choline-rich foods include egg yolks, soy, and organ meats (especially liver), and many vegetables contain choline in smaller amounts. Adequate daily intakes of this micronutrient have been established by the Food and Nutrition Board of the Institute of Medicine of the National Academy of Sciences and are reported to be between 425 and 550 mg/day for adults (Veenema *et al.*, 2008), or between 5 and 6.4 mg/kg/day.

Lecithin has been researched as naturopathic treatment for a variety of conditions, and is also covered in Chapter 7 of this book. Choline has similarly been researched and has been shown to offer some potential benefit in treating symptom of ADHD (as discussed in Chapter 5). In addition, Polinsky *et al.* (1980) reported good efficacy when using choline to treat symptoms of TD, and Moldofsky and Sandor (1983), in a small open trial, found that lecithin did not improve symptoms of TD. Still, both lecithin and choline have shown some efficacy in treating symptoms of motor disturbances associated with the use of antipsychotic medications and other motor disturbances (Gelenberg *et al.*, 1990). In addition, individuals with TD have been shown to have reduced levels of choline in various regions of the basal ganglia (DeVito *et al.*, 2005), although this does not necessarily indicate that supplementation with choline will be effective. Risks of lecithin and choline supplementation, however, are very limited, and the supplements are generally well tolerated. Consequently, it is reasonable to attempt a trial for managing symptoms of TD if other methods have failed.

As a supplement, lecithin and choline are generally sold in capsules, and lecithin is also available in liquid, and granulated forms. Little is known about the pharmacokinetics of lecithin and choline. Following ingestion, the lipid is absorbed from the small intestine and may enter the lymph system, as well as systemic blood circulation. It is taken up by cell membranes and becomes involved in a number of metabolic processes, including the conversion of acetylcholine. Lecithin and choline are absorbed and metabolized rapidly. The half-life is unknown, and the supplement have been dosed in varying regimens, from once to three times per day.

Lecithin supplements are not usually dosed by body weight, and adequate intake (AI) levels have been established for various ages. These range from 200 mg/day for children under age 4, to 375 mg/day for adolescents, although supplementation to manage symptoms of clinical disorders usually needs to exceed those ranges (Medical Economics, 2008a). It is best to start low and gradually titrate the dose in accordance with response and onset of any adverse effects. No upper limit for lecithin ingestion has been established, but dosage in adults has not been studied beyond 30 g/day.

Doses of 3 mg/day of choline have been studied with adults and produced few side effects (Medical Economics, 2008a). Usual effective doses are 425–550 mg/day for adults, and 250–350 mg/day for children. Choline is generally regarded as safe, and pregnant mothers are sometimes encouraged to take choline to aid the brain development of the fetus. The most common side effects are nausea, diarrhea, and loose stools. High doses of choline have sometimes resulted in hypotension and increases in depressive symptoms.

Lecithin and choline are generally well tolerated. Since many commercially available supplements are derived from soy, those who are allergic to soy or its byproducts should not take lecithin. Otherwise, few adverse effects are reported, except for mild gastrointestinal symptoms, such as looser stools, or transient nausea. Higher doses (at 25 g/day or more) have been associated with acute gastrointestinal distress, sweating, salivation, and anorexia (Potter et al., 2009), and these are most often evident in supplements with a high percentage of choline.

Vitamin B6

The B family of vitamins contains eight vitamins that play important physiological functions in the body. These include B1 (thiamine), B2 (riboflavin), B3 (niacin), B5 (pantothenic acid), Vitamin B6 (pyridoxine), B7 (biotin), B9 (folic acid), and B12 (cobalamins). B vitamins are involved in cellular metabolism and, like all other vitamins, must be obtained from the diet.

Vitamin B6, in particular, is an important co-enzyme involved in many biochemical reactions, including amino acid metabolism, and it is vital for proper protein synthesis. After proteins are ingested, they are broken down into their constituent amino acids, and those must then be degraded during digestion and are then taken up by the cells to form individual protein molecules. The presence of the vitamin B6 is essential for this process.

Vitamin B6 is widely available in foods, including meat, vegetables (especially potatoes, avocados, Brussels sprouts, cauliflower, and tomatoes), whole grain products, fruit (especially, bananas and apples), peanuts, and sunflower seeds (Hingle, 2007). Supplemental vitamin B6 is available in capsules and tablets, in a wide range of doses. B6 is also commonly included in B complex preparations. Dietary reference intakes (DRI) have been established for vitamin B6, and range from 0.05 mg/day for infants to 1.3–1.7 mg/day for adults. In addition, upper intake levels have also been established, and these range from 30 mg/day for infants to 100 mg/day for adults (Medical Economics, 2008a). However, when used clinically, the typical dose is 100–200 mg/day, and lowest observed adverse effect level has been established at 500 mg/day (Medical Economics). It is clear that children and adolescents should receive much lower doses.

Supplementation with vitamin B6 has been shown to have some beneficial effects in reducing symptoms of TD. Anecdotal evidence has long existed supporting its use, and some empirical studies have confirmed its efficacy. For example, Garcia-López et al. (2008), performed an open trial with children aged 7–14 years diagnosed with TD and found that doses of 2 mg/kg per day, combined with magnesium at doses of 0.5 mEq/kg per day (about 6 mg/kg per day) were effective in significantly reducing the tics. The same results were obtained in a follow-up, double-blind, placebo-controlled study (Garcia-López et al., 2009). Other research also confirmed these results, although focused more specifically on the role of magnesium (Grimaldi, 2002). In addition, supplementation with vitamin B6 has been shown to block the therapeutic effects of L-dopa, a dopamine agonist used to treat symptoms of Parkinson's (Medical Economics, 2008a). Taken together, these results suggest that a trial of vitamin B6 may be warranted in children and adolescents with symptoms of TD.

Following ingestion, vitamin B6 undergoes hydrolysis in the small intestine and is absorbed in the jejunum. The vitamin is well absorbed, even at high doses, enters systemic circulation, and is delivered to various tissues in the body, and is easily taken up by the muscles. Depending on the form of vitamin B6 supplements, and interpersonal variations among patients, sometimes magnesium may assist in the absorption, and the two supplements are sometimes taken together.

Vitamin B6 is generally well tolerated, especially at doses that do not exceed upper intake limits. When supplemented above these limits, adults who take vitamin B6 at 200 mg per day usually tolerate the dose well, and adverse effects are rare. Children and adolescents should start vitamin B6 supplementation at the upper intake limits listed above, and increase weekly to the 2 mg/kg per day that has been shown to be effective in clinical studies. At high doses, some individuals develop nausea, vomiting, abdominal pain, loss of appetite, and sensory neuropathies, and rare cases of photosensitivity have also been reported (Medical Economics, 2008a).

Scullcap

Scullcap (*Scutellaria lateriflora*), sometimes spelled skullcap, and also known as American skullcap, is an herb that has sometimes been presumed to be effective for hysteria, nervous tension, epilepsy, chorea, and other psychological disorders. Although some have presumed that it may be effective as a hypnotic, a review of literature concluded that scullcap is not effective as a sleep aid (Morin *et al.*, 2007). Another review concluded that its psychogenic effects fall into the category of 'unproven uses' (Medical Economics, 2007, p. 739). However, anecdotal evidence has long existed that scullcap may be effective for treatment of muscle spasms (Kurnakov, 1957), and some herbal references report anecdotal evidence that scullcap may be useful to treat 'mild' symptoms of TD (Newall *et al.*, 1996; Miller & Murray, 1998), alone, or in combination with other sedative herbs, like valerian (Moore, 2003).

The pharmacology of scullcap is poorly understood, but it is presumed to exert its sedating effects by interacting with the benzodiazepine receptors in the brain (Medina, 1997). Consequently, its clinical effects may be produced by neuromodulating the action of GABA and increasing the opening of chloride channels on cell membranes. As more chloride flows into the cell, neuronal firing is reduced overall and an inhibitory effect is evident.

Scullcap is sold in capsules, and powder and liquid extracts are also available. Raw leaves are also used to brew a tea. Various strands of scullcap are available and Chinese skullcap (usually spelled with a 'k') is considered to be most potent, but may also exert less psychoactive properties. Adult doses of scullcap range from 1–2 g per day, which converts to about 11.6–23.25 mg/kg per day, usually in divided doses (two to three times per day). Children and adolescents may be dosed similarly. Herbal enthusiasts often prefer to brew scullcap into a tea-like beverage, which is done by pouring one cup of boiling water over one teaspoon of the dried herb, and steeped for 20–30 minutes. When brewed, children under age 3 may be given a quarter cup three times per day, children age 3–6 may be given a half a cup three times per day, children age 7–11 may be given three-quarters of a cup three times per day, and children 12 or older may be given the low range of adult dose (one cup three times per day). In addition, it is recommended that steeping time is reduced when the tea will be given to young children. Although this form of preparation may be easier to administer, inconsistencies in the brewing methods are likely, and therefore whenever possible, use of capsules is preferred.

Scullcap is generally well tolerated and few side effects are expected (Medical Economics, 2007). Because scullcap seems to act on benzodiazepine receptors, a tolerance to the psychological effect may develop. In addition, scullcap has in the past been adulterated with germander (teucrium), a group of plants known to cause liver problems. Although most recently this has been less of a problem, consumers are advised to purchase scullcap from reliable and trusted sources. In high doses, scullcap may produce mental confusion, irregular heartbeat, and twitching. Consequently, when used to treat symptoms of TD, if partial response is evident, and an increase in dose causes an increase of tics, the dosage should be reduced. Scullcap should not be used during pregnancy, and therefore it is necessary to assure that teenage females who take scullcap use redundant forms of contraception to assure the prevention of pregnancy.

Vitamin E

Vitamin E is a name that is commonly given to a family of substances known as tocopherols and tocotrienols, eight of which occur naturally. Of these, alpha-tocopherol is considered to be the most important in human physiology, although the other forms may be indirectly important – for example, they may play a role in the absorption and metabolism of alpha-tocopherol. Vitamin E must be obtained from the diet and is widely available in unrefined vegetable oils (including olive, safflower, and canola), meat (especially, the fatty portion), cereal grains, fruit, nuts, and vegetables. Supplemental vitamin E is available in caplets, in a wide range of doses. Dietary reference intakes (DRI) range from 6 mg/day for infants to 15 mg/day for adults. In addition, upper intake levels have also been established, and these range from 200 mg/day for infants to 1000 mg/day for adults (Medical Economics, 2008a).

Vitamin E is well known as an antioxidant and anticoagulant. In addition, it has important functions as a cell membrane stabilizer, and may also be neuroprotective. Oxidative stress is presumed to play a role in a number of neurological disorders, and vitamin E seems to exert protective effects, and these may especially be evident in the cerebellum (Medical Economics, 2008a). Vitamin E may be involved in signal transduction, and may alter the permeability of cell membranes, thus changing the action potential of the neurons.

Supplementation with vitamin E has been shown to have some beneficial effects in reducing muscle spasms and various motor side effects associated with the use of conventional antipsychotics. Although not all studies have shown consistent results, benefit in improving extrapyramidal symptoms has been shown in many studies (Connor & Meltzer, 2006). Consequently, herbal and naturopathic references often recommend a trial of vitamin E to manage symptoms of TD. Although these suggestions are only based on anecdotal evidence, vitamin E is generally well tolerated and side effects are rare, and consequently a trial of vitamin E may be reasonable if all other treatment options have not produced good results.

Following ingestion, vitamin E is emulsified with other lipids and absorbed in the small intestine. Absorption is low and variable, and improves significantly with the intake of food. For this reason, supplementation with vitamin E is usually recommended to be taken with meals. The lipids are then transported to the liver, which excretes vitamin E in very low density lipoproteins. Alpha-tocopherol is then transported to the central nervous system where it crosses the blood–brain barrier and enters the neurons. Some suggest that the absorption of alpha-tocopherol is further assisted by the presence of other tocopherols and tocotrienols, and consequently some of the preparations on the market contain various tocopherols and tocotrienols, in varying amounts. However, it is not clear whether such a combination is better absorbed, and research findings suggest that only alpha-tocopherol is maintained in human plasma (Medical Economics, 2008a).

Vitamin E is generally well tolerated, especially at doses that do not exceed upper intake limits. When supplemented above these limits, children who take vitamin E at doses ranging from 1 mg/kg to 100 mg/day usually tolerate the dose well, and adverse effects are rare (Connor & Meltzer, 2006). Children and adolescents should start vitamin E supplementation at the upper intake limits listed above, and increase weekly to 1 mg/kg per day (or 100 mg, whichever is lower). At high doses, some individuals develop fatigue, muscle soreness, gastrointestinal disturbances, and altered serum levels of lipids. Very rarely, thyroid problems have been reported (Medical Economics, 2008a). Because vitamin E is an anticoagulant, supplementation should not be done with individuals who take other blood thinning medications (for example, aspirin).

SUPPLEMENTS NOT LIKELY TO BE EFFECTIVE

It is not possible to review all compounds that have been presumed to reduce tics. However, herbal and naturopathic sources, especially those on the Internet, sometimes recommend the use of various compounds, despite the lack of evidence of efficacy. Clinicians who seek to practice in the area of naturopathic psychopharmacology should be aware of these compounds and choose those supplements that are most likely to be effective. The compounds listed below are not likely to offer any benefit in managing symptoms of TD.

GABA

As discussed in Chapter 4, GABA is a major neurotransmitter in the central nervous system that is ubiquitous and affects the firing of all neurons by increasing membrane polarization. Most GABA receptors are ionotropic and regulate the influx of chloride into the cell. As chloride levels increase in the cell, the negative charge also increases, and the cell becomes more and more difficult to stimulate.

A number of medications target GABA neurotransmission and have been shown to be effective in treating mood disturbance (especially mania and agitation), anxiety, and tics. Consequently, naturopaths sometimes recommend GABA supplementation, and various forms of GABA tablets and capsules are available on the market.

Unfortunately, these are of very limited value. GABA does not easily cross the blood–brain barrier (Foster & Kemp, 2006), and the majority of GABA becomes metabolized and/or excreted before it can enter the brain. Although some peripheral effects have been observed, like muscle relaxation, few psychogenic effects seem evident. When administered at high doses (at 1000 mg or higher), supplemental GABA does, in fact, appear to begin to cross the blood–brain barrier, but surprisingly, the effects are not the inhibition that is expected, and a mix of increased relaxation as well as increased anxiety becomes evident (Abdou *et al.*, 2006). Thus far, there has been no empirical research investigating the effect of GABA supplements on tics, but judging from its lack of effect in treating symptoms of anxiety, GABA supplements are not likely to be beneficial in treating symptoms of TD.

Iron

Iron is a chemical element involved in the anabolism of catecholamines. Iron is present throughout the body and is converted into amino acids. The vast majority of necessary iron intake is derived from the normal diet, and many iron-rich foods are commonly consumed in meats, cereals, fruit, and vegetables. Some members of at-risk populations may require iron supplementation – for example, those who are malnour-ished, infants who are not breast-fed, or individuals who have lost a lot of blood. However, iron supplementation in patients who are not iron deficient is dangerous. Careful RDA limits must be observed and excess iron intake has been associated with serious toxic effects, including death. Children are especially at risk for these problems, and iron sup-plementation should only be undertaken under the supervision (and rec-ommendation) of a physician (Medical Economics, 2008a).

Ferritin is a complex protein and serves as the primary storage of iron within the body. Serum ferritin level correlates highly with total body storage of iron; and therefore measuring serum ferritin is a convenient way to estimate levels of iron within the body. Some studies have found that peripheral ferritin levels were significantly lower in subjects with TD than in healthy comparison subjects, and ferritin correlates with the volumes of the sensorimotor, midtemporal, and subgenual cortices (for example, Gorman *et al.*, 2006). In addition, iron is hypothesized to have impact on the dopaminergic systems and therefore may be involved in dopaminergic abnormalities associated with symptoms of TD.

Unfortunately, although iron levels may play a role in the patho-physiology of TD, there are no studies confirming any benefits of iron supplement in reducing tics. In addition, iron supplements are very risky and iron overdose is the leading cause of poisoning among small children, including many deaths reported each year. Given the risks of iron supplementation, clinicians should stay away from this practice unless it can be confirmed that the patient exhibits iron deficiency, and any iron supplementation should be given under close supervision of a physician.

SUMMARY

In order to help clinicians select the compounds that are most likely to be effective, an algorithm was developed and is presented in Figure 10.1. This diagram takes into account the amount of research support available for each compound, as well as the specific mechanism of action of each supplement and its applicability to the treatment of the symptoms of TD (as well as CTD, if these symptoms are deemed sig-nificant enough to warrant pharmacological treatment).

Initially, clinicians should determine whether the symptoms of TD or CTD are comorbid with symptoms of OCD or ADHD. If the patient, unmedicated, concurrently presents symptoms of combined TD (or CTD) with ADHD or OCD, clinicians should proceed by initially treating

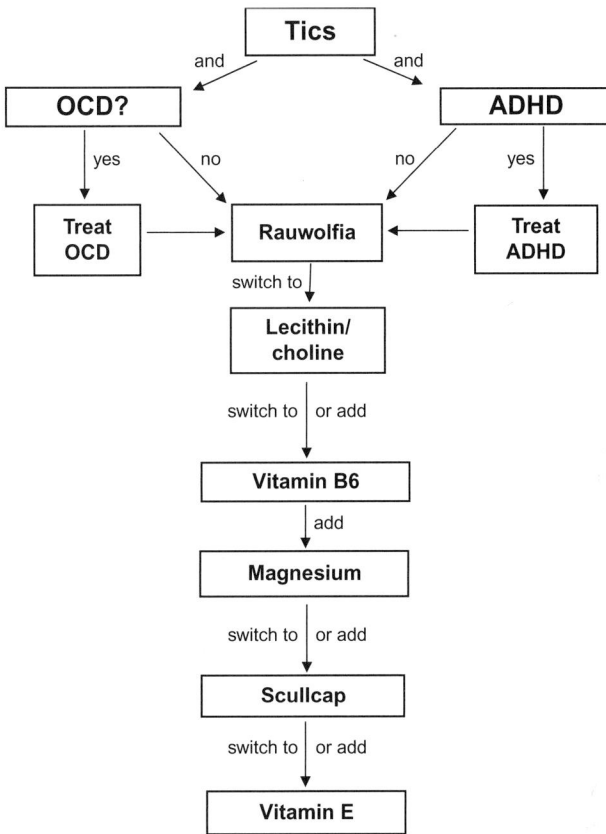

FIGURE 10.1 Algorithm for treatment of Tourette's (or chronic tic) disorder with naturopathic supplements.
© Elsevier 2009.

ADHD (as discussed in Chapter 5) or OCD (Chapter 8) and monitoring whether all symptoms (including the tics) improve.

If not, then TD-specific treatments should be attempted, as discussed in this chapter. Although not specifically researched in treatment of TD, the pharmacological mechanism of action of rauwolfia suggests that it is most likely to be effective, but adverse effects may become difficult to tolerate. If insufficient response is obtained, or side effects are too significant, rauwolfia should be discontinued and lecithin or choline supplement should be attempted.

If insufficient response is still evident, vitamin B6 should be used as an adjunct or monotherapy, with the addition of magnesium if it becomes necessary to augment the effect. As a last resort, scullcap and/or vitamin E supplements can be utilized.

Chapter 11

Psychosis

It has long been recognized that, in a small group of children, symptoms of psychosis may develop. Cases of childhood psychosis have been reported for at least 200 years (Walk, 1964), and more than 100 years ago researchers started to expect that children with psychotic symptoms were exhibiting a childhood version of the disorder we now know as schizophrenia (Asarnow & Asarnow, 2003). Gradually, it became apparent that psychotic symptoms may be present in children and adolescents with various disorders. The symptoms of childhood schizophrenia became differentiated from adult schizophrenia, and for a time they were presumed to co-occur with autism and other developmental delays. Today, we understand that childhood psychosis may be present as a core feature of some disorders, or as an adjunct group of symptoms in severe variants of some other disorders (for example, bipolar or major depression).

The prevalence of childhood psychosis is difficult to establish. Childhood schizophrenia is rare in children and increases in frequency with adolescence (Remschmidt, 1993). One study estimated the prevalence rate of 0.19 per 10,000 children (Burd & Kerbeshian, 1987), and another suggested that one in 10,000 children can be expected to develop schizophrenia (Remschmidt *et al.*, 1994). There is no data available about the prevalence of other psychotic disorders (for example, schizophreniform or schizoaffective) among children and adolescents. The prevalence of psychosis as a symptom accompanying other disorders is equally difficult to estimate. Although bipolar disorder is present in about 1 percent of children (Verlhurst *et al.*, 1997), only a small portion of them exhibit symptoms of psychosis. Similarly, less than 1 percent of preschoolers (Kashani & Carlson, 1987) and about 3 percent of preadolescents (Fleming & Offord, 1990) exhibit symptoms of a depressive disorder, and only a small fraction of these exhibit symptoms severe enough to include psychosis. By adolescence, however, up to 14 percent may develop major depression (Hammen & Rudolph, 2003), a rate that is similar to epidemiological rates in adults. Thus, it can be expected that childhood psychosis is rare, its prevalence increases with age, and rates in adolescents may be similar to those observed in adults.

SYMPTOMS OF PEDIATRIC PSYCHOSIS

In adults, core symptoms of psychosis may include both positive and negative symptoms. In children and adolescents, however, the profile of symptoms may be different. In addition, there are many other symptoms that are commonly associated with psychosis, including social withdrawal and difficulties in school.

Core Symptoms

When psychotic disorders occur in adults, the disturbance almost always includes positive symptoms of psychosis, and in some cases negative symptoms may also be apparent. This is especially true in cases where the psychotic disorder lasts for many years, since negative symptoms usually exacerbate with the duration of the disorder. In children, however, the profile of symptoms may be different, and negative symptoms may be less common. When present, negative symptoms may be expressed somewhat differently.

Positive Symptoms

Positive symptoms of psychosis are usually called 'positive' because they constitute an addition to, and excess of, normal perceptual experiences. Normally, we experience perceptual states when our senses are stimulated – we hear when our ears detect a sound, we see when light rays stimulate our retina, etc. Positive symptoms of psychosis include experiences during which we experience perceptual states in absence of sensory stimulation – in other words, we see something that is not there, hear a voice that does not exist, etc. These experiences are called hallucinations.

Although hallucinations may technically be connected to all of our senses, in reality the most common hallucinations include visual and auditory – seeing or hearing something that is not there. Visual hallucinations may include human, monster-like, or animal figures, as well as (more rarely) inanimate objects. Auditory hallucinations include a variety of sounds, but may also include voices that talk to the patient. In some cases, these voices instruct the patient to perform an action, a phenomenon known as command hallucinations. Although visual and auditory hallucinations may occur together – for example, when a child sees a figure that is speaking to him – they may also occur separately.

In more severe cases, hallucinations may include other senses, including olfactory, somatic, and even gustatory. When these experiences are evident, they represent an extreme deviation from norm that usually is preceded by other forms of hallucinations. However, in some cases, these experiences may signal other problems (for example, a seizure), and therefore cases where these unusual experiences are evident should comprehensively be evaluated by a physician.

Positive symptoms may also include delusions – strongly held beliefs that are obviously discrepant with reality but tightly held on to by the patient. These may include non-bizarre content – for example, suspecting that others are plotting against the patient – or bizarre content – for instance, believing that one has turned into a monster. The severity of these delusions often correlates with the severity of the hallucinations, although sometimes delusions may be more evident than hallucinations (as is the case with paranoid schizophrenia).

As discussed in the DSM, in addition to delusions and hallucinations, symptoms of psychosis may also include disorganized speech (including thought derailment and incoherence), and motor disturbances (like catatonia). Some clinicians also consider these as positive symptoms of psychosis (Stahl, 2008).

Negative Symptoms

Negative symptoms are usually called 'negative' because they constitute a deficit in normal functioning. Normally, we are able to communicate in a manner where cognitions are connected logically and flow consistently when formulating or communicating a thought. When alogia is present, thoughts seem disjointed and communications become derailed, lacking a clear goal. While this may be similar to disorganized speech discussed above, when alogia is present, the clinical character is one of significant impoverishment of thought content and a clear deficit in the ability to express an idea, whereas disorganized speech is usually characterized by expressing many ideas, although these seem disjointed and may be incoherent.

Similarly, affective blunting is considered to be a negative symptom, and a person who exhibits this problem seems emotionally flat. As discussed below, this must be differentiated from flatness that commonly occurs during symptoms of major depression. However, when flatness is a negative symptom, it is present in absence of prominent mood disturbance. Negative symptoms may also be apparent in significant avolition and lack of motivation. Again, it is necessary to determine whether this occurs with or without prominent mood disturbance.

Secondary Symptoms

Children and adolescents who present with symptoms of psychosis are likely to exhibit a variety of other disturbances. Although a very young child may not be able to differentiate internal and external stimuli, by preschool years, most children are able to tell whether the sight or sound they just experienced took place in reality. When they realize that they experienced a hallucination, many children become scared, and view this in a similar manner to a nightmare. Thus, when children begin to experience symptoms of psychosis, it is not unusual for these to co-occur with significant anxiety and withdrawal, and they may worry about whether these voices or sight will hurt them.

Along with anxiety, children who experience delusion and hallucinations are also likely to become depressed. Since they recognize that they are experiencing something unusual and abnormal, they may be scared that something is wrong with them. In addition, situations they find stressful may precipitate more psychotic symptoms, and therefore they may shy away from others, avoid contact with peers, become clingy with primary caretakers, etc.

Children with psychosis are likely to exhibit serious difficulties in school. They may refuse to attend school, exhibit significant distractibility in class, display problems with learning and retaining information, and reveal poor academic performance. When they experience a hallucination, they are not likely to complete academic tasks and may also exhibit symptoms of agitation. Some, especially adolescents, may display significant acting out that may include substantial aggression and violence. As a result, it often becomes hard to maintain these children and adolescents in regular education settings, and many attend special education placements.

In social settings, youth with delusions and hallucinations are likely to be withdrawn, defensive and, unpopular. Because they feel very different, they feel that they do not belong among others and some may seek out alternative peer groups. To compensate for feelings of inadequacy, some may become involved in mischief and criminal activity. Adolescents with psychosis are also likely to turn to drugs to self-medicate.

DIAGNOSTIC CONSIDERATIONS, RULE-OUTS, AND COMORBID DISORDERS

Before an appropriate treatment plan can be developed, clinicians must consider whether the symptoms of psychosis constitute the central features of the disorder. If so, then treatment with antipsychotic compounds will become the main focus of treatment. However, several other disorders may also present symptoms of psychosis, and in those cases the other symptoms must be the main focus of treatment and an antipsychotic compound may be used as an adjunct. In order to differentiate these situations, comprehensive differential diagnosis must be performed.

Psychotic Disorders

There are disorders in which psychosis is the central feature of the symptoms. This means that if anxiety or depression are present, these are secondary to the psychosis and constitute the child's reaction to the hallucinations, or the hallucinations were once accompanied by mood disturbance but now persist after mood disturbance has resolved. In these cases, clinicians must recognize that the pharmacological treatment must focus, first and foremost, on alleviating the symptoms of psychosis.

Schizophrenia

Schizophrenia is considered to be the most severe of all psychotic disorders. Although the onset of psychotic symptoms usually occurs in early adulthood, in some cases the initial psychotic break may come during adolescence. In rare cases, the onset of schizophrenia may occur in childhood. To be diagnosed with schizophrenia, the child or adolescent must exhibit hallucinations and/or delusions, continuously for at least 6 months, and the symptoms must impair social/occupational (or academic) functioning (APA, 2000).

Although person-to-person presentation varies, schizophrenia usually is a severe disorder and its symptoms are likely to be debilitating. In most cases, schizophrenia is a progressive disorder that exacerbates with the duration of the illness. This is especially true in children. Early onset of schizophrenia is usually associated with much more significant severity of symptoms later in life, and children with schizophrenia show a greater severity of premorbid symptoms than those who develop schizophrenia later in life (Hollis, 2003).

In most cases, schizophrenia begins with positive symptoms and negative symptoms gradually come on and exacerbate as the disorder progresses. For this reason, children with schizophrenia are less likely to exhibit negative symptoms and positive symptoms are more common. However, in some cases this pattern may not be evident. Since children with schizophrenia often exhibit significant disturbance prior to the onset of psychosis, it may be difficult to determine when prodromal symptoms progress into a full-blown disorder (Asarnow & Asarnow, 2003). Thus, some children with schizophrenia may exhibit significant negative symptoms.

When a diagnosis of schizophrenia is made, the focus of pharmacological treatment should primarily be on the symptoms of psychosis, and antipsychotic compounds need to be used first and foremost. If ancillary symptoms of depression or anxiety are present, these are presumed to be secondary to the psychosis, and therefore should resolve as the psychosis improves. In some cases, an anxiolytic or an antidepressant may be used as an adjunct, but usually should not be administered until at least some response to the antipsychotic is evident.

Schizoaffective Disorder

Schizoaffective disorder may only be diagnosed in individuals who have a documented history of a severe mood episode – depressive or manic. Thus, patients with schizoaffective disorder usually can be easily differentiated from those with schizophrenia because they will have a history of major depression or bipolar disorder. In the usual presentation, the patient experiences a mood disorder with severe presentation of symptoms that includes psychosis – depression with psychosis or mania ('classic' or mixed) with psychosis – and during an uninterrupted period of symptomatic disturbance, the mood symptoms resolve but the psychosis persists, in absence of prominent mood symptoms, for a period of at least 2 weeks (APA, 2000).

When a patient is diagnosed with schizoaffective disorder, the symptoms of mood disturbance have already resolved, at least temporarily. This may be because the patient was treated with an antidepressant or mood stabilizer, or the patient was untreated but mood symptoms resolved spontaneously, as part of the cyclical progression of the mood disorder. In these cases, pharmacological treatment should focus on the remaining symptoms of psychosis. It may be desirable to use a maintenance dose of an antidepressant or a mood stabilizer as an adjunct in order to diminish the likelihood of another mood episode. As discussed in Chapters 6 and 7, there are some compounds that may have efficacy in simultaneously treating symptoms of psychosis and mood disturbance. Naturally, these may be preferred when treating patients with schizoaffective disorder.

Other Psychotic Disorders

Schizophrenia and schizoaffective disorder account for the vast majority of patients diagnosed with a psychotic disorder. However, on very rare occasions, some patients may exhibit psychosis that is not part of schizophrenic, schizoaffective, major depressive, or bipolar presentation. For example, patients who exhibit symptoms of psychosis for a brief period of time may be diagnosed with brief psychotic disorder (if the symptoms last less than a month), or schizophreniform disorder (if the symptoms last more than 1 month but less than 6 months). In these cases, symptoms may progress into schizophrenia, but since in the majority of patients symptoms resolve spontaneously, no treatment is usually needed.

Delusional disorder is another rare psychotic disorder. It is characterized by symptoms of nonbizarre delusions, in absence of hallucinations or negative symptoms, for at least 1 month. This disorder is mostly associated with late onset, and so childhood presentation is very uncommon. Anyone suspected of this disorder should undergo an in-depth assessment to clarify the diagnosis. If confirmed, treatment with an antipsychotic may be attempted, but because delusional disorder is so rare, little is known about effective treatments.

Mood Disorders

When mood disturbance is present with psychosis, clinicians need to determine whether psychosis is the primary disturbance and mood symptoms are secondary to the positive or negative symptoms, or whether the mood disturbance is primary and psychosis merely accompanies mood disturbance. Depending on which diagnosis becomes the primary focus of treatment, antipsychotic, antidepressant, or mood stabilizing compounds will be primary in treating all the symptoms.

Major Depression

As discussed in Chapter 6, symptoms of major depression may be accompanied by psychotic features. In such a presentation, depression usually comes on gradually, and as it becomes more severe, psychosis may eventually become evident. In such cases, hallucinations are more likely than delusions, and the content is less likely to be bizarre. Instead, self-deprecating auditory hallucinations may be present, and they may sometimes command the patient to self-mutilate or commit suicide. When symptoms of depression are deemed to constitute the primary disturbance, an antidepressant compound should initially be attempted. As the depression resolves, it is likely that the psychosis will as well. If residual symptoms of psychosis are still present while the mood is resolving, an adjunct antipsychotic may be added to the regimen.

Conversely, if the psychosis appears to have come on first, and the depression appears secondary to the patient's reaction to the psychosis, the patient is likely to need pharmacological with antipsychotic compounds first and foremost, and the depression is expected to begin to resolve as the psychosis diminishes, although some delay in reduction of depression may be evident. If needed, an antidepressant compound may be administered as an adjunct to the antipsychotic.

When clinicians need to simultaneously manage symptoms of depression and psychosis, contents of Chapter 6 should be cross-referenced with the compounds discussed in this chapter to determine whether any supplement is known to be effective in managing both sets of symptoms. Such compounds exist (for example, Omega-3), and may be a good first-line treatment of this combination of symptoms.

Bipolar Disorder

As discussed in Chapter 7, manic episodes may be accompanied by psychosis. In those cases, symptoms of mania are likely to come on first and progress gradually. Clinicians should especially look for symptoms of mixed mania, since this presentation is more common in children and adolescents. As manic symptoms exacerbate, psychosis may become apparent. Depending on severity, symptoms may include both hallucination and delusions, but bizarre content is less common. Significant agitation may accompany the mood disturbance, and the content of the hallucinations may be self-deprecating, including command hallucinations to self-mutilate or commit suicide. When symptoms of mania are deemed to constitute the primary disturbance, treatment with a mood stabilizer should initially be attempted. As the mood disturbance resolves, it is likely that the psychosis will as well. If residual symptoms of psychosis are still present while the mood is improving, an adjunct antipsychotic may be added to the regimen.

Conversely, if the psychosis appears to have come on before the agitation, and the anger appears secondary to the patient's reaction to the psychosis, the patient is likely to need pharmacological with antipsychotic compounds first and foremost, and the mood reaction is expected to begin to resolve as the psychosis diminishes, although some delay may be evident. If needed, a mood stabilizer may be administered as an adjunct to the antipsychotic.

When clinicians need to simultaneously manage symptoms of depression and psychosis, contents of Chapter 7 should be cross-referenced with the compounds discussed in this chapter to determine whether any supplement is known to be effective in managing both sets of symptoms. Such compounds exist (for example, Omega-3), and may be a good first-line treatment of this combination of symptoms.

Adjustment and Trauma

Children and adolescents who have undergone traumatic experiences are much more likely to exhibit a variety of difficulties, although psychosis is not likely unless the stress is unusually severe.

Post-Traumatic Disorders

Children and adolescents who have been exposed to severe trauma may exhibit symptoms of acute stress disorder (ASD) or post-traumatic stress disorder (PTSD). Youngsters with ASD or PTSD usually exhibit substantial anxiety and hypervigilance, sleep disturbance and nightmares (which do not necessarily need to contain trauma-related content), reliving the event through play (or other forms of flashbacks), and avoidance of (and/or detachment from) trauma-related stimuli. In rare cases, psychosis may accompany these symptoms. When it can be verified that the onset of the symptoms, including psychosis, occurred after the trauma, it is likely that a post-traumatic reaction is responsible for the symptoms.

When clinicians encounter children or adolescents with ASD or PTSD, all symptom groups must be managed. Intensive psychological and pharmacological treatment is likely to be necessary, and psychosis should not be treated in isolation. While using an antipsychotic may be helpful, it is not likely to be effective unless the other symptoms are also being addressed. Unfortunately, this will usually mean that multiple supplements will need to be used, and such cases should be approached with extreme caution, since the use of multiple supplements has rarely been researched, especially in the pediatric population.

Dissociative Identity Disorder

Perhaps the most severe reaction to trauma is evident when symptoms of dissociative identity disorder (DID) are present. In this disorder, the trauma that the child experienced was so severe that the personality became fragmented and various components that normally become integrated throughout development begin to coexist independently. Separate identities often take on different names, although this may not be apparent when symptoms begin during early childhood. When these 'alters' take over the 'host' personality, the patient exhibits distinct changes in attitude, behavior, and demeanor, and these differences are much more pronounced than those evident during normal mood changes. Severe anxiety is often present and may be connected with specific settings, people, or situations. In rare and severe cases, psychosis may co-occur, especially during times of intense anxiety and dissociation.

DID is rare in adults and extremely rare in children. Although the vast majority of cases seen in adulthood are thought to begin in childhood, as a result of severe child abuse, the symptoms associated with this syndrome are rarely evident in childhood, and prodromal disturbance may be evident, characterized by anxiety, moodiness, fear and avoidance of certain people or settings, and other disturbances (for example, sleep problems). The pattern characteristic of DID (distinct switching of alters that take over the host's body) is not usually recognizable until late adolescence or adulthood.

As with ASD or PTSD, when clinicians encounter children or adolescents who present symptoms that may be characteristic of DID, all symptom groups must be managed. Intensive psychological and pharmacological treatment is likely to be necessary, and psychosis should not be treated in isolation. While using an antipsychotic may be helpful, it is not likely to be effective unless the other symptoms are also being addressed. Unfortunately, this will usually mean that multiple supplements, in addition to intense psychotherapy, will need to be used, and such cases should be approached with extreme caution.

Neurological Disorders

In addition to psychological disorders, psychosis is sometimes associated with some medical conditions. These may be secondary to neurodevelopmental delays, brain damage, and a variety of other etiologies. Because these need to be treated medically, it is necessary to carefully perform a differential diagnosis and rule out these disorders.

Epilepsy

Some forms of psychosis are closely linked to seizures. Since epilepsy is more common in children than it is in adults, the association between psychosis and seizures may be even stronger in the pediatric population. In relation to epilepsy, psychosis is most often classified according to the time when episodes occur. Postictal psychosis may affect between 6 and 10 percent of people with epilepsy (Kanner, 2000). In this presentation, psychosis occurs within a few days after a seizure or seizure cluster. The psychosis may also co-occur with mood disturbance. These episodes are more common after secondarily generalized tonic-clonic seizures. Sleep disturbance may precede postictal psychosis. Some studies have found that postictal psychosis is much more common in people who experience bilateral independent seizure foci (Kanner).

Ictal psychosis occurs during seizures, and is especially associated with nonconvulsive status epilepticus (Kanner, 2000). Ictal psychosis is characterized by concurrent unresponsiveness and automatic movements, but because loss of consciousness may not be evident, some may not recognize that a seizure is taking place. Individuals with a long history of severe seizures are at greatest risk for ictal psychosis. Interictal psychosis can occur at any time between seizures, with no relationship to the timing of seizures. When seen, it may indicate the presence of brain tumors. Generally, whenever psychosis is evident in children or adolescents, especially when these symptoms are accompanied by neurodevelopmental delays or other neurological symptoms, an evaluation by a neurologist is warranted.

ETIOLOGY

Our understanding of the etiology of symptoms of psychosis continues to evolve. In most disorders involving psychosis, whether the psychosis is a core or adjunct feature, positive symptoms are evident. In severe cases, mostly evident in cases of serious mental illness (such as schizophrenia), negative symptoms also become apparent. Because these two categories of symptoms are presumed to have different etiologies, they should be reviewed separately.

Positive Symptoms

For many years, it was suspected that dopaminergic overactivity in portions of the brain was responsible for the perceptual experience of hallucinations, and was also implicated in delusions. As brain circuits continued to be identified, dopaminergic pathways and their functions were clarified. As discussed in Chapter 4, dopaminergic projections originate in the upper portions of the brain stem and extend into many subcortical and cortical areas, including the frontal lobes, the limbic system, and the basal ganglia.

The mesolimbic pathway, specifically, is implicated in producing symptoms of psychosis. It is a complex pathway that stimulates portions of the limbic system, including nucleus accumbens. When overstimulated (for example, as seen when individuals abuse psychostimulants, like cocaine or methamphetamine), these circuits produce excessive perceptual experiences that may take a form of hallucinations and delusions. Although dopamine activity is presumed to play the most major role, serotonin, GABA, and glutamate may also be involved in producing these symptoms (Stahl, 2008).

Overactivation of the mesolimbic pathways has significant implications for the progression of the disorder. When cells are stimulated to fire too frequently, the refractory period necessary for the cell to reconstitute itself and become ready to fire again is abnormally shortened. As a result, the cell does not sufficiently recover after each successive action and gradually begins to deteriorate. Consequently, it has been hypothesized that individuals who experience psychosis for extended periods of time gradually experience cellular apoptosis associated with excessive cell firing, and begin to show signs of structural brain damage in later years.

Negative Symptoms

Our understanding of the etiology of the negative symptoms continues to evolve. Initially, it was presumed that negative symptoms result from the gradual destruction of dopaminergic cells in areas that regulated emotional control. Since psychosis occurs when a portion of the mesolimbic pathways is overstimulated, the mesolimbic pathway gradually deteriorates, and psychological functions associated with this pathway (such as emotional reactivity and social awareness) begin to deteriorate. Indeed, this line of reasoning was supported by the results of many brain imaging studies that revealed that the size of lateral ventricles, which are adjacent to portions of the mesolimbic pathways, increases with the length of time the patient has been diagnosed with schizophrenia, and these increases are correlated with decreases in behaviors associated with the functioning of this pathway (the results of these studies are discussed in the next section).

More recently, our understanding of the etiology of negative symptoms evolved further. It is apparent that the mechanism described above may be responsible for some of the negative symptoms, especially those that seem to come on gradually, but negative symptoms may also be secondary to deficits in the functioning of portions of the mesocortical dopaminergic pathway. Specifically, projections leading to the dorsolateral prefrontal area and the ventromedial prefrontal cortex are especially implicated in producing cognitive blunting, apathy, and avolition (Stahl, 2008). Thus, when a mix of positive and negative symptoms is apparent, the brain's dopaminergic pathways may be miswired and deficits and excesses in various dopaminergic pathways are evident at the same time.

Summary of Research Findings

Schizophrenia and other psychotic disorders have long been suspected to be caused by brain abnormalities, propensity for which is transmitted genetically. Children of patients with schizophrenia have a risk for developing this disorder that is 10– 20 times greater than the general population, and remains in the same range when the child is separated from the parents and raised by parents without schizophrenia. If both parents have schizophrenia, the risk goes up to 25–46 times the general population. In addition, a monozygotic twin of a schizophrenic has a risk of developing the disorder that is nearly 50 times the rate seen in the general population (Gottesman, 1991).

It is further notable that studies that examined other disorders that may include symptoms of psychosis similarly reveal high rates of heritability. For example, the heritability of major depression is estimated to be about 40 percent (Sutker and Adams, 2001), and the heritability of bipolar disorder has been estimated to be as high as 80 percent (Bertelsen *et al.*, 1977). Although the rates for heritability of schizoaffective disorder have not been established, it is clear that those disorders that most commonly include symptoms of psychosis (schizophrenia, major depression, and bipolar) present a substantial genetic risk of heritability.

In addition to genetic links, numerous neuroanatomical and neurophysiological studies examined the brain structure and function of patients with schizophrenia.

Neuroanatomical Abnormalities

As discussed earlier in the chapter, several decades of brain research, mostly performed with the use of CT scans, revealed that patients with schizophrenia have enlarged lateral ventricles, and several study groups obtained similar results with children with schizophrenia (Asarnow & Asarnow, 2003). On average, the brain of patients with schizophrenia is about 4 percent smaller than normal (Lawrie & Abkumeil, 1998), and studies of children with schizophrenia have reported the same brain size differences (Rapoport *et al.*, 1999). These have been found to increase with the duration of schizophrenia (Rapoport *et al.*, 1997), and the speed of the progression was found to be more rapid for children than for adults with schizophrenia (Gogtay *et al.*, 2004). Other structural abnormalities have also been revealed. Children with schizophrenia have been shown to exhibit smaller vermis and cerebellum (Jacobsen *et al.*, 1997), and *larger* basal ganglia (Blanton *et al.*, 1999), although the latter finding may be secondary to the use of neuroleptic medications with these patients.

In addition, children with schizophrenia reveal *increases* in the volume of white matter, particularly in the anterior and posterior corpus callosum (Jacobsen *et al.*, 1997). Some have interpreted these findings to be suggestive of 'white matter sparing' that may be taking place in the context of decreasing cortical volume (Asarnow & Asarnow, 2003, p. 470). Indeed, Thompson *et al.* (2001) found that children with schizophrenia reveal accelerated gray matter loss in parietal brain regions, and these progress anteriorly into the temporal lobes, gradually engulfing sensorimotor and dorsolateral prefrontal cortices. In addition, these symptoms correlated with the severity of the psychotic symptoms. Similarly, gray matter loss, nearly absent in early childhood, progressed as the disease continued. Other studies have also revealed loss of brain matter in the right temporal lobe, bilateral superior and posterior temporal gyrus, right anterior temporal gyrus, and left hippocampus. Collectively, these findings reveal that children with schizophrenia exhibit progressive reductions in neural density in gray (but not white) matter, and that the compromised areas include cortical and subcortical structures.

Neurophysiological Abnormalities

Studies that utilize functional imaging to investigate brain activity in patients with schizophrenia also report a number of abnormalities. PET scans reveal that brains of schizophrenics take up and metabolize less glucose, particularly in the frontal lobes, and schizophrenics exhibit less blood perfusion in the frontal and prefrontal cortex. In addition, when exposed to tasks that normally stimulate the prefrontal cortex, patients with schizophrenia do not reveal increases in activation that is evident in nonschizophrenics. Consequently, some have proposed that schizophrenic deficits are associated with hypofrontality (Winn, 1994). In addition, parts of the brain involved in working and associative memory, as well as those that process thought in relation to context, have been shown to be significantly underactive (Dehaene *et al.*, 1999).

Numerous brain scans focused on dopaminergic activity in the brains of patients with schizophrenia. The findings generally reveal that dopaminergic activity in portions of the frontal lobes (and surrounding areas) seems to exhibit patterns of activity consistent with the 'miswiring' hypothesis. Laruelle *et al.* (1996) found that brains of patients with schizophrenia were hypersensitive to release of dopamine, and that dopaminergic activity correlated with symptoms of psychosis. In addition, some postmortem studies also found that brains of patients with schizophrenia exhibit increases in dopaminergic receptors (Jaskiw & Kleinman, 1988), particularly in the area of the nucleus accumbens (Gurevich *et al.*, 1997), although these findings have not been consistently reported. Since most schizophrenics were treated with dopamine blockers at the time these studies were performed, it is possible that exposure to these medications underlies the lack of consistency of these findings. Indeed, Abi-Dargham *et al.* (2000) found that neuroleptics-naïve patients had more D2 receptors and extracellular dopamine than nonschizophrenic controls.

Although the dopamine hypotheses has generated the most research, and appears best supported, it does not appear to apply to everyone. Medications that are dopamine blockers seem to effectively eliminate symptoms of psychosis in most patients with schizophrenia or other psychotic disorders, but some patients do not respond well to these drugs, and instead show better response to medications that block serotonin and only have a minor impact on dopamine. In addition, recent investigations reveal that glutamate may be involved in the symptoms of psychosis, and a new class of antipsychotic medications that targets glutamatergic functions is under development (Stahl, 2007), although some studies are contradictory with regard to whether glutamate hypoactivity or hyperactivity underlies psychosis.

Results of EEG studies also reveal interesting findings. Schizophrenia is associated with abnormal EEG patterns in gamma band (30–100 Hz) oscillations. During a recent study, schizophrenics were given tasks that normally stimulate gamma-band oscillation at occipital and parietal lobes, but schizophrenics did not reveal this oscillation, and instead oscillations were elicited at sub-gamma frequencies (22–26 Hz). The gamma-wave activity presumably occurs at the frequency that cell groups use to communicate with each other when processing distinct features of an object, and neurons of patients with schizophrenia do not seem to communicate with each other with the same efficiency as normal controls. The investigators further found that the deficiency was associated with visual hallucinations, and hypothesized that hallucinations may constitute aberrant activity in the visual cortex so that false perceptions are generated. Interestingly, antipsychotic medications had no effect on the aberrant EEG manifestations (Spencer *et al.*, 2004).

SUPPLEMENTS WITH ESTABLISHED EFFICACY

At this time, it is apparent that only one naturopathic supplement has sufficiently been studied for its antipsychotic properties and reveals documented efficacy. Compounds that block the effects of dopamine are known to be effective in reducing symptoms of psychosis, and rauwolfia exerts similar effects in the brain.

Rauwolfia

Rauwolfia (*Rauwolfia serpentina*), also spelled ravolphia, is a medicinal shrub in the milkweed family. Its root is ground into a powder and packaged in this form or sold in tablets or capsules. It is a compound commonly used in Asian medicine, including traditional Ayurveda medicine native to India. Its active components are alkaloids and about 50 have been identified, although the primary psychoactive components appear to be reserpine, rescinnamine, and deserpidine (Spinella, 2001).

Supplementation with rauwolfia has been performed in western medicine since the 1950s (Spinella, 2001), primarily for the purpose of treating psychosis. At this time, atypical antipsychotic medications are used most frequently because they successfully treat symptoms of psychosis with fewer risks of motor side effects. However, rauwolfia supplements (especially those that contain reserpine) are still sometimes used as adjuncts to a prescription antipsychotic (Spinella), and use of rauwolfia may also offer some benefits in treating tic disorders (as discussed in Chapter 10), and insomnia (see Chapter 9).

Evidence of Efficacy

Evidence of the efficacy of rauwolfia to treat psychosis dates back to the early 1930s, when Sen and Bose (1931) published the first scientific report about its value as an antipsychotic. Subsequently, Kline (1954) published the first western report of its antipsychotic properties. In subsequent decades, many American and European studies confirmed these findings (López-Muñoz *et al.*, 2004), and its clinical effect has found to be to be similar to that of typical antipsychotics (Spinella, 2001). For example, Ramu *et al.* (1983) studied an herbal combination that included crude plant extract of rauwolfia and found it effective in reducing symptoms of psychosis in chronic schizophrenics, and a subsequent placebo-controlled trial confirmed this effect (Ramu *et al.*, 1999). In another controlled trial, 136 participants were randomized to one of four groups – herbal mix with rauwolfia, chlorpromazine (brand name Thorazine, a typical antipsychotic), valeriana wallichi, or placebo – and found that the groups taking rauwolfia or chlorpromazine improved the most, and both groups showed comparable reduction in symptoms (Mahal *et al.*, 1976). A similar study performed with 78 chronic schizophrenics again revealed that patients taking chlorpromazine and rauwolfia exhibited significant improvement in symptoms in comparison to the group taking placebo (Prathikanti, 2007).

In western medicine, rauwolfia supplements are usually given in the form of reserpine, one of its active ingredients, isolated from the crude extract. By contrast, in eastern medicine, crude plant extract is used, usually in a preparation called Brahmyadiyoga, a combination of six Ayuverdic herbs (Prathikanti, 2007). Cott and Misra (1999) investigated the difference in pharmacokinetics between raw rauwolfia plant extract and purified reserpine, and found some differences in the binding profile. Thus, the raw plant extract may have fewer adverse effects and address a wider range of symptoms of schizophrenia (Prathakanti).

Pharmacodynamics

Reserpine has been shown to block vesicular storage of monoamines (including dopamine). Consequently, these neurotransmitters remain longer in the cytoplasm, and are more likely to be destroyed by monoamine oxidase, the enzyme that destroys all monoamine neurotransmitters. As a result, depletion of monoamines becomes evident in central and peripheral neurons, and levels of monoamine neurotransmitters released with each neuronal action are significantly decreased. In addition, the effects of this action seem evident a few days to a few weeks after discontinuation of the supplement (Spinella, 2001).

Raw rauwolfia extract seems to have a broader binding profile, and may also be a GABA and alpha 2 noradrenergic antagonist (Cott & Misra, 1999). This appears to change its pharmacodynamics and allows the compound to address a wider variety of symptoms. This also seems to reduce the adverse effects, although this property may be the result of lower reserpine levels in raw rauwolfia extracts.

Pharmacokinetics

Little is known about the pharmacokinetics of rauwolfia or reserpine. Following administration, the compound is absorbed and enters systemic circulation, where it crosses the blood–brain barrier and is absorbed into cell bodies of monoaminergic neurons. Rates of metabolism or excretion have not been established, but effects have been known to last for days or weeks after discontinuation of the compound. Although some have hypothesized that this continued effects is evident because this is how long it takes neurons to synthesize new vesicles to store the monoamines (Spinella, 2001), it is also possible that reserpine may have active metabolites that continue to affect the neuron and take much longer to be eliminated from the body.

Dosing

Rauwolfia supplements are generally available in tablets and capsules. Whole and crude forms are also available, but because dosing is more difficult to establish and monitor, the use of these forms is not recommended.

Adult daily dose is usually 600 mg of rauwolfia or 6 mg of reserpine (Medical Economics, 2007). Thus, the daily dose may be about 7 mg/kg of rauwolfia supplement, or 0.07 mg/kg of reserpine. While this dose may be appropriate for adolescents, children should start much lower. It is preferable to purchase the tablet preparations for use with children, since these can be scored to begin with a low dose. Because rauwolfia is sedating, it may be better to take the compound at night.

Adverse Effects

Use of rauwolfia carries a risk of significant side effects. To begin with, patients who take rauwolfia (or reserpine) are at a significant risk of developing symptoms of depression, and this effect is presumed to be directly caused by the pharmacodynamic properties of the compound – the depletion of monoamine neurotransmitters. Consequently, youngsters who take rauwolfia or reserpine supplements must carefully be monitored for the onset of depressive symptoms, and rauwolfia is contraindicated in anyone with a history of depression.

Because rauwolfia exerts a significant antagonistic effect dopamine, some patients may experience unpleasant motor side effects associated with typical antipsychotic medications (like Haldol), including problems with coordination and stereotypic movements. In extreme cases, and if the compound is used for long periods of time, it is possible that it may carry a risk of tardive dyskinesia (TD) that is similar to other conventional antipsychotics, although the link between TD and use of rauwolfia (or reserpine) has not been established. However, because TD is irreversible, it is prudent to exercise extreme caution when using this compound.

In eastern medicine rauwolfia continues to be used as a tranquilizer, and the compound is approved by Commission E for the treatment of hypertension and insomnia. Rauwolfia is sedating. When administered, it reduces blood pressure and may result in dizziness. Although in low doses patients may develop tolerance to these effects, blood pressure of patients who take rauwolfia should regularly be monitored.

In addition, rauwolfia is contraindicated during pregnancy, so if it is used with adolescent females, they need to be counseled about the need to use contraception (Medical Economics, 2007).

SUPPLEMENTS WITH LIKELY EFFICACY

Although compounds that block dopamine transmission have been shown to be effective most consistently, they do not seem to work for everyone, and dopamine blockade can also result in significant adverse effects, making dopamine blockers difficult to tolerate for some patients. Consequently, other ways of treating symptoms of psychosis are being researched, and Omega-3 supplements have shown promising results in some clinical studies.

Omega-3 Polyunsaturated Fatty Acids

Effects of Omega-3 were previously discussed in Chapters 5, 6, and 7. Omega-3 fatty acids, including both eicosapentaenoic acid (EPA) and docosahexanoic acid (DHA), have been presumed to have many beneficial effects, including mood stabilization, protection against dementias (especially, Alzheimer's), and reducing risks associated with low density lipoproteins' (LDL) artery clogging effects. Some studies have also shown benefits in improving symptoms of schizophrenia.

Omega-3 supplements are generally available as caplets filled with fish oil rich in Omega-3. The pills usually contain 1000 mg, but those containing higher and lower amounts are also available. In addition, since the caplets are usually rather large, and may be difficult to swallow by some patients, other forms are also available – for example, a chewable preparation. As is the case with all supplements, there are many manufacturers, and Omega-3 supplements are sold in drug stores, supermarkets and health food stores. Many are also available through the Internet.

Omega-3 is also sold by prescription in 1000 mg tablets that contain 465 mg of eicosapentaenoic acid (EPA) and 375 mg of docosahexanoic acid (DHA). These are approved to treat hyperlipidemia and are marketed as Lovaza (formally Omacor). They are manufactured in a process that removes mercury from the fish oil, and therefore these pills are marketed as superior to other Omega-3 supplements (which usually do not remove mercury from the fish oil): the amount of mercury contained in fish oil supplements is considered to be much lower than it is in many types of fish, since the oil is not usually derived from fish known to have high amounts of mercury. In addition, plant-based Omega-3 supplements (in flax, soybean, or canola oil), also available on the market, do not contain mercury. One potential benefit of Lovaza is that, as an FDA-approved compound, its sale and manufacture is regulated, and therefore the consumer can be more certain that Lovaza really contains the ingredients that it claims to have, in the specific amount that is advertised. Consumers must balance these benefits against the added cost of this medication and the inconvenience of seeking a prescription.

Evidence of Efficacy

Omega-3's efficacy to treat symptoms of depression, bipolar disorder, and ADHD has been researched more extensively than its benefit in treating psychosis. However, case reports and small double-blind trials have begun to emerge over the last two decades. For example, Su *et al.* (2001) found that Omega-3 supplements were effective in reducing psychosis in a pregnant woman with schizophrenia. One team of researchers performed a series of small double-blind trials with schizophrenics and consistently found positive results (Mellor *et al.*, 1995; Laugharne *et al.*, 1996; Peet *et al.*, 1996). Another study found similar results in a 4 month open trial, during which a combination of EPA, DHA, and antioxidant vitamins (C and E) was found to be effective in reducing both positive and negative symptoms of schizophrenia (Arvindakshan *et al.*, 2003).

It is apparent EPA has greater antipsychotic properties than DHA. Peet *et al.* (1996) found that supplements with high ratio of EPA were more effective in reducing psychosis than those with higher ratio of DHA, and EPA supplements, taken at a dose of 2 g/day, were also found effective as adjunct to antipsychotic medications in further reducing symptoms of schizophrenia (Peet & Horrobin, 2002), but another study failed to confirm these results (Fenton *et al.*, 2001). It is apparent that augmentation with EPA may be effective when added to some antipsychotic medications, but not others.

Benefits from Omega-3 supplementation may extend to patients who present psychosis in addition to mood disturbance. Puri *et al.* (2002) reported that EPA was effective in reducing severe symptoms of depression (including psychosis) in treatment-refractory patients. In addition, Omega-3 supplements have been found to lower levels of aggression and violence (Gesh *et al.*, 2002), and is showing promising results in studies that investigated its effects as a mood stabilizer (as reviewed in Chapter 7). Consequently, Omega-3 supplements may be particularly useful in patients who present simultaneous mood disturbance and psychosis.

Pharmacodynamics

Essential Omega-3 fatty acids include a-linolenic acid (ALA), eicosapentaenoic acid (EPA), and docosahexaenoic acid (DHA). These cannot be synthesized by the body and must be ingested from food. Following ingestion, DHA inhibits lipogenesis and stimulates oxidation. ALA, EPA, and DHA undergo downconversion and retroconversion (as described below) and contribute to the metabolism of various nutrients and lipids. This is responsible for a broad-based therapeutic effect that includes changes in cardiovascular function, decrease in triglycerides, and improvement in pulmonary function. Most of these effects are directly associated with DHA, although related fatty acids may play a contributory role.

DHA is taken up by the brain at greater rates than the other fatty acids. DHA is then incorporated into the phospholipids of cell membranes. DHA contributes to proper formation and elongation of synapses. In addition, DHA-containing phospholipids improve cell function by stabilizing the membrane fluidity and changing firing rates of neurons (Horrocks & Yeo, 1999). Eicosanoids (EPA) contribute to this process. They are localized in cells and serve as catalysts for a large number of processes, including the movement of calcium in and out of the cells (Enig & Fallon, 1999). Because calcium channels are involved in the rates of firing of brain cells, regulation of these channels changes the brain's action potential. It is possible that EPA's regulation of calcium channels may contribute to DHA's influence of cell membrane phosphorization, providing a synergistic effect on the rates of neuronal firing. This may be the reason why EPA seems to show greater benefits in managing symptoms of psychosis than DHA.

Pharmacokinetics

Following ingestion, the metabolism of fatty acids begins in the small intestine by special digestive enzymes. These lipases break down fatty acids into individual chains, glycerol, and monoglycerides (glycerol with one remaining fatty acid still attached). These are then absorbed through the intestinal wall into the lymph stream. Fat molecules are then carried in the lymph system and slowly metabolized to provide gradual release of energy (Enig, 2000).

Essential fatty acids go through many conversions. ALA is converted into EPA and DHA, and these are then gradually absorbed into cell membranes. However, they also undergo complex cross-metabolism. While Omega-6, also known as linoleic acid (LA), undergoes a one-way transformation into various fatty chains, culminating in docosapentaenoic acid, ALA undergoes circular transformation that involves many steps, including the formation of EPA and DHA, and then retroconversion of EPA and DHA. It is difficult to determine how the body regulates the amounts of DHA and EPA that remain in the cells. It is likely that these are constantly transformed into each other to provide a balance of essential nutrients necessary for many metabolic processes, including membrane phosphorization.

ALA is converted into EPA and DHA, and EPA and DHA are retroconverted into each other. Consequently, when Omega-3 supplements are used to manage symptoms of some disorders (like ADHD), it may not be necessary to purchase a specific combination of these fatty acids. However, EPA has been shown in studies to have the most beneficial effects in reducing symptoms of psychosis. Thus, it may be desirable to use Omega-3 supplements with high content of EPA when the supplement is used to manage psychotic symptoms.

Optimal ratio of Omega-6 to Omega-3 in the human body is estimated to be 2:1. However, it is not uncommon for individuals in westernized countries to consume diets where the two are ingested at a ratio of about 20:1. For this reason, the majority of supplements primarily focus on delivering additional amounts of Omega-3 into the body, and any amounts of Omega-6 in the tablet may be superfluous, since the common diet already includes so many foods rich in LA. When purchasing a supplement, consumers should select one that maximizes the amount of Omega-3 and minimizes the amount of Omega-6 in the preparation.

Manufacturers of Omega-3 generally advise to take the supplements with or without food. Researchers, however, have long recognized that Omega-3 fatty acids ingested in food are better absorbed than those taken in supplements. Some studies have found that Omega-3 taken without a meal is poorly absorbed. For this reason, nutritionists generally recommend to take an Omega-3 supplement as part of a meal, so that it is absorbed together with the food that is being consumed (Neville, 2006).

In order to prevent oxidation of fatty acids before they are taken up into cell membranes, antioxidants must be present. Those whose diets are rich in antioxidant foods probably consume enough of these during a meal to prevent fatty acid oxidation. However, those who consume meals low in antioxidants may need to take an antioxidant supplement – for example, tocopherol, a form of vitamin E. For this reason, some formulations of Omega-3 supplements include a small amount of tocopherol. However, instead of (or in addition to) tocopherol, some supplements also include vitamins A and/or D. Because these vitamins do not get cleared from the body, clients should be careful with these supplements because high intake of these vitamins may lead to toxicity.

Although fatty acids are metabolized and absorbed rapidly, the onset of effect is not evident for a long time. Some have reported that the onset of clinical effect is not evident for weeks, even months, and that treatment for up to 3 months is necessary to determine the eventual clinical response (Lake, 2007). This makes it difficult to dose the supplements, since clinical effects are not likely to be immediately evident.

Dosing

Omega-3 supplements are not usually dosed by body weight. To treat symptoms of psychosis in children, the recommended starting dose is 500 mg (Potter *et al.*, 2009). Some have found doses below 1000 mg/day to be ineffective (Lake, 2007). Because Omega-3 is generally well tolerated, gradual titration is recommended. However, the maximum dose is often determined by how many tablets the child is willing to take and whether digestive effects (for example, fish burps or a fishy taste in the mouth) prevent further increase in dose. Because response will not immediately be evident, it is difficult to determine what dose will eventually be effective.

Teens are generally dosed closer to the adult dose of 2–3 g/day, and some have found doses below 2 g/day to be ineffective (Lake, 2007). As with children, dosing should gradually be increased to a maximum level that can be tolerated with minimal gastrointestinal discomfort. Again, it is difficult to determine what dose will be effective since response to the supplement may not immediately be evident.

Co-factors are necessary for metabolism of some of the fatty acids, especially EFA. Carnitine is necessary for the elongating EFA and transporting it across inner cell membranes. It is possible that some of the inconsistent findings about the efficacy of fatty acids may be secondary to carnitine deficits. For this reason, supplementation with l-carnitine has been studied and has shown promising effects in hyperactive girls with fragile X syndrome (Torrioli *et al.*, 1999). Since humans metabolize only a portion of the necessary supply of carnitine, supplementing fatty acid therapy with l-carnitine may be helpful. L-carnitine is supplied in capsules, tablets, solution, and chewable wafer. Children may take about 250 mg of l-carnitine with fatty acids, while adults may need to take about 500 mg. These doses are generally well tolerated although a small incidence of seizures has been reported (Medical Economics, 2008a). Individuals with risk factors for seizures should consider l-carnitine supplementation only under supervision of a physician.

Adverse Effects

Omega-3 oils are generally well tolerated. The most common adverse effects involve the gastrointestinal tract, including nausea and diarrhea. Because the majority of Omega-3 supplements are sold as fish oils, some individuals experience an unpleasant, 'fishy' taste in their mouth, a 'fishy' smelling breath after a meal during which Omega-3 supplement was taken, and fishy 'burps' that may last for several hours. For this reason, some manufacturers offer 'burpless' formulas manufactured by increasing the thickness of the pill's outer coating. This allows the supplement to survive the stomach acids and dissolve when it reaches the small intestine. These have been shown to effectively reduce the above problems. Omega-3 supplements are also available in non-fish based formulas that are not associated with burps or an unpleasant taste.

Because Omega-3 supplements are oil based, there is a caloric value associated with the caplet. The exact amount varies, but generally a 1000 mg pill will contain about 20 calories. For individuals who consume a low amount, an extra 20 or 40 calories per day will probably have a minimal amount on weight. However, those on higher amounts (for example, 8000 or 9000 mg per day) must remember that they are consuming an additional 160 or 180 calories. In addition, fatty acids are high density lipoproteins (HDL) and contribute to the overall HDL levels within the body. While this is generally beneficial, those on high levels of Omega-3 supplements who also consume diets rich in HDL may experience additional increases of HDL and total cholesterol, which may not always be beneficial. Individuals who take high doses of fatty acid supplements should periodically check their cholesterol profile.

Omega-3 fatty acids are associated with an antithrombotic effect. Patients who take blood thinners (like aspirin) must be careful about taking subsequent fatty acid supplements, and should consult a physician before initiating Omega-3 therapy. In addition, some patients regularly use over-the-counter non-steroidal anti-inflammatory drugs (NSAIDs, like Advil or Motrin) to manage headaches, backaches, or similar conditions. While combining fatty acids with NSAIDs has not been shown to pose a risk, many NSAIDs have some blood thinning properties, and combining NSAIDs with fatty acids has sometimes been linked to nose bleeds and easy bruising (Medical Economics, 2008a). For this reason, those who take NSAIDs daily should probably consult a physician before initiating Omega-3 therapy.

Use of fatty acid supplements has sometimes been reported to alter glucose tolerance, especially in patients with type 2 diabetes. The mechanism of this is poorly understood, and some studies have not confirmed this finding. However, because there is a risk, children and adolescents who are diabetic and take insulin should consult their physician before starting Omega-3 treatment.

SUPPLEMENTS WITH POSSIBLE EFFICACY

The two supplements discussed above have the greatest likelihood of alleviating symptoms of psychosis. If they are not effective, clinicians may look into other compounds that have shown some possible suggested benefits. However, since the data that supports the use of the following supplements is extremely limited, clinicians should proceed with caution, and consider the use of the compounds discussed in this section as experimental.

Glycine

Glycine is an amino acid commonly found in proteins. It is synthesized in the body from serine, another proteinogenic amino acid naturally synthesized within cells. As one of the 20 most common amino acids found in proteins, it serves multiple metabolic functions, but some of it is also released into synapses as a neurotransmitter.

Like glutamate and GABA, glycine is present in the nervous system and is an important building block for many chemical processes. As a neurotransmitter, it binds to several families of ionotropic and metabotropic receptors, but its primary inhibitory action seems to be the result of regulating chloride channels in a manner similar to the action of GABA. These effects are primarily seen in the spinal cord. In the brain, the effects of glycine are less predictable. For example, it seems to be involved in regulating glutamatergic neurotransmission at the NMDA glutamate ionotropic receptors that are involved in opening calcium channels and causing rapid depolarization of the post-synaptic cell. Thus, glycine may be an alosteric modulator for glutamate.

Increase in glycine function may result in effects similar to the increase of GABAergic neurotransmission (fatigue, drowsiness, etc.). However, since glycine seems to have varying effects in different parts of the brain, supplementation with glycine may also result in excitatory effects. For example, in overdose, glycine causes death by hyperexcitability of the brain. Supplementation with glycine has been shown to have some antispastic effects, and antioxidant and anti-inflammatory properties may also be evident. Some research also documented positive effects when anticonvulsants were supplemented with glycine. Very limited research exists on the benefit of glycine supplementation in the management of psychosis. In one study, high doses of glycine improved enduring negative symptoms of schizophrenia (Heresco-Levy *et al.*, 1999).

Little is known about the pharmacokinetics of glycine. The amino acid is primarily absorbed from the small intestine and transported to the liver, where some of the glycine undergoes extensive metabolism. The remaining portion enters systemic circulation and crosses the blood–brain barrier through active transport. When glycine supplements are used to augment medications (for example, anticonvulsants), 1 g/day is generally administered, in divided doses. However, much larger doses are needed when symptoms of schizophrenia are being managed, and necessary daily intake was shown to range from 40–90 g/day (46–100 mg/kg/day). In animals, doses of 3–4.5 g/kg, administered by intravenous infusion, have shown to be lethal, so the clinical range used to treat symptoms of schizophrenia is still considered to be safe in humans and no overdose with glycine has thus far been reported (Medical Economics, 2008a). However, since little research has been done, especially with children, clinicians and parents should exercise much caution.

Glycine supplementation may result in sedation, and additive effects have been shown with other sedatives (like benzodiazepines). It is unknown whether glycine changes plasma levels of, or is affected by, any other supplements or medications.

Taurine

Taurine is a non-protein organic amino sulfonic acid mainly found naturally in meat, fish, eggs, and milk. Humans also produce it from cysteine, but infants and children do so in much lower amounts, and some children lack the enzyme necessary for its metabolism. For this reason, taurine is added to most baby foods, as it is presumed to be necessary for normal retinal and brain development. Taurine has membrane stabilizing effects and consequently has been hypothesized to offer some benefit in treating symptoms of mania (as discussed in Chapter 7) and anxiety (see Chapter 8). Because taurine may activate glycine receptors (Spinella, 2001), it may therefore exert inhibitory effects similar to glycine. However, no research studies have thus far been performed and therefore its possible antipsychotic benefit may only be hypothesized from taurine's pharmacodynamic effects.

Taurine is absorbed from the small intestine and enters the brain through sodium and chloride dependent transport systems. In the cell, taurine may keep potassium and magnesium inside the cell while keeping sodium out. Thus, it may affect neuronal firing. Remaining taurine is conjugated to form the bile salts and is excreted into bile, where it is transported to the duodenum to take part in the metabolism of various lipids. Excess taurine is excreted by the kidneys.

Taurine supplements are generally available as tablets and capsules and clinical doses range from 500 mg/day to 3 g/day in adults (Medical Economics, 2008a). Child and adolescent doses may be estimated to fall around 35 mg/kg, but, as with glycine, it is possible that much higher doses may be required. Taurine supplements are usually well tolerated and no adverse effects have been reported thus far. However, pregnant and nursing mothers should only use the supplement under medical supervision.

SUPPLEMENTS NOT LIKELY TO BE EFFECTIVE

It is not possible to review all compounds that have been speculated to treat symptoms of agitation and mania. However, some of these compounds are sometimes marketed to treat symptoms of schizophrenia and psychosis, despite the lack of evidence of efficacy. In addition to being ineffective, some of these compounds may actually be dangerous when used at high doses. Clinicians who seek to practice in the area of naturopathic psychopharmacology should be aware of these compounds and the potential risks that they may pose.

Vitamin B3

Vitamin B3, also known as niacin and nicotinic acid, is an important nutrient involved in a wide variety of biological processes, including synthesis of fatty acids, production of energy, regulation of gene expression, and signal transduction. When metabolized, its metabolites serve as co-enzymes to transfer energy stored in carbohydrates, lipids, and proteins. One of these metabolites, nicotinamide adenine dinucleotide (NAD) is a precursor for ATP, a nucleotide extensively involved in cellular metabolism.

One researcher maintains that supplementation with vitamin B3 has beneficial effects in reducing symptoms of schizophrenia, and appears to have built his professional life around this claim. He has published journal articles and books about its efficacy (for example, Hoffer, 1999, 2004), and widely reports evidence of thousands of case studies that supposedly showed that symptoms of schizophrenia improved significantly with megadoses of vitamin B3, and some patients recovered with no further psychotic episodes. He conceptualizes schizophrenia as a disease caused by the accumulation of adrenochrome in the body, and claims that supplementation with vitamins B3 and C remove this toxin. To date, however, all data to support these claims comes from his research, and his findings have never been independently verified. In fact, double-blind studies have shown that B3 was not effective in reducing symptoms of schizophrenia (Wittenborn, 1973), and the American Psychiatric Association Task Force on Vitamin Therapy in Psychiatry maintains that niacin therapy is ineffective and recommends against its use (APA, 1973). More recently, Hoffer altered his views to some degree, but still maintains that niacin is effective in acute schizophrenia when used early in the progression of the disease (Hoffer, 1996). However, he provides no empirical evidence to support those claims.

Dietary reference intakes (DRI) have been established for vitamin B3, and range from 2 mg/day for infants to 18 mg/day for adults. In addition, upper intake levels have also been established, and these range from 10 mg/day for infants and toddlers to 35 mg/day for adults (Medical Economics, 2008a). However, Hoffer recommends doses of 3 g/day for children, adolescents, and adults, and maintains that lower doses are ineffective (Hoffer, 2004). Moreover, he recommends children and adolescents to stay on this dose until they turn 21, at which time the therapy can be discontinued but will have to be restarted if symptoms return, and in that case it will need to be maintained indefinitely.

Although doses of vitamin B3 that do not exceed upper intake levels are usually well tolerated and few adverse effects are apparent, megadoses of various B vitamins, including B3, may be dangerous. Doses above 1 mg/day have been associated with dermatological problems, gastrointestinal complaints, liver dysfunction, cardiac arrhythmias, hyperglycemia, and hyperuricemia (Parker *et al.*, 2006). In rare cases, high doses have resulted in blindness (Gass, 2003). In addition women who are sexually active must avoid high doses because birth defects have been associated with vitamin B3 supplementation (Parker *et al.*). All in all, it is clear that the risks of vitamin B3 supplementation, especially at the doses recommended by Hoffer, clearly outweigh potential benefits, and clinicians are advised against this method of treatment.

Dehydroepiandrosterone

Dehydroepiandrosterone (DHEA) is a natural substance produced in the brain, as well as the adrenal glands and the gonads. DHEA, and its major metabolite, dehydroepiandrosterone-3-sulfate (DHEAS) are the most abundant steroids circulating in the human body. DHEA is metabolized to various hormones, including testosterone and estrogen. In the brain, DHEA is classified as a neurosteroid and may act as a modulator of GABA A and glutamate NMDA receptors (Medical Economics, 2008a).

DHEA has been investigated as a pharmacological compound for many decades, and has been shown to have some efficacy in the treatment of lupus, asthmatic attacks, and severe burns. Supplementation with DHEA or DHEAS has been attempted in the treatment of symptoms of schizophrenia and some have reported promising results (Strauss & Stevenson, 1955). However, subsequent double-blind trials revealed no efficacy in the treatment of psychosis (Wolkowitz & Reus, 2002), although it appears to exhibit some efficacy in treatment of depression (as discussed in Chapter 6).

Use of DHEA should be cleared with a medical professional. DHEA is usually contraindicated in children and adolescents, and use of the compound in this population should generally be avoided (Medical Economics, 2008a). Supplementation with DHEA has been associated with significant adverse effects, including dermatological problems, hirsutism, and voice changes in women (which may be permanent), cardiovascular problems, hepatitis, insulin resistance, and manic symptoms. In addition, males who use DHEA may have an increased risk of prostate cancer (Medical Economics). Consequently, the risks of DHEA supplementation, especially with children and adolescents, significantly outweigh any presumed benefits, and clinicians should avoid using this compound with pediatric patients.

SUMMARY

In order to help clinicians select the compounds that are appropriate given the specific presentation of psychosis evident in each patient, an algorithm was developed and is presented in Figure 11.1. This diagram takes into account the amount of research support available for each compound, as well as the specific mechanism of action of each supplement and its applicability to the treatment of psychosis as a core feature or an additional symptom.

Patients with symptoms of psychosis that is not associated with mood disturbance may cautiously attempt treatment with rauwolfia, although dose should be kept low and the patient should closely be monitored for any adverse effects (especially including the onset of depression and motor problems). If partial response is evident, Omega-3 supplement (with high EPA content) may be used as an adjunct, or switched to as monotherapy. Vitamin C, E, and/or carnitine may be added to this regimen. When inadequate response is still evident, glycine and/or taurine may be attempted, and those compounds may be used together with Omega-3, carnitine, and vitamins C and E. However, this combination should not be used concurrently with rauwolfia.

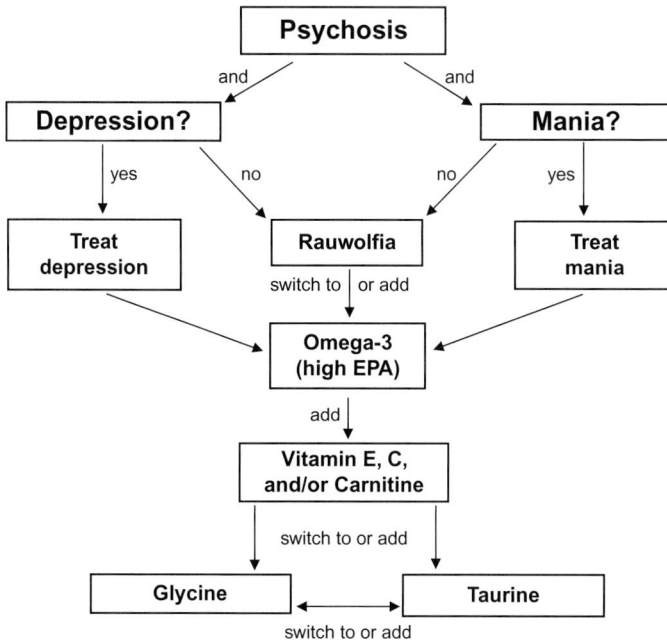

FIGURE 11.1   Algorithm for treatment of psychosis with naturopathic supplements.
© Elsevier 2009.

Patients who experience symptoms of psychosis in addition to mood disturbance should avoid rauwolfia. Instead, they should initially try treatment with Omega-3 supplements (with high EPA content), and vitamin C, E, and/or carnitine may be added. If inadequate response is evident, glycine and/or taurine may be attempted, and those compounds may be used together with Omega-3, carnitine, and vitamins C and E.

Chapter 12

Autism

Autism is one of the most controversial of all disorders evident in the pediatric population. Although historical accounts describe cases of children with symptoms similar to today's autism dating back several centuries (Wing & Potter, 2002), modern research and attempts at consistent classification only date back a few decades.

For a time, autism was presumed to represent a childhood version of schizophrenia, and symptoms of autism were thought to be similar to those of adult schizophrenia. Since the 1970s, it is recognized that autism is a separate disorder that, in most cases, does not closely resemble symptoms of schizophrenia, and therefore nowadays the two disorders are considered to be distinct.

Another controversy surrounds the question of whether autism is a diagnostic category or a specific disorder. Because individuals with autistic-like symptoms exhibit a wide range of overall level of functioning and different functional impairments, a variety of diagnostic terms have been used to describe these individuals, including autism, high-functioning autism, Asperger's disorder, and pervasive developmental disorder. Since 1994, the DSM system attempts to revolve this dispute by providing a *category* of pervasive developmental disorders (PDD) that contains several specific disorders, including autistic disorder (APA, 2000). Thus, autism is specifically differentiated from a number of other specific disorders.

Rett's disorder is a severe neuropsychiatric disorder, only evident in females, characterized by normal development up to age of 5 months and subsequent deceleration of head growth, loss of previously acquired motor skills, and severe language impairment. Similarly, childhood disintegrative disorder is a severe neuropsychiatric disorder characterized by normal development for at least the first 2 years of life, and significant loss of previously acquired motor, play, physical, social, and/or language skills occurring prior to age 10 (APA, 2000). Because of their specific developmental progression, in most cases these disorders can easily be differentiated from autism-spectrum disorders.

Within the current DSM system, three diagnoses constitute autism-spectrum disorders, and some consider these three disorders to constitute three expressions of the same etiology, with different severity of symptoms (Szatmari, 2000). Asperger's disorder is characterized by qualitative impairments in social interaction, and repetitive or stereotyped patterns of behavior, but delay in cognitive or language development is not evident. By contrast, the diagnosis of autism requires the presence of impairments in social interaction, repetitive or stereotyped pattern of behavior, *and* a qualitative impairment in communication. Finally, the diagnosis of pervasive developmental disorder not otherwise specified (PDD NOS) is generally assigned to those who exhibit some, but not all of the symptoms of the above disorders. This specifically includes what the DSM calls 'atypical autism' (APA, 2000, p. 84), a presentation of symptoms that resembles autistic disorders but does not meet diagnostic criteria because of late age at onset (to be diagnosed with autistic disorder, impairment must be evident prior to age 3), and/or atypical or subthreshold symptoms. Thus, it is evident that children with autism usually represent much higher level of impairment than children with Asperger's disorder or PDD NOS, and children with autism, rather than Asperger's or PDD NOS, are more likely to need pharmacological interventions. Consequently, this chapter will focus on the treatment of autistic disorder (as defined within the DSM-IV-TR) with nutritional and herbal supplements.

The prevalence of autism in children has been researched for several decades. Currently, it is estimated that about 30 children per 10,000 are diagnosed with any PDD, and about 15 children per 10,000 are diagnosed with autism (Fombonne, 2003). However, some have reported that several, small geographic areas seem to have prevalence rates as high as 67 per 10,000 (Bertrand *et al.*, 2001). Such findings have spawned speculations about certain environmental factors (for example, toxins from pharmaceutical companies) being involved in the development of autism. To date, however, these findings have not been confirmed by credible research, and it is equally likely that certain geographical areas attract families who have children with autism – for example, because of increased services available to these children within some local school districts – or the likelihood that some geographical regions are much better at recognizing, and reporting, cases of autism.

SYMPTOMS OF AUTISM

As with all disorders, children with autism exhibit core symptoms, as defined in the DSM classification. In addition, significant secondary symptoms usually result from the changes in their family, social, and educational development caused by the expression of the core symptoms, and additional difficulties are also frequently associated with autism.

Core Symptoms

Within the DSM classification, three sets of core symptoms are necessary in order to diagnose autistic disorder – impairment in social interaction, impairment in communication, and restricted, repetitive, stereotyped patterns of behaviors.

Impairment in Social Interaction

From early on, children who later go on to be diagnosed with autism exhibit different patterns of interaction. When held, they are often stiff, unresponsive, or 'floppy' (Prior & Ozonoff, 1998). They usually do not initiate contact with others or respond when others try to get their attention. They do not exhibit reciprocal social interaction, and often interact with people (for example, parents, siblings, or peers) as if they were inanimate objects (Klinger *et al.*, 2003). Their eye contact is very limited and they exhibit significant impairment in the use of facial expression, body posture, or gestures to regulate social interactions (APA, 2000). As a result, they develop very limited relationships with family members or peers, and do not seem to exhibit the need to share enjoyment or interests with others around them.

Impairment in Communication

Children with autism exhibit a significant delay in the development of spoken language, and do not seem to utilize other means to compensate for these delays (for example, gesturing or miming). In fact, only about half the children with autism go on to develop meaningful spoken language or other forms of communication (Klinger *et al.*, 2003). When language function starts to emerge, it is often accompanied by anomalies, such as echolalia, abnormal prosody, or pronoun disuse and/or reversal. These difficulties are especially evident in the use of personal pronouns, including the lack of appropriate use of 'me' when referring to himself/herself, and 'you' when referring to others – for example, reversing these (Lee *et al.*, 1994). Their pragmatics are also impaired and they exhibit problems using language to get a message across to another person. Because of their difficulties with reciprocity (as described above), they find it hard to conceive that others do not understand what they are trying to say and must often guess at the purpose of the communication (Tager Flushberg, 2001).

Restricted, Repetitive, and Stereotyped Behaviors

This is a broad category of symptoms that may include physical behaviors, as well as interests and participation in activities. Children with autism are often preoccupied with sameness and order – autistic children often need their rooms to be arranged a certain way, and a daily routine to be followed consistently, and become very distraught when these are disturbed. They may focus on small components of items (rather than the whole item) that spark their interests – playing with only specific parts of a stuffed animal, only the wheels of a toy car, etc. (APA, 2000). They may have unusual interests – for example, one teenager with Asperger's disorder who was previously treated by this author became extremely well versed with the Klingon language and culture (as developed by the *Star Trek* series of books, comics, and films).

Children with autism frequently also exhibit repetitious, rhythmic behaviors that usually seem to have no overt function (Nijhof *et al.*, 1998). These commonly include hand flapping, finger movements, tapping, or rocking, and may also be self-injuries (for example, head banging). Although the presence of at least some of these features is necessary for the diagnosis of autism, the degree of severity is variable, and is associated with other aspects of functioning. For example, Militerni *et al.* (2002) report that these behaviors are inversely related with intelligence – those children with severe mental retardation exhibit much more extensive stereotyped behaviors.

Secondary Symptoms

Children who present with symptoms of autism are likely to exhibit a variety of other disturbances. Most autistic children exhibit frequent and severe temper tantrums that may be severely violent. The violence may be directed at parents or siblings, especially in situations where the parent or sibling did not do what the child wanted. Their ability to understand the environment is very limited, and therefore they do not comprehend why a situation did not come out as they hoped for or planned. This severely limits their ability to tolerate frustration and accept outcomes different than their expectations. Children with autism may also exhibit self-injurious behaviors, including head banging, scratching, or biting.

Because their ability to understand the environment is so limited, children with autism frequently exhibit impulsivity and poor self-control.

Because they do not recognize many forms of danger, they may place themselves in harm's way and require close supervision (for example, when on the street or in a parking lot). The danger may similarly be evident at home – children with autism may have difficulties learning the danger of sharp objects (like knives), or a hot stove. Generally, children with autism require a high degree of supervision that often is very wearing and overwhelming for their parents.

Children with autism have difficulties with communication. This means that they have problems expressing their needs and wants. When they are hungry or cold, they may act out rather than explaining what is wrong and asking for assistance. When they want something, they may not be able to express what it is, and may tantrum when they do not get it, without understanding that they did not explain their needs. Family members and peers often find children with autism very frustrating.

In educational settings, children with autism usually present very significant challenges. They may not understand directions and their poor frustration tolerance usually results in significant acting out when they are forced to do something they do not want to (or prevented from doing something they want at the moment). Because their communication impairments are likely to be both receptive and expressive, they have difficulties learning academic skills, even when their intellectual functioning is not impaired. They usually require intensive one-on-one instruction and supervisions, and use of specialized interventions based on Applied Behavior Analysis (for example, Alberto & Troutman, 2008) or similar methods (for example, Lovaas, 1987).

In social settings, children with autism are likely to be withdrawn, aloof, and unpopular. Because they exhibit lack of interest in social interactions, they usually do not form significant friendships. When interacting with others, they are likely to tantrum regularly, because they do not understand the basics of social reciprocity, such as the need to share and jointly arrive at rules for play activities.

RULE OUTS AND COMORBID DISORDERS

Associated features of autism may involve a broad range of functional difficulties. In some cases, these problems may resemble symptoms of autism, and the diagnosis of autistic disorder may not be appropriate. In other cases, additional difficulties may be evident with symptoms of full-blown autism. In order to differentiate these situations, and determine the appropriate course of treatment, comprehensive differential diagnosis must be performed.

Psychotic Disorders

As discussed in Chapter 11, some children may exhibit psychosis. Delusions and hallucinations may co-occur with prominent mood disturbance. When psychosis is present with severe major depression, social withdrawal and isolation may likely accompany the symptoms, but because major depression is an episodic disorder, during periods of more stable mood states, better social functioning and normal reciprocity will be evident. Differentiating autism from childhood schizophrenia, however, may sometimes be more difficult.

Schizophrenia

A child with schizophrenia may, at times, appear to be isolated, aloof, emotionally flat, and, in severe cases, unresponsive. These symptoms may be secondary to the delusions and/or hallucinations, as well as the reaction of the child to these frightening experiences. Like mood disturbance, however, psychotic symptoms usually are episodic and periods without delusions and hallucinations are apparent. During those times, more normal social functioning should be apparent. In addition, children with schizophrenia typically exhibit the ability to communicate their feelings, although during states of psychosis they may too impaired or frightened to utilize those skills.

On the other hand, there are times when childhood schizophrenia and autism may co-occur. If the child exhibits a history of early onset developmental impairments sufficient for the diagnosis of autism, the DSM system states that the diagnosis of schizophrenia should be made 'only if prominent delusions and hallucinations are also present for at least a month (or less if successfully treated)' (APA, 2000, p. 312). Thus, it is clear that a child with autistic symptoms who also exhibits psychotic symptoms may be diagnosed with both disorders. In such a case, it is logical to start treatment by focusing on symptoms of psychosis, and address remaining symptoms after psychosis has subsided.

Mental Retardation

By current estimates, about two-thirds of children with autistic disorder exhibit intellectual functioning within the range of mental retardation (IQ below 70, APA, 2000). In addition, only a few exhibit intelligence higher than the borderline range (IQ of 80 or above, Gillberg & Coleman, 1996). Consequently, the vast majority of children with autism will also carry a diagnosis of mental retardation.

On the other hand, it is necessary to consider whether severe intellectual deficits already account for the symptoms associated with autism.

Individuals with profound mental retardation only reach a mental age of about 3 years, and those with severe mental retardation only reach a mental age of about 6 years (Haugaard, 2008). Consequently, children and adolescents in these two groups are likely to exhibit severe functional impairments, including limited ability to communicate and interact with others. In addition, severe and profound mental retardation is usually associated with many physical and neurodevelopmental delays (Hodapp & Dykens, 2003), and therefore children with very low intellectual functioning may also exhibit some of the motor and behavior peculiarities evident in children with autism.

When children and adolescents exhibit severe deficits in intellectual skills, the etiology is likely to include diverse factors, as is the cause with autism. However, since causal factors for both disorders may involve difficulties in the brain's integrative functions, it is reasonable to attempt to treat autism and severe mental retardation through similar pharmacological methods.

Mood Disorders

As briefly mentioned above, children with some mood states may exhibit social and communication deficits that may resemble autism. This is not likely to be evident during a manic presentation, but may be present during a major depressive episode.

Major Depression

When a child is exhibiting severe depression, he or she may be withdrawn, aloof, isolated, and uncommunicative. In rare and severe cases, the depression may also be characterized by catatonic features that may sometimes resemble behavioral disturbances characteristic of autism, such as echolalia, echopraxia, and mutism (APA, 2000, p. 418). Thus, children who present such symptoms should be assessed for possible presence of depression. In major depression, these physical states accompany mood disturbance, but once mood symptoms improve, catatonic states usually do as well. Consequently, a child with major depression may present impoverished and stereotyped movements when severely depressed (and perhaps briefly afterward), but not when more normal mood states are evident.

Anxiety Disorders

Children with autism often exhibit difficulties adjusting to new situations or changes in routine. When in a novel context, children with autism often react with significant agitation and many of them panic. Indeed, a review of research suggests that 11–84 percent of children with autism exhibit symptoms of a comorbid anxiety disorder (White *et al.*, 2009), and 16–81 percent of children with autism exhibit at least some symptoms of OCD (Klinger *et al.*, 2003). It is difficult to diagnose anxiety disorders in children with symptoms of autism because their difficulties in interacting and communication delays significantly impair their abilities to express their feelings and describe their symptoms. In addition, compulsive behaviors may resemble, and be mistaken for, repetitive and stereotypical behaviors. Some researchers suggest that anxiety disorders are especially evident among teenagers with higher-functioning forms of autistic-spectrum disorders, such as Asperger's (Kim *et al.*, 2000).

Because it is so difficult for children with autism to talk about their feelings, many parents may miss symptoms of anxiety. Clinicians should direct parents to identify significant reactions in situations that involve novel settings, disruptions of repetitive routines, and presence of strangers. When these situations seem to provoke unusually strong reactions, a comorbid anxiety disorder may be present. In such cases, clinicians should begin by treating the symptoms of anxiety (as discussed in Chapter 8), and address residual problems after anxiety has sufficiently been addressed.

Disruptive Disorders

Children with disruptive disorders are not usually mistaken for exhibiting autism. The nature of many of the core symptoms of disruptive disorders is inconsistent with autism. For example, argumentativeness assumes an interactional component, and therefore a child with autism may exhibit a violent tantrum when he does not get his way, but he is not likely to become involved in an extensive argument. However, a debate continues with regard to comorbidity – whether autism can co-occur with, and be co-diagnosed with, disruptive disorders, especially ADHD.

Attention Deficit Hyperactivity Disorder

The diagnosis and treatment of ADHD is discussed in Chapter 5 of this volume. Symptoms of ADHD include the dimensions of distractibility/ disorganization, and impulsivity/hyperactivity. The DSM specifically prevents clinicians from diagnosing both disorders simultaneously, and only allows the diagnosis of ADHD when 'symptoms do not occur exclusively during the course of a Pervasive Developmental Disorder' (APA, 2000, p. 93). The reason for this mandate stems from DSM's adherence to the principle of parsimony – symptoms should be described by as few labels as possible. Conceptually, symptoms of autism already account for the distractibility, disorganization, impulsivity, and hyperactivity that children with autism frequently exhibit, and therefore a secondary diagnosis of ADHD is not necessary. However, it is also true that some children and adolescents with autism, especially those who exhibit normal intellectual functioning and eventually develop sufficient communication skills, do not exhibit symptoms associated with ADHD. This may indicate that individuals with autistic disorder may also require a separate diagnosis of ADHD (since not all individuals with autism exhibit these symptoms), but the DSM system assumes that such variations are within the range of expression of the symptoms of autism.

Whatever the DSM approach, clinicians who treat children or adolescents with autistic disorder should consider whether the specific presentation also includes symptoms of ADHD. If so, treatment approaches described in Chapter 5 may prove helpful, and clinicians may want to consider starting with the use of those compounds. Once the impulsivity/hyperactivity and inattentiveness/disorganization improve, clinicians will be able to assess the remaining symptoms to determine further course of action.

Sleep Disorders

Sleep disturbances are common in children with autism. Studies show that between 44 and 83 percent of children with autism exhibit severe sleep problems, especially before age 8 (Klinger *et al.*, 2003). These commonly include problems with early, middle, and late insomnia (as described in Chapter 9), as well as shortened night sleep. These symptoms are especially evident in parental reports, and indicate that parents experience sleep difficulties as a troubling feature associated with symptoms of autism, even when more objective measures do not always corroborate the intensity of these problems (Schreck & Mulick, 2000). There may be many reasons for this phenomenon. For example, children with autism usually are extremely taxing and overwhelming to parents, and it is likely that parents look forward to the time after the child goes to sleep, and before the child wakes, as a break from the constant care and supervision that these children require. Whatever the reason, parents of children with autism are likely to ask mental health professionals to address sleep problems evident in their children with autism, and use of a hypnotic supplement may be necessary in those cases.

Adjustment and Trauma

Children and adolescents who have undergone traumatic experiences are much more likely to exhibit a variety of difficulties. When an adjustment disorder is evident, many aspects of functioning (for example, communication) are not impaired, although specific emotional and behavioral symptoms may be present. On the other hand, when the child has undergone severe early trauma, severe withdrawal, problems with communication, and difficulties with forming relationships may be evident.

Post-Traumatic Disorders

Children and adolescents who have been exposed to severe trauma may exhibit symptoms of acute stress disorder (ASD) or post-traumatic stress disorder (PTSD). Youngsters with ASD or PTSD usually exhibit substantial anxiety and hypervigilance, sleep disturbance and nightmares (which do not necessarily need to contain trauma-related content), reliving the event through play (or other forms of flashbacks), and avoidance of (and/or detachment from) trauma-related stimuli. In rare cases, severe withdrawal and mutism may accompany these symptoms. When it can be verified that the onset of the symptoms occurred after the trauma, and prior to the trauma the child's social and communication skills did not appear delayed, it is likely that a post-traumatic reaction is responsible for the symptoms. Conversely, when the development is characterized by delays and atypical behaviors associated with autism, it is likely that an autistic disorder is present, which may co-occur with a post-traumatic reaction.

When clinicians encounter children or adolescents with ASD or PTSD, all symptom groups must be managed. Intensive psychological and pharmacological treatment is likely to be necessary and multiple supplements will likely need to be used. Such cases should be approached with extreme caution, since the use of multiple supplements has rarely been researched, especially in the pediatric population.

Reactive Attachment Disorder

Reactive attachment disorder (RAD) is evident when a child exhibits symptoms of markedly disturbed and developmentally inappropriate social relatedness, which may include 'persistent failure to initiate or respond in a developmentally appropriate fashion to most social interactions, as manifest by excessively inhibited, hypervigilant, or highly ambivalent and contradictory responses' (APA, 2000, p. 130). This often includes significant avoidance and resistance to comforting that may be similar to symptoms of autism. However, the ability to communicate is less likely to be impaired, and peculiar behaviors associated with autism are absent.

RAD cannot be diagnosed when the above symptoms are presumed to be secondary to developmental delays, such as mental retardation and any PDD. In addition, RAD can only be diagnosed when evidence of pathogenic care is verified, including upbringing in an environment characterized by persistent disregard of the child's physical or emotional needs (such as comfort or affection), or repeated changes in caregivers that prevented the formation of a stable attachment. Thus, when these criteria are present, it is likely that symptoms of RAD are evident and intense psychological treatment will be necessary. Conversely, when significant developmental delays are present that meet the criteria for mental retardation or PDD, a diagnosis of RAD cannot be given, even if pathogenic care seemed present.

Neurological Disorders

Autism is associated with a number of neuropsychiatric conditions. Because most of these need to be treated medically, it is necessary to carefully perform a differential diagnosis and rule out these disorders.

Epilepsy

About one-quarter to one-third of patients with autism also exhibit seizures (Connor & Meltzer, 2006). While symptoms of the two are not likely to be confused, parents and clinicians should carefully track whether the child suspected of autism exhibits consistent periods of withdrawal, aloofness, and unusual behaviors, or whether these periods seem to come and go. Since petit mal seizures may not involve convulsions, it is possible that some of the times when behavioral disturbances exacerbate may be related to seizure activity. As a rule, whenever a child is suspected of symptoms of autism, a neurological evaluation should be performed.

Genetic Abnormalities

About 10–15 percent of children with autism have an identifiable chromosomal abnormality or another genetic syndrome (Folstein & Rosen-Sheidley, 2001). These genetic problems are usually associated with many medical problems, and require regular monitoring. The genetic disorder most commonly occurring with autism is tuberous sclerosis, and about 20 percent of children with tuberous sclerosis meet the diagnostic criteria for autism (Connor & Meltzer, 2006). Tuberous sclerosis or tuberous sclerosis complex (TSC) is a multisystem genetic disorder that causes non-malignant tumors to grow in the brain, kidneys, heart, eyes, lungs, and skin of the affected patients. Additional symptoms may also include seizures. Because TSC often causes significant medical problems, and in some cases death (usually, from renal disease, brain tumor, or lung disease), it is necessary to diagnose and begin to manage this disorder and all its associated problems as early as possible.

ETIOLOGY

Etiology of autism is among the most complex and poorly understood of all etiologies of mental health disorders. Whereas the etiology of symptoms of most other disorders has focused on understanding specific portions of the brain, symptoms of autism are very broad and may involve most basic abilities to process information and recognize social cues.

For example, Baron-Cohen *et al.* (1985) suggested that children with autism exhibit an impairment in the development of a 'theory of mind' – the ability to understand that other people have beliefs, desires, and intentions that are different from one's own. Subsequent research also identified significant deficits in executive functions (planning, problem solving, and mental flexibility) and semantic memory (Klinger *et al.*, 2003). Individuals with autism may also have difficulties processing environmental stimuli and may focus on parts of a stimulus instead of the whole stimulus, suggesting problems with integrative processes (Frith & Happe, 1994). These deficits suggest that many brain areas may be involved in producing the symptoms of autism.

Summary of Research Findings

Many studies have confirmed that genetic factors seem to play a role in the development of autism. Frequency of autism in siblings of autistic children is about 30 times greater than the prevalence of autism in the general population (Klinger *et al.*, 2003), and when other autistic-spectrum disorders are included, the risk increases almost twofold (Szatmari, 1999). Concordance rates among monozygotic twins is reported to range from 36–91 percent, and is about 30–40 times greater than concordance rates for dizygotic twins (Bailey *et al.*, 1995). At this time, it is estimated that autism involves at least 5–10 genes, and the risk of developing autism depends on the number of genes inherited (Pickles *et al.*, 1995). A specific genetic abnormality on chromosome 7 has been confirmed by three different studies, and additional genes have also been identified on chromosomes 1, 2, 13, 16, and 19, although these have not been consistently replicated (Klinger *et al.*, 2003).

In addition, subclinical abnormalities resembling characteristics from the three main categories of autistic symptoms have been identified in relatives (including parents) of individuals with autism at much higher rates than in individuals without family history of autism (Pickles *et al.*, 2000). Collectively, these results suggest that a 'broader autism phenotype' is apparent in individuals at risk for autism (Klinger *et al.*, 2003). Bailey *et al.* (1996) proposed a two-level mechanism of genetic factors. Those who inherit level 1 genetic predisposition exhibit subclinical symptoms characteristic of the 'broader autism genotype.' Then, a subset of those with level 1 vulnerability is affected by another set of factors, perhaps involving additional genetic abnormalities or environmental events (like a prenatal insult), greatly increasing their risk for developing the full-blown disorder.

Much has been hypothesized about the nature of the prenatal (or postnatal) insult that may contribute to the development of autism. Some have implicated childhood immunizations as responsible for many cases of autism, and a variety of mechanisms has been proposed. Thimerosal, a preservative added to immunizations around the world since early twentieth century, was presumed to contribute to autism, and subsequently has been withdrawn from use in the US and most countries in the European Union. Since 2001, childhood injections in the US do not contain thimerosal, but rates of autism have not decreased. Others have proposed that the immune reaction that the child's body undergoes when he or she is exposed to simultaneous measles, mumps, and rubella (MMR) immunizations may be responsible for subsequent brain changes that lead to autism (Wakefield *et al.*, 1998). However, much research has disproved this theory. For example, a retrospective study of over 20,000 children born between 1980 and 1994 tracked rates of autism and MMR immunizations, and found that rates of MMR remained stable, while rates of autism gradually increased (Dales *et al.*, 2001). At this time, most health care professionals recognize that the age of onset of initial symptoms correlates with the age when children receive vaccinations, but this correlation does not imply a causal relationship and theories that vaccines cause autism lack convincing scientific evidence and are considered biologically implausible (Doja & Roberts, 2006). Unfortunately, continued parental concern about vaccines and autism has led to lower rates of childhood immunizations and higher rates of measles (European Centre for Disease Prevention and Control, 2008).

In addition to genetic links discussed above, numerous neuroanatomical and neurophysiological studies examined the brain structure and function of patients with autism.

Neuroanatomical Abnormalities

Brain imaging techniques, brain autopsies, and animal models have revealed neuroanatomical abnormalities that seem to correlate with symptoms of autism. Collectively, it is apparent that autism is associated with the enlargement of some brain areas, and reduction in others. Conceptually, this is consistent with theories proposed for other serious psychopathology (for example, schizophrenia) that suggest that abnormal cell growth may be associated with autism. In normal brains, proliferation of brain cells eventually leads to gradual pruning as needed pathways are strengthened and unneeded ones decay. In autism, this process may be disturbed, leaving too many neurons in some areas and too few in others (Minshew, 1996).

Several studies have shown brain enlargement in patients with autism. This enlargement seems especially evident in occipital, parietal, and temporal regions, but not in the frontal lobes. Results of autopsy studies also confirm these findings (Klinger et al., 2003). In addition, malformations in the cortical lobes have also been identified, revealing that abnormal neuronal proliferation and pruning seem to take place inconsistently in the cerebral cortex (Piven et al., 1990). Indeed, other research has confirmed these malformations, especially in the occipital lobes (Courchesne et al., 1993). In addition, studies have also found evidence of reduced side of corpus callosum in patients with autism, suggesting that impaired communication between brain regions may be involved in the symptoms (Piven et al., 1997).

Similarly, brain imaging and autopsy studies also revealed abnormalities in the cerebellum of patients with autism. Cereberal hypoplasia in vermal lobules VI and VII of the cerebellum has been identified, and seems unconnected to other brain regions in the area. These portions of the cerebellum are involved in regulating attention, sensory modulation, autonomic reactivity, and motor and behavior initiation, and therefore the changes in the cerebellum seem to correlate with problems commonly seen in patients with autism (Klinger et al., 2003). In addition, brain imaging studies have also revealed Purkinje and granule cell loss in the neocerebellum of patients with autism, and a brain tissue study also found decreased amounts of key proteins in the cerebellum (Fatemi et al., 2001).

Social skill impairments in autism may be secondary to problems in the functioning of the limbic system. Autopsy studies revealed that individuals with autism exhibit reduced neuronal cell size and increased cell-packaging density in portions of the limbic system, especially the amygdala and hippocampus (Bauman & Kemper, 1988), although some MRI studies have not confirmed these findings (Klinger et al., 2003). In a provocative study, Bachevalier (1994) damaged the amygdala, the hippocampus, or both structures in monkeys and found that those with lesions in either structure exhibited notable but subclinical symptoms associated with autism, while those with damage to both structures revealed blank facial expressions, poor body language, lack of eye contact, motor stereotypies, and failure to develop social relationships. Thus, the most severe forms of autism, including severe symptoms and mental retardation, may involve deficits in both amygdala and hippocampus.

Neurophysiological Abnormalities

Cortical EEG studies revealed that hemispheric laterality is abnormal in patients with autism. When presented with language tasks, individuals with autism appear to exhibit greater right than left activation (Dawson et al., 1983), a reverse of what is seen in normal brains (especially in males). Similarly, during alert resting states, individuals with autism do not reveal typical brain asymmetry, and children with autism have been found to exhibit reduced EEG power in frontal and temporal regions, but in the parietal region, and these differences were especially prominent on the left side (Dawson et al., 1995). In addition, during a social task, some EEG brain patterns seem to correlate with the degree of the impairment – those with most pronounced passivity and least social interaction revealed significantly *increased* amount of activity in the brain's frontal region, as opposed to children with autism who exhibited less impaired social interactions (Dawson et al. 1995). It is possible that autistic children with most severe social impairment struggle the most when attempting to process social contexts.

Studies have also investigated neurotransmitter activity in patients with autism. Results of several studies reveal that between 25 and 50 percent of patients with autism exhibit increases in levels of serotonin that are estimated to fall at the top 5 percent of levels found in the normal population (Leboyer et al., 1999). Interestingly, similar findings were observed in parents and siblings of patients with autism, suggesting that some of the hypothesized brain abnormalities may indeed be evident in relatives of patients with autism. Similar studies were performed to investigate levels of dopamine, norepinephrine, and endogenous opioids, and results of various investigations produced mixed and inconsistent results (Klinger et al., 2003).

The mirror neuron system is a series of recently discovered structures that fire when an action is performed and also when the individual witnesses the same action being performed by others. Thus, the functioning of these neurons is presumed to play a key role in empathy and the processing of social situations, and has been hypothesized to play a role in the symptoms of autism (Dapretto, 2006). In humans, brain activity consistent with mirror neurons has been found in the premotor cortex and the inferior parietal cortex, and studies have revealed that individuals with autism exhibit structural and functional abnormalities in these regions (Iacoboni & Dapretto, 2006). In addition, a brain-imaging study also found that children with autism reveal abnormal patterns in the activation of the cingulate cortex (Chiu *et al.*, 2008), an area of the brain extensively involved in social and emotional processing, possibly reflecting a disturbance of self-referential thought (Broyd *et al.*, 2009). Overall, the results of neuroanatomical and neurophysiological research support many of the hypothesized functional deficits evident in individuals with autism, and it is evident that a broad and complex pathology, including both structural and functional changes, is involved in producing the symptoms of autism.

SUPPLEMENTS WITH LIKELY EFFICACY

Treating symptoms of autism is different than treating all the disorders described in this book. Because of the wide range of symptoms, no single compound (allopathic or naturopathic) has been found to be effective in reducing the symptoms of autism. In addition, individuals with autism present problems from various symptom groups, and in varying amounts, and therefore the uniqueness of the presentation of the symptoms evident in each individual further complicates the selection of appropriate interventions.

For these reasons, symptoms of autism are usually treated by identifying categories of problems that are best candidates for pharmacological treatment, and selecting compounds to treat those symptom groups. Research literature reveals that some prescription medications have been found to be effective in treating various symptoms in children with autism, and some are FDA approved for this population of patients. Psychostimulants have been shown to be effective in reducing ADHD-like symptoms (hyperactivity/impulsivity and distractibility), atypical antipsychotics and mood stabilizers have been shown to reduce aggression and agitation, hypnotics have been shown to improve problems with sleep, and anxiolytics have been shown to improve symptoms of anxiety and compulsive behaviors (Connor & Meltzer, 2006). For this reason, it is recommended that clinicians identify the symptom groups that most urgently require treatment and select those compounds that are best suited to address these problems.

ADHD-Like Symptoms

Stimulants have been shown to be effective in reducing hyperactivity, impulsivity, and inattention in children with autism, and consequently it is sensible to attempt to treat those symptoms with naturopathic supplements that have also been shown effective to treat those symptoms. Although it is apparent that those compounds have not been researched in children with autism, it is likely that the same level of efficacy obtained with children and adolescents with ADHD may be expected in children with autism that present ADHD-like symptoms.

As discussed in Chapter 5, caffeine has been shown to be the most effective non-prescription compound, and supplements with likely efficacy include Omega-3, and SAM-e. Inositol, DMAE/choline, pycnogenol, and rhodiola may also have some efficacy, although the use of these compounds is considered experimental. Readers should consult Chapter 5 for guidelines about the use of these supplements, including dosage recommendations and cautions about possible adverse effects.

Aggression and Agitation

Mood stabilizers have been shown to be effective in reducing agitation, aggression, and violence in children with autism, and consequently it is sensible to attempt to treat those symptoms with naturopathic supplements that have also been shown effective to treat those symptoms. Although those compounds have not been researched in children with autism, it is likely that the same level of efficacy obtained with children and adolescents with mania and agitation may be expected in children with autism that present similar symptoms.

As discussed in Chapter 7, Omega-3 and lecithin are likely to be effective in managing symptoms of agitation and aggression, and melatonin, magnesium, theanine, and taurine may also be effective, although the use of these compounds is considered experimental. Readers should consult Chapter 7 for guidelines about the use of these supplements, including dosage recommendations and cautions about possible adverse effects.

Anxiety and Compulsions

Anxiolytics have been shown to be effective in reducing symptoms of anxiety, including obsessions and compulsions, in children with autism, and consequently it is sensible to attempt to treat those symptoms with naturopathic supplements that have also been shown effective to treat those symptoms. Although those compounds have not been researched in children with autism, it is likely that the same level of efficacy obtained with children and adolescents with anxiety disorders may be expected in children with autism that present similar symptoms.

As discussed in Chapter 8, kava appears to be best supported, but, because of risks of hepatotoxicity, it is probably best not to use it in children with autism. However, inositol is also likely to be effective in managing symptoms of anxiety, and St. John's Wort, tryptophan (or 5-HT), valerian, theanine, ginger, taurine, passion flower, and chamomile may also be effective, although the use of these compounds is considered experimental. Readers should consult Chapter 8 for guidelines about the use of these supplements, including dosage recommendations and cautions about possible adverse effects.

Sleep Difficulties

Although research on the use of hypnotics with autistic children is sparse, these medications have been shown to be effective in reducing sleep problems in children with a variety of psychological disorders, including anxiety and mood disorders. Consequently, even though the use of naturopathic hypnotics has not been researched in children with autism, it is sensible to attempt to treat sleep difficulties with naturopathic supplements that have been shown to be effective in a wide range of disorders, and it can be expected that the efficacy obtained with children and adolescents with sleep problems may be similar when these compounds are used with children with autism that present similar symptoms.

As discussed in Chapter 9, melatonin has been found to be most effective. However, melatonin is produced from serotonin and children with autism have sometimes been found to exhibit unusually high levels of serotonin. It is not clear what significance this may have for treatment recommendations. On the one hand, whether high levels of serotonin may also indicate high levels of melatonin, but it is possible that serotonin function is altered in some children with autism and high levels of serotonin may not correlate with high melatonin release. Indeed, there is research that suggests that melatonin supplementation may be effective in treating sleep difficulties in children with autism (Chamberlain & Herman, 1990). For this reason, it may be sensible to follow the recommendations outlined in Chapter 9 and begin with melatonin, and switch to valerian and then tryptophan if improvement is not noted. If these are ineffective, phenibut, hops or rauwolfia may be tried, although the use of these compounds is considered experimental. Readers should consult Chapter 9 for guidelines about the use of these supplements, including dosage recommendations and cautions about possible adverse effects.

SUPPLEMENTS WITH POSSIBLE EFFICACY

In addition to the treatment strategies discussed above, a few compound have shown some promise in the treatment of symptoms of autism. Since the data that supports its use is extremely limited, clinicians should proceed with caution, and consider the use of these compounds as experimental.

Vitamin B6

The B family of vitamins contains eight vitamins that play important physiological functions in the body. These include B1 (thiamine), B2 (riboflavin), B3 (niacin), B5 (pantothenic acid), Vitamin B6 (pyridoxine), B7 (biotin), B9 (folic acid), and B12 (cobalamins). B vitamins are involved in cellular metabolism and, like all other vitamins, must be obtained from the diet.

Vitamin B6, in particular, is an important co-enzyme involved in many biochemical reactions, including amino acid metabolism, and it is vital for proper protein synthesis. After proteins are ingested, they are broken down into their constituent amino acids, and those must then be degraded during digestion and are then taken up by the cells to form individual protein molecules. The presence of the vitamin B6 is essential for this process.

Vitamin B6 is widely available in foods, including meat, vegetables (especially potatoes, avocados, Brussels sprouts, cauliflower, and tomatoes), whole grain products, fruit (especially bananas and apples), peanuts, and sunflower seeds (Hingle, 2007). Supplemental vitamin B6 is available in capsules and tablets, in a wide range of doses. B6 is also commonly included in B complex preparations. Dietary reference intakes (DRI) have been established for vitamin B6, and range from 0.05 mg/day for infants to 1.3–1.7 mg/day for adults. In addition, upper intake levels have also been established, and these range from 30 mg/day for infants to 100 mg/day for adults (Medical Economics, 2008a). However, when used clinically, the typical dose is 100–200 mg/day, and lowest observed adverse effect level has been established at 500 mg/day (Medical Economics). It is clear that children and adolescents should receive much lower doses.

The benefits of vitamin B6 supplementation with children with autism have been researched for some 20 years. While anecdotal evidence has long existed supporting its use, empirical studies are scarcer and do not reveal consistent results. For example, a review by Pfeiffer *et al.* (1995) revealed that studies performed thus far have not revealed efficacy, but more recently Kuriyama *et al.* (2002) reported improvement in cognitive and social functioning in eight children treated with vitamin B6 and magnesium. Similarly, Mousain-Bosc *et al.* (2006) found, in an open study of 33 children, that treatment with magnesium and vitamin B6 improved symptoms of autism. Thus, it is possible that supplementation with vitamin B6 and magnesium may offer some benefits for children with autism.

Following ingestion, vitamin B6 undergoes hydrolysis in the small intestine and is absorbed in the jejunum. The vitamin is well absorbed, even at high doses, enters systemic circulation, and is delivered to various tissues in the body, and is easily taken up by the muscles. Magnesium may assist in the absorption, and the two supplements are often taken together.

Vitamin B6 is generally well tolerated, especially at doses that do not exceed upper intake limits. When supplemented above these limits, adults who take vitamin B6 at 200 mg/day usually tolerate the dose well, and adverse effects are rare. Children and adolescents should start vitamin B6 supplementation at the upper intake limits listed above, and increase weekly to the 2 mg/kg per day that has been shown to be effective in clinical studies. At high doses, some individuals develop nausea, vomiting, abdominal pain, loss of appetite, and sensory neuropathies, and rare cases of photosensitivity have also been reported (Medical Economics, 2008a).

Carnosine

Carnosine is a dipeptide comprising beta-alanine and histidine. It is commonly found in proteins, and has been marketed as a meat-substitute extract since the 1800s. It is present in significant concentrations in muscle tissues in beef, turkey, pork, and in lower concentrations in chicken.

Carnosine is involved in a series of metabolic reactions in the body. It is presumed to have antiglycating properties, which may prove beneficial in diabetes and Alzheimer's disorder, although research support thus far has not proven this benefit. It may also exert antioxidant activity and has been shown to inhibit lipid oxidation, including the oxidation of LDL, and may be a free radical scavenger. It seems to have the ability to buffer pH activity, and appears to delay muscle fatigue. Its hypothesized psychogenic effects may be due to neurotransmitter activity, although specific receptors have not been identified. However, carnosine has been found to protect against reactive oxygen reactions that degrade polyunsaturated lipids into malondialdehyde (MDA), and MDA is presumably involved in cellular toxicity that may underlie Alzheimer's disorder as well as autism. Glutamate may also regulate glutamatergic neurotransmission, thus preventing cellular apoptosis (Medical Economics, 2008a). Indeed, one small study found that use of 800 mg/day of carnosine supplements was effective in improving expressive and receptive vocabulary over an 8 week trial in 31 children with autism (Chez *et al.*, 2002).

Carnosine supplements are generally available in tablets at strengths between 100 and 500 mg. Carnosine is easily absorbed from the gastrointestinal tract and enters portal circulation, where it is hydrolyzed into beta-alanine and histidine. Unmetabolized portions enter systemic circulation and are gradually transported into the muscles and other tissues. At the same time, carnosine is also hydrolyzed in the kidneys and excreted. Thus, although specific half-life of carnitine has not been established, it is presumed to be short, and intravenous doses have shown excretion after 90 minutes (Medical Economics, 2008a).

Little is known about the effects of carnosine supplementation. Some have found that high doses are activating, but generally the compound is well tolerated and no adverse reactions have been reported. Similarly, no upper limits of intake have been established, and overdosage has been reported (Medical Economics, 2008a). However, because so little is known about the effects of carnitine supplementation, clinicians are advised to exercise much caution when using carnitine with children or adolescents.

SUPPLEMENTS NOT LIKELY TO BE EFFECTIVE

Of all of the disorders discussed in this book, autism is treated most frequently with the use of complementary and alternative medicine (CAM).

Studies have shown that up to 50 percent of children with autism are treated with CAM methods (Davis & Darden, 2003), and some consider this figure to be an underestimate (Levy & Hyman, 2008). This trend may reflect the wild speculation that has surrounded the causes of autism, including the suspicions that child immunizations, dietary allergies (for example, those to gluten or casein), reactions to sugar or food additives, or causes involving heavy metals are to blame. Just like these theories have been disproven by a significant amount of research, most naturopathic approaches have also been shown to be ineffective, and some are potentially harmful. It is not possible to review all of those treatments, but some supplements that are most frequently attempted, and those that pose the most potential harm must be identified to help clinicians steer parents away from these alternatives.

Vitamin B9

Vitamin B9, also known as folate or folic acid, is a vitamin found in green leafy vegetables, fruit, fortified foods (especially cereal and bread), and organ meats. Folate is presumed to have many effects within the body, including antioxidant and cardioprotective benefits. It has been hypothesized that oxidative stress may cause neuronal insult and lead to the neuroanatomical and neurophysiological difficulties associated with autism, including the disruption of normal cellular development. Thus, proponents of the use of folate to treat autism expect that its antioxidant properties may correct underlying oxidative pathology.

Indeed, abnormal levels of antioxidants have been reported in children with autism (Pardo & Eberhart, 2007), and James *et al.* (2004) described abnormal metabolic profiles in 20 children with autism consistent with presumed methylation impairments. Following administration of folate (supplemented by betaine), laboratory findings normalized, but behavioral presentation did not improve. Thus, at this time there clearly is a lack of evidence of any behavioral or psychological benefit of use of folate supplements in children with autism.

Folate is generally well tolerated, but high doses may produce flushing, rash, disturbed sleep, and gastrointestinal symptoms (Hingle, 2007). In addition, high doses of folate supplements may change levels of vitamin B12, and mask vitamin B12 deficiency. This may lead to severe problems, including anemia, irreversible damage to the nervous system, and a degeneration of the spinal cord. Thus, given these risks and the lack of benefits of folate supplementation with children in autism, clinicians are advised against attempting treatment with folate supplements.

Secretin

Secretin is a hormone, primarily found in the gastrointestinal tract. Its primary role is to regulate the pH of the duodenal contents via the control of gastric acid secretion. Intravenous, transdermal and oral administration has been attempted, and one early study reported that some 200 individuals with autism improved after taking supplemental secretin (Balch, 2006). Unfortunately, no plausible mechanism for the effectiveness of secretin was ever elucidated, although some speculation has been forwarded that secretin may be involved in the regulation of monoamine neurotransmission (Rimland, 1998). To date, over a dozen controlled trials, many of which followed the randomized placebo-controlled design, revealed lack of any benefit (Levy & Hyman, 2008). More importantly, two studies have revealed that individuals given secretin were at higher risk for developing seizures, even with no risk factors evident before trying to supplement (Hayward, 2000). On balance, it is clear that the benefits from attempting supplementation with secretin are unlikely and the risks of dangerous consequences may be significant.

Chelation

Intoxication with heavy metals, especially mercury, has long been hypothesized to underlie autism, and some medical reports have given at least some credence to this theory (Bernard et al., 2001). Proponents of this approach suggest that heavy metals are poorly eliminated by children with autism and interfere with immune function, causing the development of autism. Unfortunately, despite the fact that meta-analyses revealed the contrary (Ng et al., 2007) and several epidemiological studies failed to find a link (Levy & Hyman, 2008), speculations about the role of mercury in the pathology of autism continue to abound. To correct this presumed metal poisoning, chemical chelation treatments are a popular intervention.

Medical chelation is the process of administering one of two medications that bind heavy metals and facilitate their elimination from the body. No controlled studies have examined the safety or efficacy of prescription chelation regimens for children with autism, and few doctors agree to perform this procedure. It is a dangerous process and deaths have been reported from hypocalcemia.

Unfortunately, naturopathic chelation is sometimes attempted by using compounds such as cysteine, livoic acid, chlorella, and brand name products like Livaplex and Antronex, and proponents of chelation suggest that in order to remove all dangerous metals from the body, treatment usually must last several years (Vibrant Life, 2008). These compounds affect many parts of the body, including liver function, respiration, calcium levels, and dermatological problems. It is clear that the limited, if any, benefits from using these compounds is significantly outweighed by the risks.

SUMMARY

Treatment of the symptoms of autism is different than the treatment of the other disorders discussed in this book, and no medications or naturopathic compounds have been shown to be effective in addressing all symptoms of autism. However, since children and adolescents with autism commonly exhibit symptoms that resemble those seen in other disorders, clinicians can attempt treating various symptom groups with compounds that have previously been shown to be effective in the pediatric population.

To guide clinicians in selecting appropriate supplements, an algorithm was developed and is presented in Figure 12.1. Clinicians should first determine whether the child or adolescent is exhibiting symptoms of anxiety, sleep difficulties, aggression, or distractibility/hyperactivity. If any of these symptoms are present, clinicians should begin treating the groups of symptoms that are most severe and debilitating, and consult relevant chapters in this book for guidance about selecting the compound, establishing the dosage, and monitoring patient's response. Management of ADHD-like symptoms is discussed in Chapter 5, agitation is discussed in Chapter 7, anxiety is discussed in Chapter 8, and sleep difficulties are discussed in Chapter 9.

If insufficient improvement is noted after those symptoms have been addressed, or if the patient does not present these problems and only exhibits social and communication delays and stereotypical behaviors, treatment with vitamin B6 (augmented by magnesium) or carnosine may be attempted. These compounds may be used together, and may also be added to other compounds that have been implemented to treat other groups of symptoms.

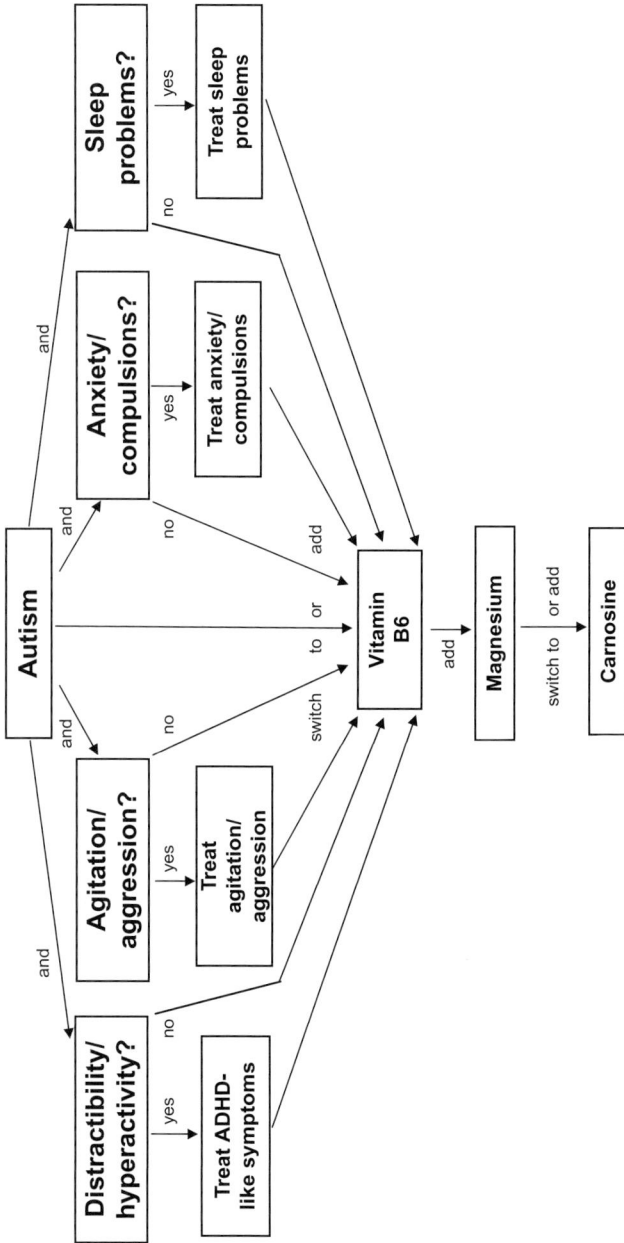

FIGURE 12.1   Algorithm for treatment of autism with naturopathic supplements.
© Elsevier 2009.

Chapter 13

Concluding Remarks

Interest in the use of naturopathic interventions continues to increase, and a wide variety of supplements is freely available on the market, especially over the Internet. Vendors often utilize aggressive marketing strategies that promote supplements that often lack any reasonable evidence of efficacy, and sometimes may not be safe, especially when given to children and adolescents. Clinicians need to be armed with accurate, research-based information to guide parents about which naturopathic compounds may be safe and effective, and which are not likely to offer much benefit. However, results of studies that research the use of naturopathic compounds are not easily accessible, and many of these studies are completed outside the US. This handbook set out to synthesize the results of available research and, based on the results of this research, offer guidance to mental health clinicians about the use of many naturopathic supplements.

While it is not possible to cover the vast array of naturopathic supplements that have been presumed to be useful in treating mental health disorders, this handbook focuses on those compounds that are most widely available and recommended by naturopaths and supplement vendors. Table 13.1 summarizes the compounds that are discussed in this book, and the amount of available evidence to support their use when treating symptoms of mental health disorders that commonly occur in children and adolescents.

At this time, it is evident that very few compounds have been researched sufficiently to consider their efficacy as established. The use of caffeine appears to be helpful in reducing symptoms of ADHD (although the benefits appear less significant than those seen with the use of prescription medications), the use of St. John's Wort and SAMe seems to be helpful in addressing symptoms of depression, the use of melatonin appears to improve sleep problems, and the use of rauwolfia is supported in reducing symptoms of psychosis (although clinicians must consider whether the adverse effects of this herb may outweigh

Nutritional and Herbal Therapies for Children and Adolescents

TABLE 13.1 Summary table for naturopathic supplements discussed in the book

Compound	ADHD Ch. 5	Depression Ch. 6	Mania Ch. 7	Anxiety Ch. 8	Sleep Ch. 9	Tics Ch. 10	Psychosis Ch. 11	Autism Ch. 12	Remarks
Adenosine	0	0	0	0	0	0	0	0	Including camp and ATP – see Chapter 4
Caffeine	3	0	0	0	0	0	0	*	
Carnosine	0	0	0	0	0	0	0	1	
Chamomile	0	0	0	1	0	0	0	*	Also see Chapter 9
Chelation	0	0	0	0	0	0	0	0	See Chapter 12
Chromium	0	1	0	0	0	0	0	0	
Coenzyme Q10	0	0	0	0	0	0	0	0	See Chapter 9
DHEA	0	0	0	0	0	0	0	0	See Chapter 6 and 11
DMAE/Choline	1	0	0	0	0	1	0	*	Also see Chapter 4
Dopamine	0	0	0	0	0	0	0	0	See Chapter 4
Ephedrine	0	0	0	0	0	0	0	0	See Chapter 4
GABA	0	0	0	0	0	0	0	0	See Chapters 4, 8, and 10
Ginger	0	1	1	1	0	0	0	*	
Ginkgo	0	0	0	0	0	0	0	0	See Chapter 8
Glutamine	0	0	0	0	0	0	0	0	See Chapter 4
Glycine	0	0	0	0	0	0	1	0	Also see Chapter 4
Hops	0	0	0	0	1	0	0	*	

(Continued)

TABLE 13.1 (Continued)

Compound	ADHD Ch. 5	Depression Ch. 6	Mania Ch. 7	Anxiety Ch. 8	Sleep Ch. 9	Tics Ch. 10	Psychosis Ch. 11	Autism Ch. 12	Remarks
Inositol	1	2	0	2	0	0	0	*	
Iron	0	0	0	0	0	0	0	0	See Chapters 5, 6, and 10
Kava	0	0	0	2	0	0	0	0	Also see Chapter 9
Lecithin	0	0	2	0	0	1	0	*	
Lemon balm	0	0	0	0	0	0	0	0	See Chapter 9
Magnesium	0	0	1	0	0	0	0	*	
Melatonin	0	0	1	0	3	0	0	*	Also see Chapter 4
Norepinephrine	0	0	0	0	0	0	0	0	See Chapter 4
Omega-3	2	2**	2	0	0	0	2***	*	May be augmented by Vitamin E and/or carnitine; also see Chapter 4
Passion flower	0	0	0	1	0	0	0	*	Also see Chapter 9
Phenibut	0	0	0n	0	1	0	0	*	
Phenylalanine	0	1	0	0	0	0	0	0	Phenylethylamine may be preferred
Pycnogenol	1	0	0	0	0	0	0	*	
Rauwolfia	0	0	0	0	1	2	3	*	
Rhodiola	1	1	0	0	0	0	0	*	

(Continued)

TABLE 13.1 (Continued)

Compound	ADHD Ch. 5	Depression Ch. 6	Mania Ch. 7	Anxiety Ch. 8	Sleep Ch. 9	Tics Ch. 10	Psychosis Ch. 11	Autism Ch. 12	Remarks
SAM-e	2	3	0	0	0	0	0	*	May be augmented by vitamin B complex
Scullcap	0	0	0	0	0	0	0	0	
Secretin	0	0	0	0	0	0	0	0	See Chapter 12
Serine	0	0	0	0	0	0	0	0	See Chapter 4, 6, and 8
Serotonin	0	0	0	0	0	0	0	0	See Chapter 4
St. John's Wort	0	3	0	1	0	0	0	*	Also see Chapter 4
Taurine	0	0	1	1	0	0	1	*	
Theanine	0	0	1	1	0	0	0	*	
Tryptophan	0	1	0	1	2	0	0	*	5-HTP may be preferred for depression and anxiety
Tyrosine	0	0	0	0	0	0	0	0	See Chapter 4
Uridine	0	0	0	0	0	0	0	0	See Chapter 4
Valerian	0	0	0	1	2	0	0	*	
Vitamin B3	0	0	0	0	0	0	0	0	See Chapter 11
Vitamin B6	0	0	0	0	0	1	0	1	May be augmented by magnesium
Vitamin B9	0	2	0	0	0	0	0	0	
Vitamin E	0	0	0	0	0	1	0	0	

Notes: * consult chapter for applications; ** instead of augmenting with carnitine, use of acetyl-l-carnitine (ALC) may be more effective; *** use high EPA content; may also be augmented by vitamin C.
0 = no efficacy and/or too dangerous; 1 = possible efficacy; 2 = likely efficacy; 3 = established efficacy.

potential clinical benefits). As is evident, this is truly a 'short list,' and there currently are no naturopathic treatments for mania, anxiety, tics, or autism that can be considered to have well-established efficacy.

On the other hand, there are many compounds that show promise in research studies and are likely to be effective, although further research is still needed. These include inositol for anxiety and/or depression, kava for anxiety (although the possible risk of liver damage must carefully be considered), lecithin for mania/agitation, Omega-3 for ADHD, depression, mania, and psychosis, rauwolfia for management of tics (keeping in mind the risk of side effects), SAMe for ADHD, tryptophan and valerian for sleep problems, and vitamin B9 for depression. This means that there is enough research support to recommend a cautious trial of these compounds with children and adolescents.

In addition, there are many compounds that appear to have some, although very limited, research support. These include carnosine for symptoms of autism, chamomile for anxiety, chromium for depression, DMAE/choline for ADHD and tics, ginger for depression and anxiety, glycine for psychosis, hops for sleep problems, inositol for ADHD (especially with comorbid anxiety), lecithin for tics, magnesium and melatonin for mania, passion flower for anxiety, phenibut for sleep problems, phenylalanine/PEA for depression, pycnogenol for ADHD, rauwolfia for sleep problems (in very low doses, while carefully monitoring adverse effects), rhodiola for ADHD and depression, scullcap for tics, St. John's Wort for anxiety, taurine for mania, anxiety, and psychosis, theanine for mania and anxiety, tryptophan/5-HTP for depression and anxiety, valerian for anxiety, vitamin B6 for tics and symptoms of autism, and vitamin E for tics. Although the majority of these supplements is safe, their efficacy is poorly established and their use must be considered experimental.

Finally, review of current literature suggests that there are several compounds that are not effective for symptoms of any psychological disorder, and/or are too dangerous to use with children and adolescents. These include adenosine, chelation compounds, coenzyme Q10, DHEA, dopamine, ephedrine, GABA, ginko, glutamine, iron, lemon balm, norepinephrine, secretin, serine, serotonin, tyrosine, uridine, or vitamin B3. Clinicians are discouraged from recommending the use of these supplements.

There are several categories of compounds that have not been included in this review. The handbook focuses primarily on individual compounds, rather than multi-compound cocktails. For this reason, the majority of Ayurvedic and Chinese medicines have not been included, since they usually utilize combinations of many ingredients, most of which have not been researched. In addition, so-called homeopathic compounds have specifically been excluded. Homeopathy is a controversial branch of health services that commonly utilizes unusual chemicals, many of which are potentially dangerous (for example, lung pus), distilled to a level where the original ingredient is no longer discernible on most laboratory tests. Most mental health professionals consider this practice to offer dubious benefits.

Because this handbook primarily focuses on using specific compounds as monotherapy, the use of combinations of supplements has generally not been addressed. Naturopathic polypharmacy is an area where there truly is a dearth of evidence, and very few studies exist that have researched a combination of naturopathic compounds. At the end of each chapter, some preliminary remarks have been made about combining the supplements discussed in that chapter, based on available evidence about their pharmacokinetic and pharmacodynamic properties. Combining compounds from various chapters may be necessary when treatment of various categories of symptoms is needed (for example, treatment of anxiety and depression, perhaps with coexisting sleep problems). In those situations, supplements should be used that may simultaneously address various symptom groups. When this approach does not produce sufficient effects, combining compounds across categories may carefully be attempted, but clinicians who want to do so must remember that they truly are venturing into 'uncharted territory' and much caution is needed.

Preparing this manuscript, the author has reviewed hundreds of studies from many countries and several continents. Even though such a broad range of research publications was consulted, one lasting impression still remains – the use of herbal and nutritional supplements is not researched nearly as much as the use of prescription medications. In some cases, naturopathic compounds may offer a viable alternative to medications, but the scarcity of research supporting their use greatly curtails the level of confidence with which these compounds may be recommended. In addition, in the United States, the sale and marketing of naturopathic supplements is almost completely unregulated, and consumers and clinicians are at the mercy of an industry that receives no oversight and has no standards to uphold. This unfortunate situation further limits the extent to which consumers and mental health clinicians can put their trust in naturopathic supplements.

References

Abdou AM, Higashiguchi S, Horie K, Kim M, Hatta H, Yokogoshi H. Relaxation and immunity enhancement effects of gamma-aminobutyric acid (GABA) administration in humans. *Biofactors*. 2006;26:201–208.

Abi-Dargham A, Rodenhiser J, Prints D, Zea-Ponce Y, Gil R, Kegeles LS, Weiss R, Cooper TB, Mann JJ, Van Heertum RL, Gorman JM. Increased baseline occupancy of D2 receptors by dopamine in schizophrenia. *Proc Natl Acad Sci*. 2000;97:8104–8109.

Adler CM, Adams J, DelBello MP. Evidence of white matter pathology in bipolar disorder adolescents experiencing their first episode of mania: A diffusion tensor imaging study. *Am J Psychiatry*. 2006;163:322–324.

Agranoff BW, Stephen K. Inositol, lithium, and the brain. *Psychopharmacol Bull*. 2001;35:5–18.

Akhondzadeh S, Naghavi HR, Vazirian M, Shayeganpour A, Rashidi H, Khani M. Passionflower in the treatment of generalized anxiety: A pilot double-blind randomized controlled trial with oxazepam. *J Clin Pharm Ther*. 2001;26:369–373.

Albano AM, Chorpita BF, Barlow DH. Childhood anxiety disorders. In: Mash EJ, Barkley RA, eds *Child Psychopathology*. 2nd ed. New York: Guilford; 2003:279–329.

Alberto PA, Troutman AC. Applied Behavior Analysis for Teachers. 8th ed. New York: Prentice Hall; 2008.

Allen AJ, Leonard HL, Swedo SE. Case study: A new infection-triggered, autoimmune subtype of pediatric OCD and Tourette's syndrome. *J Am Acad Child Adolesc Psychiatry*. 1995;34:307–311.

Almeida Montes LG, Ontiveros Uribe MP, Cortes Sotres J. Treatment of primary insomnia with melatonin: A double-blind, placebo-controlled, crossover study. *J Psychiatry Neurosci*. 2003;28:191–196.

Alpert J, Mischoulon D, Rubenstein G. Folinic acid (leucovorin) as an adjunctive treatment from SSRI-refractory depression. *Ann Clin Psychiatry*. 2002;14:33–38.

Altshuller LL, Bookheimer SY, Townsend J, Proenza MA, Eisenberger N, Sabb F, Mintz J, Cohen MS. Blunted activation in orbitofrontal cortex during mania: A functional magnetic resonance imaging study. *Biol Psychiatry*. 2005;58:763–769.

Alvarado A, Diaz L, Sucre Z, Perez R, Veracoechea G, Hernandez M, Alvarado M. H Magnetic Resonance Spectroscopy (MRS) assessment of the effects of eicosapentaenoic-docosahexaenoic acids and choline-inositol supplementation on children with attention deficit hyperactivity disorder. *Acad Biomédica Digit*. 2004;20. Retrieved June 15, 2008, from http://www.vitae.com.

American Academy of Child and Adolescent Psychiatry. Practice parameters for the assessment and treatment of children and adolescents with bipolar disorder. *J Am Acad Child Adolesc Psychiatry*. 1997;36:138–157.

American Psychiatric Association. *Megavitamin and orthomolecular therapy in psychiatry*. Washington, DC: Author; 1973.

American Psychiatric Association. *Diagnostic and statistical manual of mental disorders*. 4th ed., text revision. Washington, DC: Author; 2000.

Andreatini R, Leite JR. Effect of valepotriates on the behavior of rats in the elevated plau-maze during diazepam withdrawal. *Eur J Psychopharmacol*. 1994;260:233–235.

Angst J, Woggon B, Schoepf J. The treatment of depression with L-5-hydroxytryptophan versus imipramine: Results of two open and one double-blind study. *Archiv fur Psychiatrie und Nervenkranheiten*. 1977;224:175–186.

Anke J, Ramzan I. Pharmacokinetic and pharmacodynamic drug interactions with kava (Piper methysticum Forst. f). *J Ethnopharmacol*. 2004;93:153–160.

Antonijevic I. HPA axis and sleep: Identifying subtypes of major depression. *Stress*. 2008;11:15–27.

Arnold LE. Treatment alternatives for attention deficit hyperactivity disorder. In: Jensen PS, Cooper JR, eds. *Attention Deficit Hyperactivity Disorder: State of the Science, Best Practices*. Kingston, NJ: Civic Research Institute; 2002:13–29.

Arvindakshan M, Ghate M, Ranjekar PK. Supplementation with a combination of omega-3 fatty acids and antioxidants (vitamins E and C) improves the outcome of schizo-phrenia. *Schizophr Res*. 2003;62:195–204.

Asarnow JR, Asarnow RF. Childhood-onset schizophrenia. In: Mash EJ, Barkley RA, eds *Child Psychopathology*. 2nd ed. New York: Guilford; 2003:455–485.

Axelson DA, Birmaher B. Relation between anxiety and depressive disorders in child-hood and adolescence. *Depress Anxiety*. 2001;14:67–78.

Azuma J, Hasegawa H, Sawamura A. Therapy of congestive heart failure with orally administered taurine. *Clin Ther*. 1983;5:398–408.

Bachevalier J. Medial temporal lobe structures and autism: A review of clinical and experimental findings. *Neuropsychologia*. 1994;32:627–648.

Bailey A, Le Couteur A, Gottesman I, Bolton P. Autism as a strongly genetic disorder: Evidence from a British twin study. *Psychol Med*. 1995;25:63–77.

Bailey A, Phillips W, Rutter M. Autism: Towards an integration of clinical, genetic and neuropsychological and neurobiological perspectives. *J Child Psychol Psychiatry*. 1996;37:89–126.

Balch PA. *Prescription for Nutritional Healing*. 4th ed. New York: Avery Publishers; 2006.

Barkai AI, Dunner DL, Gross HA, Mayo P, Fieve RR. Reduced myo-inositol levels in cerebrospinal fluid from patients with affective disorder. *Biol Psychiatry*. 1978;13:65–72.

Barkley RA. ADHD and The *Nature of Self Control*. New York: Guilford Press; 1997.

Barkley RA. *Attention-Deficit Hyperactivity Disorder: A Handbook for Diagnosis and Treatment*. 3rd ed. New York: Guilford Press; 2006.

Baron-Cohen S, Leslie AM, Frith U. Does the autistic child have a 'theory of mind?'. *Cognition*. 1985;21:37–46.

Bauman M, Kemper T. Limbic and cerebellar abnormalities: Consistent findings in infan-tile autism. *J Neuropathol Exp Neurol*. 1988;47:369–370.

Beck JS. *Cognitive Therapy: Basics and Beyond*. New York: Guilford Publications; 1995.

Becker S. Tourette's syndrome and Chinese medicine: Treatment possibilities. *J Chin Med*. 2003. Retrieved April 19, 2009, from http://www.thefreelibrary.com.

Bella R, Biondi R, Raffaele R. Effect of acetyl-L-carnitine on geriatric patients suffering from dysthymic disorders. *Int J Clin Pharmacol Res*. 1990;10:355–360.

Bell-Dolan D, Brazeal TJ. Separation anxiety disorder, overanxious disorder, and school refusal. *Child Adolesc Psychiatr Clin N Am*. 1993;2:563–580.

Belmaker RH, Benjamin J, Stahl Z. Inositol in the treatment of psychiatric disorders. In: Mischoulon D, Rosenbaum JF, eds. *Natural Medications for Psychiatric Disorders: Considering the Alternatives*. Philadelphia, PA: Lippincott, Williams & Wilkins; 2002:111–122.

Belmaker RH, Yuly B, Galila A. How does lithium work on manic depression? Clinical and psychological correlates of the inositol theory. *Annu Rev Med*. 1996;47:47–56.

Benjamin J, Levine J, Fux M. Double-blind, placebo-controlled crossover trial of inositol treatment for panic disorder. *Am J Psychiatry*. 1995;152:1084–1086.

Bent S, Padula A, Moore D. Valerian for sleep: A systematic review and meta-analysis. *Am J Med*. 2006;119:1005–1012.

Benton D, Buts JP. Vitamin/mineral supplementation and intelligence. *Lancet*. 1990; 335:1158–1160.

Benton D, Cook R. Vitamin and mineral supplements improve the intelligence scores and concentration of six-year-old children. *Pers Individ Dif*. 1991;12:1151–1158.

Benton D, Haller J, Fordy J. Vitamin supplementation for 1 year improves mood. *Neuropsychobiology*. 1995;32:98–105.

Bernard S, Enayati A, Redwood L. Autism: A novel form of mercury poisoning. *Med Hypotheses*. 2001;56:462–471.

Berriman M. Depression and nutrition. *New Vegetarian Nat Health*. 2004;74:14–19.

Bersani G, Alessandra G. Melatonin add-on in manic patients with treatment resistant insomnia. *Prog Neuropsychopharmacol Biol Psychiatry*. 2000;24:185–191.

Bertelsen A, Harvald B, Hauge M. A Danish twin study of manic-depressive disorders. *Br J Psychiatry*. 1977;130:330–351.

Bertrand J, Mars A, Boyle C, Bove E, Yeargin-Allsopp M, Decoufle P. Prevalence of autism in the United States population: The Brick Township, New Jersey, investigation. *Pediatrics*. 2001;108:1155–1161.

Bezchlibnyk-Butler KZ, Jeffries JJ. *Clinical handbook of psychotropic drugs*. 17th ed Seattle: Hogrefe & Huber; 2007.

Bezchlibnyk-Butler KZ, Virani AS. *Clinical handbook of psychotropic drugs for children and adolescents*. Seattle: Hogrefe & Huber; 2004.

Biederman J, Faraone S, Mick E, Wozniak J, Chen L, Oulette C, Marrs A, Moore P, Garcia J, Mennin D, Lelon E. Attention-deficit hyperactivity disorder and juvenile mania: An overlooked comorbidity? *J Am Acad Child Adolesc Psychiatry*. 1996;35: 997–1008.

Biederman J, Mick E, Faraone S, Spencer T, Wilens T, Wozniak J. Pediatric mania: A developmental subtype of bipolar disorder? *Biol Psychiatry*. 2000;48:458–466.

Biederman J, Newcorn J, Sprich S. Comorbidity of attention deficit hyperactivity disorder with conduct, depressive, anxiety, and other disorders. *Am J Psychiatry*. 1991;148: 564–577.

Birmaher B, Ryan ND, Williamson DE, Brent DA, Kaufman J, Dahl R. Childhood and adolescent depression: A review of the past 10 years, part I. *J Am Acad Child Adolesc Psychiatry*. 1996;35:1427–1439.

Bittner A, Egger HL, Erkanli A, Costello E, Foley DL, Angold A. What do childhood anxiety disorders predict? *J Child Psychol Psychiatry*. 2007;48:1174–1183.

Blanton RE, Levitt J, Thompson PM, Badrtalei S, Capetillo-Cunliffe L, Toga AW. Average 3-dimensional caudate surface representations in a case of juvenile-onset schizophrenia. *Arch Gen Psychiatry*. 1999;53:617–624.

Blumberg HP, Kaufman J, Martin A, Whiteman R, Gore JC, Charney DS, Krystal JH, Peterson BS. Amygdala and hippocampus volumes in adolescents and adults with bipolar disorder. *Arch Gen Psychiatry*. 2003;60:1201–1208.

Blumenthal M. Kava. In: Goldberg A, Kunz T, Dinda K, eds *ABC Clinical Guide to Herbs*. Austin, TX: American Botanical Council; 2003:259–272.

Boerner RJ, Sommer H, Berger W. Kava-kava extract LI 150 is as effective as opipramol and buspirone in generalized anxiety disorder: An 8-week randomized, double-blind multicenter clinical trial in 129 outpatients. *Phytomedicine*. 2003;10(suppl.): 38–49.

Bolton S, Null G. Caffeine: Psychological effects, use and abuse. *Orthomolecular Psychiatry*. 1981;10:202–211.

Bourin M, Bougerol T, Guitton B, Broutin E. A combination of plant extracts in the treatment of outpatients with adjustment disorder with anxious mood: Controlled study versus placebo. *Fundamentals Clin Pharmacol*. 1997;11:127–132.

Boylan K, Vaillancourt T, Boyle M, Szatmari P. Comorbidity of internalizing disorders in children with oppositional defiant disorder. *Eur Child Adolesc Psychiatry*. 2007;16:484–494.

Bradley PR, ed. *British herbal compendium, vol. 1*. Bournemouth, UK: British Herbal Medicine Association; 1992.

Brenesova V, Oswald L, Loudon J. Two types of insomnia: Too much waking or not enough sleep. *Br J Psychiatry*. 1975;126:439–445.

Bressa G. S-adenosyl-L-metionine (SAMe) as antidepressant: Meta-analysis of clinical studies. *Acta Neurol Scand*. 1994;154:7–14.

Bronson PJ. Mood biochemistry of women at mid-life. *J Orthomolecular Med*. 2001;16:13–46.

Brown RP, Gerberg P, Bottiglieri T. S-Adenosylmethionine (SAMe) for depression. *Psychiatric Ann*. 2002;32:29–44.

Broyd SJ, Demanuele C, Debener S, Helps SK, James CJ, Sonuga-Barke EJ. Default-mode brain dysfunction in mental disorders: A systematic review. *Neurosci and Biobehavioral Rev*. 2009;33:279–296.

Brzezinski A, Vangel MG, Wurtman RJ. Effects of exogenous melatonin on sleep: A meta-analysis. *Sleep Med Rev*. 2005;9:41–50.

Burattini MG, Amendola F, Aufierio T, Spano M, DiBitonto G, Del Vecchio GC, De Mattia D. Evaluation of the effectiveness of gastro-protected proteoferrin in the therapy of sideropenic anemia in childhood. *Minerva Pediatrica*. 1990;42:343–347.

Burd L, Kerbeshian J. A North Dakota prevalence study of schizophrenia presenting in childhood. *J Am Acad Child Adolesc Psychiatry*. 1987;26:347–350.

Burns GL, Walsh JA. The influence of ADHD-hyperactivity/impulsivity symptoms on the development of oppositional defiant disorder symptoms in a 2-year longitudinal study. *J Abnorm Child Psychol*. 2002;30:245–256.

Bursztajn HJ. Melatonin therapy: from benzodiazepine-dependent insomnia to authenticity and autonomy. *Arch Intern Med*. 1999;159:2393–2395.

Butterweck V. Mechanisms of action of St. John's wort: What is known? *CNS Drugs*. 2003;17:539–562.

Byerley W, Risch S. Depression and serotonin metabolism: Rationale for neurotransmitter precursor treatment. *J Clin Psychopharmacol*. 1985;5:191–206.

Campo JV, McNabb J, Perel J, Mazariegos GV, Hasegawa SL, Reyes J. Kava-induced fulminant hepatic failure. *J Am Acad Child Adolesc Psychiatry*. 2002;41:631–632.

Carney M, Sheffield B. Associations of subnormal serum folate and vitamin B12 values and effects of replacement therapy. *J Nervous Mental Dis.* 1970;150:404–412.

Cecil KM, DelBello MP, Morey R. Frontal lobe differences in bipolar disorder as determined by proton MR spectroscopy. *Bipolar Disord.* 2002;4:357–365.

Chamberlain RS, Herman BH. A novel biochemical model linking dysfunction in the brain melatonin, proopiomelanocortin peptides, and serotonin in autism. *Biol Psychiatry.* 1990;28:773–793.

Chatterjee SS, Bhattacharya SK, Wonnemann M, Singer A, Muller WE. Hyperforin as a possible antidepressant component of hypericum extracts. *Life Sci.* 1998;63: 499–510.

Chez MG, Buchanan CP, Aimonovitch MC. Double-blind, placebo-controlled study of L-carnosine supplementation in children with autistic spectrum disorders. *J Child Neurol.* 2002;17:833–837.

Child and Adolescent Bipolar Foundation Work Group. Consensus guidelines for diagnosis and treatment of bipolar disorder in children. *J Am Acad Child Adolesc Psychiatry.* 2005;44:213–239.

Chinevere TD, Sawyer RD, Creer AR, Conlee RK, Parcell AC. Effects of L-tyrosine and carbohydrate ingestion on endurance exercise performance. *J Appl Physiol.* 2002;93:1590–1597.

Chiu PH, Kayali MA, Kishida KT. Self responses along cingulate cortex reveal quantitative neural phenotype for high-functioning autism. *Neuron.* 2008;57:463–473.

Chojnacka-Wójcik E, Hano J, Sieroslawska J, Sypniewska M. Pharmacological properties of gamma-aminobutyric acid and its derivatives, IV: Aryl gaba derivatives and their respective lactams. *Archivum Immunologiae et Therapiae Experimentalis.* 1975;23:733–746.

Coffey B, Frazier J, Chen S. Comorbidity, Tourette syndrome, and anxiety disorders. *Adv Neurol.* 1992;58:95–104.

Cohen BM, Joseph IF, Altesman RI. Lecithin in the treatment of mania: Double-blind, placebo-controlled trials. *Am J Psychiatry.* 1982;139:1162–1164.

Cohen BM, Miller AL, Lipinski JF. Lecithin in mania: A preliminary report. *Am J Psychiatry.* 1980;137:242–243.

Colter AL, Cutler C, Meckling KA. Fatty acid status and behavioural symptoms of attention deficit hyperactivity disorder in adolescents: A case-control study. *Nutrition J.* 2008;7:8.

Comings DE. *Tourette syndrome and human behavior.* Duarte, CA: Hope Press; 1990.

Comings DE. Attention-deficit/hyperactivity disorder with Tourette's syndrome. In: Brown TE, ed. *attention-Deficit Disorders and Comorbidities in Children Adolescents, and Adults.* Washington, DC: American Psychiatric Press; 2000:363–392.

Commentz J, Uhlig H, Henke A, Hellwege M, Willig R. Melatonin and 6-hydroxymelatonin sulfate excretion is inversely correlated with gonadal development in children. *Hormonal Res.* 1997;47:97–101.

Conners CK. *Feeding the Brain.* New York: Da Capo Press; 2001.

Connor DF, Meltzer BM Pediatric Psychopharmacology: Fast Facts. New York: W. W. Norton; 2006.

Connor KM, Davidson RT. Homeopathy, kava, and other herbal treatments for anxiety. In: Mischoulon D, Rosenbaum JF, eds. *Natural Medications for Psychiatric Disorders: Considering the Alternatives.* Philadelphia, PA: Lippincott, Williams & Wilkins; 2002:125–131.

Coppen A, Bailey J. Enhancement of the antidepressant action of fluoxetine by folic acid: A randomized, placebo controlled trial. *J Affect Disord*. 2000;60:121–130.

Coppen A, Bolander-Gouaille C. Treatment of depression: Time to consider folic acid and vitamin B12. *J Psychopharmacol*. 2005;19:59–65.

Coppen A, Chaudhry S, Swade C. Folic acid enhances lithium prophylaxis. *J Affect Disord*. 1986;10:9–13.

Cott J, Misra R. Medicinal plants: A potential source for new psychotherapeutic drugs. In: Kanba S, Richelson E, eds. *Herbal Medicines for Neuropsychiatric Diseases: Current Development and Research*. Philadelphia, PA: Brunner/Mazel; 1999: 51–70.

Courchesne E, Press GA, Yeung-Courchesne R. Parietal lobe abnormalities detected with magnetic resonance in patients with infantile autism. *Am J Roentgenol*. 1993;160: 387–393.

Currie BJ, Clough AR. Kava hepatotoxicity with western herbal products: Does it occur with traditional kava use? *Med J Aust*. 2003;178:421–422.

Dales L, Hammer SJ, Smith NJ. Time trends in autism and in MMR immunization coverage in California. *J Am Med Assoc*. 2001;285:2852–2853.

Dapretto M. Understanding emotions in others: Mirror neuron dysfunction in children with autism spectrum disorders. *Nat Neurosci*. 2006;9:28–30.

Darbinyan V, Aslanyan G, Amroyan E, Gabrielyan E, Malmström C, Panossian A. Clinical trial of rhodiola rosea L. extract SHR-5 in the treatment of mild to moderate depression. *Nord J Psychiatry*. 2007;61:343–348.

Davanzo P, Yue K, Thomas A, Belin T, Mintz J, Venkatraman TN, Santoro E, Barnett S, McCracken J. Proton magnetic resonance spectroscopy of bipolar disorder versus intermittent explosive disorder in children and adolescents. *Am J Psychiatry*. 2003;160:1442–1452.

David OJ, Hoffman SP, Sverd J, Clark J, Voeller K. Lead and hyperactivity – behavioral response to chelation: A pilot study. *Am J Psychiatry*. 1976;133:1155–1158.

Davidson JR, Connor KM. St. John's wort in generalized anxiety disorder: Three case reports. *J Clin Psychopharmacol*. 2001;21:635–636.

Davis MP, Darden PM. Use of complementary and alternative medicine by children in the United States. *Arch Pediatr Adolesc Med*. 2003;157:393–396.

Davison J, Abraham K, Connor K. Effectiveness of chromium in atypical depression: A placebo-controlled trial. *Biol Psychiatry*. 2003;53:261–264.

Daviss WB. A review of co-morbid depression in pediatric ADHD: Etiologies, phenomenology, and treatment. *J Child Adolesc Psychopharmacol*. 2008;18:565–571.

Davydov L, Stirling AL. Stevens-Johnson syndrome with Gingko biloba. *J Herb Pharmacother*. 2001;1:65–69.

Dawson G, Klinger LG, Panagiotides H, Lewy A, Castelloe P. Subgroups of autistic children based on social behavior display distinct patterns of brain activity. *J Abnorm Child Psychol*. 1995;23:569–583.

Dawson G, Warrenburg S, Fuller P. Hemisphere function and motor imitation in autistic persons. *Brain Cogn*. 1983;2:346–354.

De Bellis MD, Casey BJ, Dahl RE. A pilot study of amygdala volumes in pediatric generalized anxiety disorder. *Biol Psychiatry*. 2000;48:51–57.

DeBattista C, Schatzberg AF. *Black book of psychotropic dosing and monitoring*. New York: MBL Communications; 2006.

Dedmon R. Tourette syndrome in children: Knowledge and services. *Health Soc Work*. 1990;15:107–115.

Dehaene S, Jonides J, Smith EE, Spitzer M. Thinking and problem solving. In: Zigmond MJ, Bloom FE, Landis SC, Roberts JL, Squire LR, eds. *Fundamental Neuroscience*. San Diego, CA: Academic Press; 1999:1543–1564.

Delle Chiaie R, Pancheri P, Scapicchio P. Efficacy and tolerability of oral and intramuscular S-adenosyl-L-metionine 1,4-butanedisulfonate (SAMe) in the treatment of major depression: Comparison with imipramine in 2 multicenter studies. *Am J Clin Nutr*. 2002;76(suppl):1172S–1176S.

DeVito TJ, Drost DJ, Pavlosky W, Neufeld RW, Rajakumar N, McKinlay BD, Williamson PC, Nicolson R. Brain Magnetic Resonance Spectroscopy in Tourette's disorder. *J Am Acad Child Adolesc Psychiatry*. 2005;44:1301–1308.

Dews PB. Behavioral effects of caffeine. In: Dews PB, ed. *Caffeine: Perspectives from Recent Research*. Berlin: Springer-Verlag; 1984:86–103.

Doja A, Roberts W. Immunizations and autism: A review of the literature. *Can J Neurol Sci*. 2006;33:341–346.

Dolberg OT, Hirchmann S, Grunhaus L. Melatonin for the treatment of sleep disturbances in major depressive disorder. *Am J Psychiatry*. 1998;155:1119–1121.

Drevets W. Neuroimaging and neuropathological studies of depression. *Curr Opin Neurobiol*. 2001;11:240–249.

Durlach J, Durlach V, Bac P. Magnesium and therapeutics. *Magnes Res*. 1994;7:313–328.

Egashira N, Hayakawa K, Osajima M. Involvement of GABA (A) receptors in the neuroprotective effect of theanine on focal cerebral ischemia in mice. *J Pharmacol Sci*. 2007;105:211–214.

Eley T. Contributions of behavioral genetics research: Quantifying genetic, shared environmental and nonshared environmental influences. In: Vasey M, Dadds M, eds. *The Developmental Pathology of Anxiety*. Oxford, UK: Oxford University Press; 2001: 49–59.

Eli Lilly and Company. *Final Labeling: Sarafem Fluoxetine Hydrochloride*. Indianapolis: Author; 2000 Retrieved April 18, 2009, from http://www.fda.gov.

Ellinoy BJ, Lake JH, Hobbs C. Patient Safety. In: Lake JH, Spiegel D, eds. *Complementary and Alternative Treatments in Mental Health Care*. Washington, DC: American Psychiatric Publishing; 2007:37–62.

Enig MG. *Know Your Fats: The Complete Primer for Understanding the Nutrition of Fats, Oils and Cholesterol*. Silver Spring, MD: Bethesda Press; 2000.

Enig MG, Fallon S. Tripping lightly down the prostaglandin pathways. *Price-Pottenger Nutr Found Health J*. 1999;20:574–577.

Ernst M, Rumsey JM, eds. *Functional Neuroimaging in Child Psychiatry*. New York: Cambridge University Press; 2000.

Ernst M, Kimes AS, London ED, Matochik JA, Eldreth D, Tata S. Neural substrates of decision making in adults with attention deficit hyperactivity disorder. *Am J Psychiatry*. 2003;160:1061–1070.

European Centre for Disease Prevention and Control. Measles once again endemic in the United Kingdom. *Eurosurveillance*. 2008;13:7–9.

Evans SM, Griffiths RR. Caffeine tolerance and choice in humans. *Psychopharmacology*. 1992;108:51–59.

Facchinetti F, Borella P, Sances G. Oral magnesium successfully relieves premenstrual mood changes. *Obstet Gynecol*. 1991;78:177–181.

Faraone SV, Biederman J, Wozniak J, Mundy E, Mennin D, O'Donnell D. In comorbidity with ADHD a marker for juvenile mania? *J Am Acad Child Adolesc Psychiatry*. 1997;36:1046–1055.

Fatemi SH, Stary JM, Halt AR, Realmuto GM. Dysregulation of Reelin and Bcl-2 proteins in autistic cerebellum. *J Autism Dev Disord.* 2001;31:529–535.

Fenton WS, Dickerson E, Boronow J. A placebo-controlled trial of omega-3 fatty acid (ethyl eicosapentaenoic acid) supplementation for residual symptoms and cognitive impairment in schizophrenia. *Am J Psychiatry.* 2001;158:2071–2074.

Findling RL, McNamara NK, O'Riordan MA, Reed MD, Demeter CA, Branicky LA, Blumer JL. An open-label pilot study of St. John's wort in juvenile depression. *J Am Acad Child Adolesc Psychiatry.* 2003;42:908–914.

Fisher E, Spatz H, Saavedra J. Urinary elimination of phenylethylamine. *Biol Psychiatry.* 1972;5:139–147.

Fleming JE, Offord DR. Epidemiology of childhood depressive disorders: A critical review. *J Am Acad Child Adolesc Psychiatry.* 1990;29:571–580.

Foa EB, Costello EJ, Franklin M, Kagan L, Kendall P, Klein R. Anxiety disorders. In: Evans DL, Foa EB, Gur RE, eds. *Treating and Preventing Adolescent Mental Health Disorders.* Oxford, UK: Oxford University Press; 2005:161–256.

Fokkema MR, van Rieke HM, Bauermann OJ, Smit EN, Muskiet FA. Short-term carnitine supplementation does not augment LCP3 status of vegans and lacto-ovo-vegetarians. *J Am Coll Nutr.* 2005;24:58–64.

Folstein M, Liu T, Peter I, Buel J, Arsenault L, Scott T, Qiu WW. The homocysteine hypothesis of depression. *Am J Psychiatry.* 2007;164:861–867.

Folstein SE, Rosen-Sheidley B. Genetics of autism: Complex aetiology for a heterogeneous disorder. *Nat Rev Genet.* 2001;2:943–955.

Fombonne E. Epidemiological surveys of autism and other pervasive developmental disorders: An update. *J Autism Dev Disord.* 2003;33:365–377.

Food and Drug Administration. FDA issues consumer advisory that kava products may be associated with severe liver injury. *Lett to Health Care Professionals.* 2002 25. Retrieved April 15, 2009, from http://www.cfsan.fda.gov/dms/supplmnt.html.

Forbes EE, Hariri AR, Martin SL, Silk JS, Moyles DL, Fisher PM, Brown SM, Ryan ND, Birmacher B, Axelson DA, Dahl RE. Altered striatal activation predicting real-world positive affect in adolescent major depressive disorder. *Am J Psychiatry.* 2009;166:64–73.

Foster AC, Kemp JA. Glutamate- and GABA-based CNS therapeutics. *Curr Opin Pharmacol.* 2006;6:7–17.

Francis AJ, Dempster RJ. Effect of valerian, Valeriana edulis, on sleep difficulties in children with intellectual deficits: Randomized trial. *Phytomedicine.* 2002;9:273–279.

Franklin M, Odontiatis J. Effects of treatment with chromium picolinate on peripheral amino acid availability and brain monoamine function in the rat. *Pharmacopsychiatry.* 2003;36:176–180.

Fredericksen KA, Cutting LE, Kates WR. Disproportionate increases of white matter in right frontal lobe in Tourette syndrome. *Neurology.* 2002;58:85–99.

Fredholm BB, IJzerman AP, Jacobson KA, Klotz KN, Linden J. International Union of Pharmacology, XXV: Nomenclature and classification of adenosine receptors. *Pharmacology Rev.* 2001;53:527–552.

Frith U, Happe F. Autism: Beyond 'theory of mind.' *Cognition.* 1994;50:115–132.

Fujita T, Ando K, Noda H, Ito Y, Sato Y. Effects of increased adrenomedullary activity and taurine in young patients with borderline hypertension. *Circulation.* 1987;75:525–532.

Fux M, Levine J, Aviv A, Belmaker RH. Inositol treatment of obsessive–compulsive disorder. *Am J Psychiatry.* 1996;153:1219–1221.

Garber J. Classification of childhood psychopathology: A developmental perspective. *Child Dev*. 1984;55:30–48.

García-López R, Perea-Milla E, Garcia CR, Rivas-Ruiz F, Romero-Gonzalez J, Moreno JL, Faus V, Aguas Gdel C, Diaz JC. New therapeutic approach to Tourette syndrome in children based on a randomized placebo-controlled double-blind phase IV study of the effectiveness and safety of magnesium and vitamin B6. *Trials*. 2009;10:10–16.

García-López R, Romero-González J, Perea-Milla E, Ruiz-García C, Rivas-Ruiz F, de Las Mulas Béjar M. An open study evaluating the efficacy and security of magnesium and vitamin B(6) as a treatment of Tourette syndrome in children. *Med Clin*. 2008;131: 689–692.

Garfinkel D, Zisapel N, Wainstein J, Laudon M. Facilitation of benzodiazepine discontinuation by melatonin. *Arch Intern Med*. 1999;159:2456–2460.

Garoufi AJ, Prassouli AA, Achilleas VA, Konstantinos AV, Katsarou ES. Homozygous MTHFR C677T gene mutation and recurrent stroke in an infant. *Pediatr Neurol*. 2006;35:49–51.

Garrett BE, Griffiths RR. The role of dopamine in the behavioral effects of caffeine in animals and man. *Pharmacolo, Biochem and Behav*. 1997;57:533–541.

Gass JD. Nicotinic acid maculopathy. *Retina*. 2003;23(Suppl.):500–510.

Gelenberg AJ, Dorer DJ, Wojcik JD. A crossover study of lecithin treatment of tardive dyskinesia. *J Clin Psychiatry*. 1990;51:149–153.

Gerard E, Peterson BS. Developmental processes and brain imaging studies in Tourette syndrome. *J Psychosom Res*. 2003;55:13–22.

Gesh CB, Hammond SM, Hampson SE. Influence of supplementary vitamins, minerals and essential fatty acids on the antisocial behavior of young adult prisoners: Randomised, placebo-controlled trial. *Br J Psychiatry*. 2002;181:22–28.

Gillberg C, Coleman M. Autism and medical disorders: A review of the literature. *Dev Med Child Neurol*. 1996;38:191–202.

Godfrey P, Crellin R, Toone BK. Enhancement of recovery from psychiatric illness by methylfolate. *Br J Psychiatry*. 1992;161:126–127.

Gogtay N, Sporn A, Clasen LS, Nugent TF, Greenstein D, Nicolson R, Giedd JN, Lenane M, Gochman P, Evans A, Rapoport JL. Comparison of progressive grey matter loss in childhood-onset schizophrenia with that in childhood-onset atypical psychoses. *Arch Gen Psychiatry*. 2004;61:17–22.

Golan ROptimal Wellness. New York: Ballantine Books; 1995.

Gold MSThe Good News about Depression. New York: Bantam Books; 1993.

Goldman W. Is there a shortage of psychiatrists?. *Psychiatr Serv*. 2001;52:1587–1589.

Gorman DA, Zhu H, Anderson GM, Davies MP, Peterson BS. Ferritin levels and their association with regional brain volumes in Tourette's syndrome. *Am J Psychiatry*. 2006;163:1264–1272.

Gorman J, Kent JM, Sullivan GM, Coplan JD. Neuroanatomical hypothesis of panic disorder, revised. *Am J Psychiatry*. 2000;157:493–505.

Gottesman ISchizophrenia Genesis: The Origins of Madness. New York: Freeman; 1991.

Graybiel AM, Rauch SI. Toward a neurobiology of obsessive–compulsive disorder. *Neuron*. 2000;28:343–347.

Gregory PJ. Seizure associated with Gingko biloba. *Ann Intern Med*. 2001;134. 344–344.

Griffiths RR, Mumford GK. Caffeine: A drug of abuse?. In: Bloom FE, Kupfer DJ, eds. *Psychopharmacol: The Fourth Generation of Progress*. New York: Raven Press; 1995:1699–1713.

Grimaldi BL. The central role of magnesium deficiency in Tourette's syndrome: Causal relationships between magnesium deficiency, altered biochemical pathways and symptoms relating to Tourette's syndrome and several reported comorbid conditions. *Med Hypotheses.* 2002;58:47–60.

Growdon JH, Cohen EL, Wurtman RJ. Treatment of brain disease with dietary precursors of neurotransmitters. *Ann Intern Med.* 1977;86:337–339.

Gurevich EV, Bordelon V, Shapiro RM, Arnold SE, Gur RE, Joyce JN. Mesolimbic dopamine D3 receptors and use of antipsychotics in patients with schizophrenia: A postmortem study. *Arch Gen Psychiatry.* 1997;54:225–232.

Halperin JM, Newcorn JH, Koda VH, Pick L, McKay KE, Knott P. Noradrenergic mechanisms in ADHD children with and without reading disabilities: A replication and extension. *J Am Acad Child Adolesc Psychiatry.* 1997;36:1688–1697.

Hamazaki T, Sawazaki S, Itomura M. The effect of docosahexaenoic acid on aggression in young adults: A placebo-controlled double-blind study. *J Clin Investig.* 1996;97: 1129–1133.

Hammen C, Rudolph KD. Childhood mood disorders. In: Mash EJ, Barkley RA, eds. *Child Psychopathology.* 2nd ed. New York: Guilford; 2003:233–278.

Harpold TL, Wozniak J, Kwon A, Gilbert J, Wood J, Smith L, Biederman J. Examining the association between pediatric bipolar disorder and anxiety disorders in psychiatrically referred children and adolescents. *J Affect Disord.* 2005;88:19–26.

Haugaard JJChild Psychopathology. Boston, MA: McGraw-Hill; 2008.

Hayward A. *Secretin.* San Diego, CA: Autism Research Institute; 2000 Retrieved May 11, 2009, from http://www.mugsy.org/asa_faq/treatments/secretin.shtml.

Heiman SW. Pycnogenol for ADHD? *J Am Acad Child Adolesc Psychiatry.* 1999;38: 357–358.

Heresco-Levy U, Javitt DC, Ermilov M. Efficacy of high-dose glycine in the treatment of enduring negative symptoms of schizophrenia. *Arch Gen Psychiatry.* 1999;56: 29–36.

Hibbeln JR, Linnoila M, Umhau JC. Essential fatty acids predict metabolites of serotonin and dopamine in cerebrospinal fluid among healthy control subjects and early- and late-onset alcoholics. *Biol Psychiatry.* 1998;44:235–242.

Hibbeln JR, Umhau JC, Linnoila M, George DT, Ragan PW, Shoaf SE, Vaughan MR, Rawlings R, Salem N Jr. Essential fatty acids predict metabolites of serotonin and dopamine in cerebrospinal fluid among healthy control subjects, and early- and late-onset alcoholics. *Biol Psychiatry.* 1998;44:243–349.

Hingle M. Nutrition. In: Lake JH, Spiegel D, eds. *Complementary and Alternative Treatments in Mental Health Care.* Washington, DC: American Psychiatric Publishing; 2007:275–299.

Hirayama S, Hamazaki T, Terasawa K. Effect of docosahexaenoic acid-containing food administration on symptoms of attention-deficit/hyperactivity disorder: A placebo-controlled double-blind study. *Eur J Clin Nutr.* 2004;58:467–473.

Hobson JA. Sleep and dreaming. In: Zigmond MJ, Bloom FE, Landis SC, Roberts JL, Squire LR, eds. *Fundamental Neuroscience.* San Diego, CA: Academic Press; 1999:1207–1227.

Hodapp RM, Dykens EM. Mental retardation (intellectual disabilities). In: Mash EJ, Barkley RA, eds. *Child Psychopathology.* 2nd ed. New York: Guilford; 2003:486–519.

Hoffer A. The vitamin paradigm wars. *Townsend Let for Doctors and Patients.* 1996 June:56–60.

Hoffer A. *Vitamin B-3 and Schizophrenia: Discovery, Recovery, Controversy*. Dallas, TX: Quarry Press; 1999.

Hoffer A. *Healing Schizophrenia: Complementary Vitamin and Drug Treatments*. Toronto, Canada: Canadian College of Naturopathic Medicine (CCNM) Press; 2004.

Hollis C. Developmental precursors of child- and adolescent-onset schizophrenia and affective psychoses: Diagnostic specificity and continuity with symptom dimensions. *Br J Psychiatry*. 2003;182:37–44.

Hong KE, Ock SM, Kang MH. The segmented regional volumes of the cerebrum and cerebellum in boys with Tourette syndrome. *J Korean Med Sci*. 2002;17:530–536.

Horrocks LA, Yeo YK. Health benefits of docosahexaenoic acid. *Pharm Res*. 1999;40: 211–225.

Houenou J, Wessa M, Douaud G, Leboyer M, Chanraud S, Perrin M, Poupon C, Martinot J-L, Paillere-Martinot M-L. Increased white matter connectivity in euthymic bipolar patients: Diffusion tensor tractography between the subgenual cingulate and the amygdalo-hippocampal complex. *Mol Psychiatry*. 2007;12:1001–1010.

Hübner WD, Kirste T. Experience with St John's wort (hypericum perforatum) in children under 12 years with symptoms of depression and psychovegetative disturbances. *Phytother Res*. 2001;15:367–370.

Huebscher R, Shuler PA. *Natural, Alternative and Complementary Health Care Practices*. New York: Mosby Publishers; 2003.

Hypericum Depression Trial Study Group. Effect of Hypericum perforatum (St John's wort) in major depressive disorder: A randomized controlled trial. *J Am Med Assoc*. 2002;287:1807–1814.

Iacoboni M, Dapretto M. The mirror neuron system and the consequences of its dysfunction. *Nat Rev Neurosci*. 2006;7:942–951.

Ivy J, Portman R. *Nutrient Timing*. Laguna Beach, CA: Basic Health Publications; 2004.

Jacobsen JG, Smith LH. Biochemistry and Physiology of taurine and taurine derivatives. *Physiol Rev*. 1968;48:424–511.

Jacobsen LK, Giedd JN, Rajapakse JC, Hamburger SD, Vaituzis AC, Frazier JA, Lenane MC, Rapoport JL. Quantitative magnetic resonance imaging of the corpus callosum in childhood onset schizophrenia. *Psychiatry Res*. 1997;68:77–86.

Jadresic D. Tourette's syndrome and the amygdaloid complex. *Br J Psychiatry*. 1993; 162:851–852.

James JJ. *Caffeine and Health*. London: Academic Press; 1991.

James SJ, Cutler P, Melnyk S. Metabolic biomarkers of increased oxidative stress and impaired methylation capacity in children with autism. *Am J Clin Nutr*. 2004;80:1611–1617.

Janicak PG, Davis JM, Preskorn SH, Ayd FJ, Marder SR, Pavuluri MN. *Principles and practice of psychopharmacotherapy*. Philadeplphia, PA: Lippincott, Williams & Wilkins; 2006.

Jaskiw G, Kleinman J. Postmortem neurochemistry studies in schizophrenia. In: Schulz SC, Tamminga CA, eds. *Schizophrenia: A Scientific Focus*. New York: Oxford University Press; 1988:264–273.

Jia F, Yue M, Chandra D, Keramidas A, Goldstein PA, Homanics GE, Harrison NL. Taurine is a potent activator of extrasynaptic GABA(A) receptors in the thalamus. *J Neurosci*. 2008;28:106–115.

Johnson M, Ostlund S, Fransson G, Kadesjo B. Omega-3/omega-6 fatty acids for attention deficit hyperactivity disorder: A randomized placebo-controlled trial in children and adolescents. *J Atten Disord*. 2009;12:394–401.

Julien RMA. *Primer of Drug Action*. 11th ed. New York: Worth Publishers; 2008.

Juneja LR, Chu DC, Okubo T. L-teanine – a unique amino acid of green tea and its relaxation effect in humans. *Trends Food Sci Tech*. 1999;10:199–204.

Kahn R, Westenberg H. L-5-hydroxytryptophan in the treatment of anxiety disorders. *J Affect Disord*. 1985;8:197–200.

Kahn R, Westenberg H, Verhoven W. Effect of a serotonin precursor and uptake inhibitor in anxiety disorders: A double-blind comparison of 5-hydroxytryptophan, clomipramine and placebo. *Int Clin Psychopharmacol*. 1987;2:33–45.

Kakuda T, Nozawa A, Unno T. Inhibiting effects of theanine on caffeine stimulation evaluated by EEG in the rat. *Biosci Biotechnol Biochem*. 2000;64:287–293.

Kanner AM. Psychosis of epilepsy: A neurologist's perspective. *Epilepsy and Behav*. 2000;1:219–227.

Kaplan BJ, Crawford SG, Field CJ. Vitamins, minerals, and mood. *Psychol Bull*. 2007;133:747–760.

Kashani JH, Carlson GA. Seriously depressed preschoolers. *Am J Psychiatry*. 1987;144:348–350.

Keeley ML, Storch EA, Dhungana P, Geffken GR. Pediatric obsessive–compulsive disorder: A guide to assessment and treatment. *Issues Ment Health Nurs*. 2007;28:555–574.

Kemper KJ, Shannon S. Complementary and alternative medicine therapies to promote healthy moods. *Pediatr Clin North Am*. 2007;54:901–926.

Kempster PA, Wahlqvist ML. Dietary factors in the management of Parkinson's disease. *Nutr Rev*. 1994;52:51–58.

Kersten H, Randis T, Giardino A. Evidence-Based Medicine in Pediatric Residency Programs: Where Are We Now? *Ambul Pediatr*. 2003;5:302–305.

Khalsa DSBrain Longevity. New York: Warner Books; 1997.

Kim J, Gorman J. The psychobiology of anxiety. *Clin Neurosci Res*. 2005;4:335–347.

Kim J, Szatmari P, Bryson S, Streiner D, Wilson F. The prevalence of anxiety and mood problems among children with autism and Asperger's syndrome. *Autism*. 2000;4:117–132.

Kimura K. L-Theanine reduces psychological and physiological stress responses. *Biol Psychol*. 2007;74:39–45.

Kimura K, Ozeki M, Juneja L, Ohira H. L-Theanine reduces psychological and physiological stress responses. *Biol Psychol*. 2007;74:39–45.

Kinzler E, Kromer J, Lehmann E. Effect of a special kava extract in patients with anxiety, tension, and excitation states of non-psychotic genesis: Double-blind study with placebos over 4 weeks. *Arzneimittel Forsch*. 1991;41:584–588.

Klein RG. Pharmacotherapy of childhood hyperactivity: An update. In: Meltzer HY, ed. *Psychopharmacol: The Third Generation of Progress*. New York: Raven Press; 1987:1215–1224.

Kline NS. Use of Rauwolfia serpentina in neuropsychiatric conditions. *Ann N Y Acad Sci*. 1954;59:107–132.

Klinger LG, Dawson G, Renner P. Autistic disorder. In: Mash EJ, Barkley RA, eds. *Child Psychopathology*. 2nd ed. New York: Guilford; 2003:409–454.

Kovacs M. Affective disorders in children and adolescents. *Am Psychol*. 1989;44:209–215.

Kovacs M, Goldston D, Gatsonis C. Suicidal behaviors and childhood-onset depressive disorders: A longitudinal investigation. *J Am Acad Child Adolesc Psychiatry*. 1993;32:8–20.

Kovacs M, Paulauskas S, Gatsonis C, Richards C. Depressive disorders in childhood, III: A longitudinal study of comorbidity with and risk for conduct disorders. *J Affect Disord*. 1988;15:205–217.

Kowalchick C, Hylon WH. *Rodale's Illustrated Encyclopedia of Herbs*. Emmaus, PA: Rodale Press; 1987.

Kuriyama S, Kamiyama M, Watanabe M. Pyridoxine treatment in a subgroup of children with pervasive developmental disorders. *Dev Med Child Neurol*. 2002;44:284–286.

Kurnakov BA. Pharmacology of skullcap. *Farmakologia i Toksikologia*. 1957;20:79–80.

Lake JH. Omega-3 essential fatty acids. In: Lake JH, Spiegel D, eds. *Complementary and Alternative Treatment in Mental Health Care*. Washington, DC: American Psychiatric Publishing; 2007:151–167.

Lake JH, Spiegel D, eds. *Complementary and Alternative Treatment in Mental Health Care*. Washington, DC: American Psychiatric Publishing; 2007.

Lange C, Irle E. Enlarged amygdala volume and reduced hippocampal volume in young women with major depression. *Psychol Med*. 2004;34:1059–1064.

Lapin I. Phenibut (beta-phenyl-GABA): A tranquilizer and nootropic drug. *CNS Drug Rev*. 2001;7:471–481.

Laruelle M, Abi-Dargham A, Van Dyck CH, Gil R, D'Souza CD, Erdos J, McCance E, Rosenblatt W, Fingado C, Zoghbi SS, Baldwin RM, Seibyl JP, Krystal JH, Charney DS, Innis RB. Single photon emission computerized tomography imaging of amphetamine-induced dopamine release in drug-free schizophrenic subjects. *Proc Natl Acad Sci*. 1996;93:9235–9240.

Larzelere MM, Wiseman P. Anxiety, depression, and insomnia. *Prim Care*. 2002;29: 339–360.

Laugharne JD, Mellor JE, Peet M. Fatty acids and schizophrenia. *Lipids*. 1996; 31(suppl):S163–S165.

Laurent J, Potter KI. Anxiety-related difficulties. In: Watson TS, Gresham FM, eds. *Handbook of Child Behavior Therapy*. New York: Kluwer; 1998:371–392.

Lawrie SM, Abkumeil SS. Brain abnormality in schizophrenia: A systematic and quantitative review of volumetric magnetic resonance imaging studies. *Br J Psychiatry*. 1998;172:110–120.

Leboyer M, Philippe A, Boouvard M, Guilloud-Bataille M, Bondoux D, Tabuteau F, Feingold J, Mouren-Simeoni M, Launay J. Whole blood serotonin and plasma beta-endorphin in autistic probands and their first degree relatives. *Biol Psychiatry*. 1999;45:158–163.

Lee A, Hobson R, Chait S. I, you, me, and autism: An experimental study. *J Autism Dev Disord*. 1994;24:155–176.

Lee R, Yee PS, Naing G. Western Herbal Medicines. In: Lake JH, Spiegel D, eds. *Complementary and Alternative Treatments in Mental Health Care*. Washington, DC: American Psychiatric Publishing; 2007:87–114.

Leibenluft E, Feldman NS, Turner EH. Effects of exogenous melatonin administration and withdrawal in five patients with rapid-cycling bipolar disorder. *J Clin Psychiatry*. 1997;58:383–388.

Leon MR. Effects of caffeine on cognitive, psychomotor, and affective performance of children with attention-deficit/hyperactivity disorder. *J Atten Disord*. 2000;4:27–47.

Leonard BE. Neurotransmitter receptors, endocrine responses, and the biological substrates of depression: A review. *Hum Psychopharmacol*. 1986;1:3–21.

Leonard BE, Myint A. The psychoneuroimmunology of depression. *Hum Psychopharmacol: Clin Exp*. 2009;24:165–175.

Leuschner J, Muller J, Rudmann M. Characterisation of the central nervous depressant activity of a commercially available valerian root extract. *Arzneimittelforschung*. 1993; 43:638–641.

Levine J. Controlled trials of inositol in psychiatry. *Eur Neuropsychopharmacol.* 1997; 7:147–155.

Levine J, Gonsalves M, Babur I. Inositol 6 gm daily may be effective in depression but not in schizophrenia. *Hum Psychopharmacol.* 1993;8:49–53.

Levine J, Mishori A, Susbisky M, Martin M, Belmaker RH. Combination of inositol and serotonin reuptake inhibitors in the treatment of depression. *Biol Psychiatry.* 1999;45:270–273.

Levy SE, Hyman SL. Complementary and alternative medicine treatments for children with autism spectrum disorders. *Child Adolesc Psychiatr Clin N Am.* 2008;17: 803–820.

Lieberman HR, Corkin S, Spring BJ, Wurtman RJ, Growdon JH. The effects of dietary neurotransmitter precursors on human behavior. *Am J Clin Nutr.* 1985;42: 366–370.

Lin PY, Su KP. A meta-analytic review of double-blind, placebo-controlled trials of antidepressant efficacy of omega-3 fatty acids. *J Clin Psychiatry.* 2007;68:1056–1061.

Lindenberg D, Pitule-Schodel H. D,L-kavain in comparison with oxazepam in anxiety disorders: A double-blind study of clinical effectiveness. *Fortschritte der Medizin.* 1990;108:49–54.

Lombardo JA. Stimulants and athletic performance: Amphetamines and caffeine. *Physician and Sports Med.* 1986;14:128–140.

López-Muñoz F, Bhatara VS, Alamo C, Cuenca E. Historical approach to reserpine discovery and its introduction in psychiatry. *Actas Españolas de Psiquiatría.* 2004;32:387–395.

Lovaas OI. Behavioral treatment and normal education and intellectual functioning in young autistic children. *J Consult Clin Psychol.* 1987;55:3–9.

Lu K, Gray MA, Oliver C, Liley DT, Harrison BJ, Bartholomeusz CF, Phan KL, Nathan PJ. The acute effects of L-theanine in comparison with alprazolam on anticipatory anxiety in humans. *Hum Psychopharmacol.* 2004;19:457–465.

Lynam DR. Early identification of the fledgling psychopath: locating the psychopathic child in the current nomenclature. *J Abnorm Psychol.* 1998;107:566–575.

Lyoo IK, Lee HK, Jung JH, Noam GG, Renshaw PF. White matter hyperintensities on magnetic resonance imaging of the brain in children with psychiatric disorders. *Compr Psychiatry.* 2002;43:361–368.

MacMaster FP, Mirza Y, Szeszko PR, Kmiecik LE, Easter PC, Taormina SP, Lynch M, Rose M, Moore GJ, Rosenberg DR. Amygdala and hippocampal volumes in familial early onset major depressive disorder. *Biol Psychiatry.* 2008;63:385–390.

Mahal AS, Ramu NG, Chaturvedi D. Double-blind controlled study of brahmyadioga and tagara in the management of various types of unmada (schizophrenia). *Indian J Psychiatry.* 1976;18:283–292.

Malsch U, Kieser M. Efficacy of kava-kava in the treatment of non-psychotic anxiety, following pretreatment with benzodiazepines. *Psychopharmacology.* 2001;157: 277–283.

Marangell LB, Martinez JM, Zboyan HA. A double-blind, placebo-controlled study of the omega-3 fatty acid docosahexaenoic acid in the treatment of major depression. *Am J Psychiatry.* 2003;160:996–998.

Mash EJ, Barkley RA, eds. *Treatment of Childhood Disorders.* New York: Guilford Press; 2006.

Masi G, Mucci M, Millepiedi S. Separation anxiety disorder in children and adolescents: Epidemiology, diagnosis and management. *CNS Drugs.* 2001;15:93–104.

Mason R. (n.d.). *Adenosine Triphosphate, the Energy of Life*. Channel Islands, UK: International Antiaging Systems; n.d. Retrieved March 15, 2009, from http://www. smart-drugs.net.

McLeod M, Golden R. Chromium treatment of depression. *Int J Neuropsychopharmacol.* 2000;3:311–314.

McLeod M, Gaynes B, Golden R. Chromium potentiation of antidepressant pharmacotherapy for dysthymic disorder in 5 patients. *J Clin Psychiatry.* 1999;60:237–240.

Medical Economics. *PDR for Herbal Medicines.* 4th ed. Montvale, NJ: Author; 2007.

Medical Economics. *PDR for Nutritional Supplements.* 2nd ed. Montvale, NJ: Author; 2008a.

Medical Economics. *Physician's Desk Reference.* 62nd ed. Montvale, NJ: Author; 2008b.

Medina M. Flavonoids: A new family of benzodiazepine receptor ligands. *Neurochem Res.* 1997;22:419–421.

Mellor JE, Laugharne JD, Peet M. Schizophrenic symptoms and dietary intake of omega-3 fatty acids. *Schizophr Res.* 1995;18:85–86.

Menzies L, Williams GB, Chamberlain SR, Ooi C, Fineberg N, Suckling J, Sahakian BJ, Robbins TW, Bullmore ET. White matter abnormalities in patients with obsessive–compulsive disorder and their first-degree relatives. *Am J Psychiatry.* 2008;165: 1308–1315.

Milak MS, Parsey RV, Keilp J, Oquendo MA, Malone KM, Mann JJ. Neuroanatomic correlates of psychopathologic components of major depressive disorder. *Arch Gen Psychiatry.* 2005;62:397–408.

Militerni R, Bravaccio C, Falco C, Fico C, Palermo MT. Repetitive behaviors in autistic disorder. *Eur Child Adolesc Psychiatry.* 2002;11:210–218.

Millan MJ. The neurobiology and control of anxious states. *Prog Neurobiol.* 2003;70: 83–244.

Miller JA. *The Childhood Depression Sourcebook.* Los Angeles, CA: Lowell House; 1998.

Miller LG, Murray WJ, eds. *Herbal Medicinals: A Clinician's Guide.* New York: Pharmaceutical Products Press; 1998.

Mink JW. The basal ganglia and involuntary movements. *Arch Neurol.* 2003;60: 1365–1368.

Minshew NJ. Brief report: Brain mechanisms in autism: Functional and structural abnormalities. *J Autism Dev Disord.* 1996;26:205–209.

Mirsky AF. Behavioral and psychophysiological markers of disordered attention. *Environ Health Perspect.* 1987;74:191–199.

Mischoulon D. Update and critique of natural remedies as antidepressant treatments. *Psychiatr Clin North Am.* 2007;30:51–68.

Miyasaka L, Atallah A, Soares B. Passiflora for anxiety disorder. *Cochrane Database Syst Rev.* 2007;24. CD004518. Retrieved May 17, 2009, from http://mrw.interscience. wiley.com.

Moldofsky H, Sandor P. Lecithin in the treatment of Gilles de la Tourette's syndrome. *Am J Psychiatry.* 1983;140:1627–1629.

Moore M. *Medicinal Plants of the Mountain West.* Santa Fe, NM: Museum of New Mexico Press; 2003.

Morin AK, Jarvis CI, Lynch AM. Therapeutic options for sleep-maintenance and sleep-onset insomnia. *Pharmacotherapy.* 2007;27:89–110.

Morita K, Hamano S, Oka M, Teraoka K. Stimulatory actions of bioflavonoids on tyrosine uptake into cultured bovine adrenal chromaffin cells. *Biochem Biophys Res Commun.* 1990;171:1199–1204.

Morlion BJ, Stehle P, Wachtler P, Siedhoff HP, Koller M, Konig W, Furst P, Puchstein C. Total parenteral nutrition with glutamine dipeptide after major abdominal surgery: A randomized, double-blind, controlled study. *Ann Surg*. 1998;227:302–308.

Morris D, Trivedi MH, Rush AJ. Folate and unipolar depression. *J Altern Complement Med*. 2008;4:277–285.

Mousain-Bosc M, Roche M, Polge A. Improvement of neurobehavioral disorders in children supplemented with magnesium-vitamin B6 – II: Pervasive developmental disorder and autism. *Magnes Res*. 2006;19:53–54.

Muller WE, ed. *St. John's Wort and its Active Principles in Depression and Anxiety*. Boston, MA: Birkauser Publishers; 2005.

Nathan PE, Gorman JM, eds. *A Guide to Treatments That Work*. 2nd ed. New York: Oxford University Press; 2002.

Nathan PJ, Lu K, Gray M, Oliver C. The neuropharmacology of L-theanine(N-ethyl-L-glutamine): A possible neuroprotective and cognitive enhancing agent. *J Herb Pharmacother*. 2006;6:21–30.

National Center for Health Statistics. Obesity still on the rise, new data show. *HHS News*. 2002 October 8. Retrieved March 15, 2009, from http://www.hhs.gov.

Neckelmann D. Chronic insomnia as a risk factor for developing anxiety and depression. *Sleep*. 2007;30:873–880.

Nehlig A, Daval JL, Debry G. Caffeine and the central nervous system: Mechanisms of action, biochemical, metabolic and psychostimulant effects. *Brain Res Rev*. 1992;17:139–170.

Nemets B, Stahl Z, Belmaker RH. Addition of omega-3 fatty acid to maintenance medication treatment for recurrent unipolar depressive disorder. *Am J Psychiatry*. 2002;159:477–479.

Nemets H, Nemets B, Apter A, Bracha Z, Belmaker RH. Omega-3 treatment of childhood depression: A controlled, double-blind pilot study. *Am J Psychiatry*. 2006;163:1098–1100.

Nemzer E, Arnold LE, Votolato NA, McConnell H. Amino acid supplementation as therapy for attention deficit disorder (ADD). *J Am Acad Child Adolesc Psychiatry*. 1986;25:509–513.

Neumeister A, Nugent AC, Waldeck T, Geraci M, Schwarz M, Bonne O, Bain EE, Luckenbaugh DA, Herscovitch P, Charney DS, Drevets WC. Neural and behavioral responses to tryptophan depletion in unmedicated patients with remitted major depressive disorder and controls. *Arch Gen Psychiatry*. 2004;61:765–773.

Neville K. Can omega-3 supplements help you reel in the health benefits of fish? *Environ Nutr*. 2006 April;23. Retrieved April 15, 2009, from http://www.environmentalnutrition.com.

Newall C, Anderson L, Phillipson J. *Herbal Medicines: A Guide for Health-Care Professionals*. London, UK: Pharmaceutical Press; 1996.

Ng DK, Chan CH, Soo MT. Low-level chronic mercury exposure in children and adolescents: Meta-analysis. *Pediatr Int*. 2007;49:80–87.

Nierenberg AA, Mischoulon D, DeCecco L. St. John's wort. In: Mischoulon D, Rosenbaum JF, eds. *Natural Medications for Psychiatric Disorders: Considering the Alternatives*. Philadelphia, PA: Lippincott, Williams & Wilkins; 2002:3–12.

Nijhof G, Joha D, Pekelharing H. Aspects of stereotypic behaviour among autistic persons: A study of the literature. *Br J Dev Disabil*. 1998;44:3–13.

Nofzinger et al., 2005 Nofzinger EA, Buysse DJ, Germain A. A comparison of regional cerebral metabolism across waking and NREM sleep between primary insomnia and major depression. *Program and Abstracts of the Associated Professional Sleep Societies 19th Annual Meeting*, Denver, CO; 2005, June, abstract no. 0691.

Nurmand LB, Otter MI, Vasar EE. Effect of structural analogs of gamma-aminobutyric acid on serotonin- and dopaminergic mechanisms. *Farmakologia et Toksikologia.* 1980;43:288–291.

Nutt DJ. Neurobiological mechanisms in generalized anxiety disorder. *J Clin Psychiatry.* 2001;62(suppl 11):22–27.

Office of the Surgeon General. *The Surgeon General's Call to Action to Prevent Suicide.* Washington, DC: Author; 1999.

Olanow JP. Oxidative stress and the pathogenesis of Parkinson's disease. *Neurology.* 1996;47(Suppl):S161–S170.

Olfson M, Marcus SC, Weissman MM, Jensen PS. National trends in the use of psychotropic medications by children. *J Am Acad Child Adolesc Psychiatry.* 2002;41:514–521.

Paavonen EJ, Nieminen T, Vanhala R, Aronen ET, von Wendt L. The effectiveness of melatonin in the treatment of sleep disturbances in children with Asperger syndrome. *J Child Adolesc Psychopharmacol.* 2003;13:83–96.

Palumbo DR. New directions in the treatment of comorbid attention deficit hyperactivity disorder and Tourette's syndrome. In: Kurlan R, ed. *Handbook of Tourette's Syndrome and Related Tic and Behavioral Disorders.* New York: Informa Health Care; 2004:89–108.

Pancheri P, Racagni G, Delle Chiaie RD. Recent experimental and clinical findings of the efficacy and safety of adementionine (SAMe) in the pharmacological treatment of depression. *Giornale Italiano di Psicopatologia.* 1997;3:1–23.

Pancheri P, Scapicchio P, Delle Chiaie RD. A double-blind, randomized parallel-group, efficacy and safety study of intramuscular S-adenosyl-L-metionine 1,4-butanedisulfonate (SAMe) versus imipramine in patients with major depressive disorder. *Int J Neuropsychopharmacol.* 2002;5:287–294.

Panijel M. Therapy of symptoms of anxiety. *Therapiewoche.* 1985;41:4659–4668.

Papakostas GI, Petersen T, Mischoulon D, Ryan JL, Nierenberg AA, Bottiglieri T, Rosenbaum JF, Alpert JE, Fava M. Serum folate, vitamin B-sub-1-sub-2, and homocysteine in major depressive disorder, part 1: Predictors of clinical response in fluoxetine-resistant depression. *J Clin Psychiatry.* 2004;65:1096–1098.

Pardo CA, Eberhart CG. The neurobiology of autism. *Brain Pathol.* 2007;17:434–447.

Parker K, Brunton L, Goodman LS, Lazo JS, Gilman A. *Goodman & Gilman's the Pharmacological Basis of Therapeutics.* New York: McGraw-Hill; 2006.

Peet M, Horrobin DF. E-E Multicentre Study Group: A dose-ranging exploratory study of the effects of ethyl-eicosapentaenoate in patients with persistent schizophrenic symptoms. *J Psychiatr Res.* 2002;36:7–18.

Peet M, Laugharne JD, Mellor J. Essential fatty acid deficiency in erythrocyte membranes from chronic schizophrenic patients and the clinical effects of dietary supplementation. *Prostaglandins Leukot Essent. Fatty Acids.* 1996;55:71–75.

Peterson BS, Staib L, Scahill L. Regional brain and ventricular volumes in Tourette syndrome. *Arch Gen Psychiatry.* 2001;58:427–440.

Peterson BS, Warner V, Bansal R, Zhu H, Hao X, Liu J, Durkin K, Adams PB, Wickramaratne P, Weissman MM. Cortical thinning in persons at increased familial risk for major depression. *Proc Natl Acad Sci.* 2009;106:6273–6278.

Peterson BS, Pine DS, Cohen P, Brook JS. Prospective, longitudinal study of tic, obsessive–compulsive, and attention-deficit/hyperactivity disorders in an epidemiological sample. *J Am Acad Child Adolesc Psychiatry.* 2001;40:685–695.

Pfeiffer SI, Norton J, Nelson L. Efficacy of vitamin B6 and magnesium in the treatment of autism: A methodology review and summary of outcomes. *J Autism Dev Disord.* 1995;25:481–493.

Pfiffner LJ, McBurnett K, Lahey BB, Loeber R, Green S, Frick PJ. Association of parental psychopathology to the comorbid disorders of boys with attention deficit hyperactivity disorder. *J Consult Clin Psychol*. 1999;67:881–893.

Piccirillo G, Fimognari FL, Infantino V, Monteleone G, Fimognari GB, Falletti D, Marigliano V. High plasma concentrations of cortisol and thromboxane B2 in patients with depression. *Am J Med Sci*. 1994;307:228–232.

Pickles A, Bolton P, Macdonald H, Bailey A, Le Couteur A, Sim L, Rutter M. Latent class analysis of recurrence risks for complex phenotypes with selection and measurement error: A twin and family history study of autism. *Am J Hum Genet*. 1995;57:717–726.

Pickles A, Starr E, Kazak S, Bolton P, Papanikolaou K, Bailey A, Goodman R, Rutter M. Variable expression of the autism broader phenotype: Findings from extended pedigrees. *J Child Psychol Psychiatry*. 2000;41:491–502.

Pillai JJ, Friedman L, Stuve TA, Trinidad S, Jesberger JA, Lewin JS. Increased presence of white matter hyperintensities in adolescent patients with bipolar disorder. *Psychiatry Res: Neuroimaging*. 2002;114:51–56.

Pini S, Martini C, Abelli M, Muti M, Gesi C, Montali M, Chelli B, Lucacchini A, Cassano GB. Peripheral-type benzodiazepine receptor binding sites in platelets of patients with panic disorder associated to separation anxiety symptoms. *Psychopharmacology*. 2005;181:407–411.

Pittler MH, Ernst E. Kava extract for treating anxiety. *Cochrane Database Syst Rev*. 2003;1. CD003383. Retrieved May 17, 2009, from http://mrw.interscience.wiley.com.

Pittler MH, Ernst E. Efficacy of kava extract for treating anxiety: Systematic review and meta-analysis. *J Clin Psychopharmacol*. 2000;20:84–89.

Piven J, Bailey J, Ransom BJ, Arndt S. An MRI study of the corpus callosum in autism. *Am J Psychiatry*. 1997;154:1051–1056.

Piven J, Berthier ML, Starkstein SE, Nehme E, Pearlson G, Folstein S. Magnetic resonance imaging evidence for a defect of cerebral cortical development in autism. *Am J Psychiatry*. 1990;147:734–739.

Plessen KJ, Grüner R, Lundervold A, Hirsch JG, Xu D, Bansal R, Hammar A, Lundervold AJ, Wentzel-Larsen T, Atle Lie S, Gass A, Peterson BS, Hugdahl K. Reduced white matter connectivity in the corpus callosum of children with Tourette syndrome. *J Child Psychol Psychiatry*. 2006;47:1013–1022.

Poldinger W, Calanchini B, Schwarz W. A functional-dimensional approach to depression: A serotonin deficiency as a target syndrome in a comparison of 5-hydroxytryptophan and fluvoxamine. *Psychopathology*. 1991;24:53–81.

Polinsky RJ, Ebert MH, Caine ED. Cholinergic treatment in the Tourette syndrome. *N Engl J Med*. 1980;302:1310.

Port J, Unal S, Mrazek D, Marcus S. Metabolic alterations in medication-free patients with bipolar disorder: A 3T CSF-corrected magnetic resonance spectroscopic imaging study. *Psychiatry Res: Neuroimaging*. 2004;162:113–121.

Post RM. Kindling and sensitization as models for affective episode recurrence, cyclicity, and tolerance phenomena. *Neurosci. Biobehavioral Rev*. 2007;31:858–873.

Post RM, Leverich GS, Nolen WA. A re-evaluation of the role of antidepressants in the treatment of bipolar depression: Data from the Stanley Foundation Bipolar Network. *Bipolar Disord*. 2003;5:396–406.

Potter M, Moses A, Wozniak J. Alternative treatments in pediatric bipolar disorder. *Child Adolesc Psychiatr Clin N Am.* 2009;18:483–514.

Prathikanti S. Ayurvedic treatments. In: Lake JH, Spiegel D, eds. *Complementary and Alternative Treatments in Mental Health Care.* Washington, DC: American Psychiatric Publishing; 2007:225–272.

Prior M, Ozonoff S. Psychological factors in autism. In: Volkmar FR, ed. *Autism and Pervasive Developmental Disorders.* Cambridge, UK: Cambridge University Press; 1998:64–108.

Puri BK, Counsell SJ, Richardson AJ. Eicosapentaenoic acid in treatment-resistant depression. *Arch Gen Psychiatry.* 2002;59:91–92.

Ramsay JR, Rostain AL. *Cognitive-Behavioral Therapy for Adult ADHD: An Integrative Psychosocial and Medical Approach.* New York: Routledge; 2008.

Ramu MG, Chaturvedi DD, Venkataram BS. *Ayurvedic Management of Unmade.* New Delhi, India: Central Council for Research in Ayurveda and Siddha; 1999.

Ramu MG, Senapati HM, Jankiramaiah N. A pilot study on role of brahmyadiyoga on chronic unmada (schizophrenia) patients. *Anc Sci Life.* 1983;2:205–207.

Rapoport JL, Giedd JN, Blumenthal J, Hamburger S, Jeffries N, Fernandez T. Progressive cortical change during adolescence in childhood-onset schizophrenia: A longitudinal magnetic resonance imaging study. *Arch Gen Psychiatry.* 1999;56:649–654.

Rapoport JL, Giedd JN, Kurma S, Jacobsen L, Smith A, Lee P, Nelson J, Hamburger S. Childhood-onset schizophrenia: Progressive ventricular change during adolescence. *Arch Gen Psychiatry.* 1997;54:897–903.

Reinstein DK, Lehnert H, Wurtman RJ. Dietary tyrosine suppresses the rise in plasma corticosterone following acute stress in rats. *Life Sci.* 1985;37:2157–2163.

Remschmidt HE. Schizophrenic psychoses in children and adolescents. *Triangle.* 1993;32:15–24.

Remschmidt HE, Schulz E, Martin M, Warnke A, Trott G. Childhood-onset schizophrenia: History of the concept and recent studies. *Schizophr Bull.* 1994;20:727–746.

Richardson AJ. The importance of omega-3 fatty acids for behaviour, cognition and mood. *Scand J Nutr.* 2003;47:92–98.

Richardson et al., 2005 Richardson GS, McClure TK, Meola G, Roth T. Dex-CRH test in primary insomnia. *Program and Abstracts of the Associated Professional Sleep Societies 19th Annual Meeting*; Denver, CO; 2005 June, abstract no. 0763.

Rimland B. The autism–secretin connection. *Autism Res Rev Int.* 1998;12:3–4.

Risby E. Ethnic considerations in the pharmacotherapy of mood disorders. *Psychopharmacol Bull.* 1996;32:231–234.

Ritchie MJ. The xanthines. In: Goodman LS, Gillman A, eds. *The Pharmacological Basis of Therapeutics.* London, UK: Collier-Macmillan; 1975:367–378.

Robertson JM, Shepard DS. The psychological development of boys. In: Kiselica MS, Englar-Carlson M, Horne AM, eds. *Counseling Troubled Boys: A Guidebook for Professionals.* New York: Routledge; 2008:3–29.

Robertson JM, Tanguay PE. Case study: The use of melatonin in a boy with refractory bipolar disorder. *J Am Acad Child Adolesc Psychiatry.* 1997;36:822–825.

Robertson MM. Diagnosing Tourette syndrome: Is it a common disorder? *J Psychosom Res.* 2003;55:3–6.

Rudin DO. The major psychoses and neuroses as omega-3 essential fatty acid deficiency syndrome: Substrate pellagra. *Biol Psychiatry*. 1981;16:837–850.

Sabelli H. Phenylethylamine deficit and replacement in depressive illness. In: Mischoulon D, Rosenbaum JF, eds, *Natural Medications for Psychiatric Disorders: Considering the Alternatives*. Philadelphia, PA: Lippincott, Williams & Wilkins; 2002:83–110.

Sachs G, Lafer B. Child and adolescent mania. In: Goodnick PJ, ed. *Mania: Clinical and Research Perspectives*. Washington, DC: American Psychiatric Publishing; 1998:37–60.

Saratikov AS, Krasnov EA. *Rhodiola Rosea is a Valuable Medicinal Plant*. Tomsk, Russia: Tomsk State University Press; 1987.

Savitz and Drevets, Savitz JB, Drevets WC. Imaging phenotypes of major depressive disorder: Genetic correlates. *Neuroscience*. In Press; Retrieved April 25, 2009, from http://www.pubmed.gov.

Schaller JT, Bazzan AJ. SAMe use in children and adolescents. *Eur Child Adolesc Psychiatry*. 2004;13:332–334.

Schatzberg AF, Cole JO, DeBattista C. *Manual of clinical psychopharmacology*. Washington, DC: American Psychiatric Publishing; 2007.

Schmidt B. Methylxanthine therapy for apnea of prematurity: Evaluation of treatment benefits and risks at age 5 years in the International Caffeine for Apnea of Prematurity (CAP) trial. *Neonatology*. 2005;88:208–213.

Schmidt M, Nahrstedt A. Is kava hepatotoxic?. *Dtsch Apoth Ztg*. 2002;142:58–63.

Schreck K, Mulick J. Parental report of sleep problems in children with autism. *J Autism Dev Disord*. 2000;30:127–135.

Schreier HA. Mania responsive to lecithin in a 13-year-old girl. *Am J Psychiatry*. 1981;139:108–110.

Schroeder C, Tank J, Goldstein DS. Influence of St. John's wort on catecholamine turnover and cardiovascular regulation in humans. *Clin Pharmacol Ther*. 2004;76:480–489.

Schulz V, Stolz C, Muller J. The effect of a valerian extract on sleep polygraphy in poor sleepers: A pilot study. *Pharmacopsychiatry*. 1994;27:147–151.

Seedat S, Stein DJ, Harvey BH. Inositol in the treatment of trichotillomania and compulsive skin picking. *J Clin Psychiatry*. 2001;62:60–61.

Sen G, Bose KC. Rauwolfia serpentina. *Indian Med World*. 1931;2:194–201.

Serby M, Schmeidler J, Smith J. Length of psychiatry clerkships: Recent changes and the relationship to recruitment. *Acad Psychiatry*. 2002;26:102–104.

Settle JE. Nutritional supplements. In: Lake JH, Spiegel D, eds. *Complementary and Alternative Treatments in Mental Health Care*. Washington, DC: American Psychiatric Publishing; 2007:115–149.

Sever Y, Ashkenazi A, Tyano S, Weizman A. Iron treatment in children with ADHD: A preliminary report. *Neuropsychobiology*. 1997;35:178–180.

Shelton RC. Cellular mechanisms in the vulnerability to depression and response to antidepressants. *Psychiatr Clin North Am*. 2000;23:713–729.

Shevtsov VA, Zholus BI, Shervarly VI, Vol'skij VB, Korovin YP, Khristich MP, Roslyakova NA, Wikman G. A randomized trial of two different doses of a SHR-5 rhodiola rosea extract versus placebo and control of capacity for mental work. *Phytomedicine*. 2003;10:95–105.

Shugart MA, Lopez EM. Depression in children and adolescents. *Postgrad Med*. 2002;112. Retrieved April 24, 2009, from http://www.biomedexperts.com.

Shulgina GI. On neurotransmitter mechanisms of reinforcement and internal inhibition. *Pavlov J Biol Sci*. 1986;21:129–140.

Simeon J, Nixon MK, Milin R. Open-label pilot study of St. John's wort in adolescent depression. *J Child Adolesc Psychopharmacol.* 2005;15:293–301.

Simopoulos A. The importance of the ratio of omega-6/omega-3 essential fatty acids. *Biomed Pharmacother.* 2002;56:365–379.

Singer JB. Making stone soup: Evidence-based practice for a suicidal youth with comorbid attention-deficit/hyperactivity disorder and major depressive disorder. *Brief Treat and Crisis Interv.* 2006;6:234–247.

Sitaram N, Moore AM, Gillin JC. Experimental acceleration and slowing of REM ultradian rhythm by cholinergic agonist and antagonist. *Nature.* 1978;274: 490–492.

Smits MG, van Stel HF, van der Heijden K, Meijer AM, Coenen AM, Kerkhof GA. Melatonin improves health status and sleep in children with idiopathic chronic sleep-onset insomnia: A randomized placebo-controlled trial. *J Am Acad Child Adolesc Psychiatry.* 2003;42:1286–1293.

Snider LA, Swedo SE. PANDAS: Current status and directions for research. *Mol Psychiatry.* 2004;9:900–907.

Spence SH, Rapee R, McDonald C, Ingram M. The structure of anxiety symptoms among preschoolers. *Behav Res Ther.* 2001;39:1293–1316.

Spencer KM, Nestor PG, Perlmutter R, Niznikiewicz MA, Klump MC, Frumin M, Shenton ME, McCarley RW. Neural synchrony indexes disordered perception and cognition in schizophrenia. *Proc Natl Acad Sci.* 2004;101:17,288–17,293,.

Spinella M. *The Psychopharmacology of Herbal Medicine.* Cambridge, MA: MIT Press; 2001.

Stahl SM. Beyond the dopamine hypothesis to the NMDA glutamate receptor hypofunction hypothesis of schizophrenia. *CNS Spectrum.* 2007;12:265–268.

Stahl SM. *Essential Psychopharmacology, Neuroscientific Basis and Practical Applications.* 3rd ed. New York: Cambridge University Press; 2008.

Starcevic V. Anxiety states: A review of conceptual and treatment issues. *Curr Opin Psychiatry.* 2006;19:79–83.

Stark KD, Simpson J, Schnoebelen S, Hargrave J, Glenn R, Molnar J. *Therapist's Manual for ACTION.* Broadmore, PA: Workbook Publishing; 2006.

Stevens L, Zhang W, Peck L. EFA supplementation in children with attention, hyperactivity, and other disruptive behaviors. *Lipids.* 2003;38:1007–1021.

Stevenson C, Ernst E. Valerian for insomnia: A systematic review of randomized clinical trials. *Sleep Med.* 2000;1:91–99.

Stewart MA. Hyperactive children. *Sci Am.* 1970;222:94–98.

Still GF. Some abnormal psychical conditions in children. *Lancet.* 2007;1. 1008–1012, 1077–1082, 1163–1168.

Stoll AL, Locke CA. Omega-3 fatty acids in mood disorders. In: Mischoulon D, Rosenbaum JF, eds. *Natural Medications for Psychiatric Disorders: Considering the Alternatives.* Philadelphia, PA: Lippincott, Williams & Wilkins; 2002:13–34.

Stoll A, Severus W, Freeman M. Omega-3 fatty acids in bipolar disorder: A preliminary double-blind, placebo-controlled trial. *Arch Gen Psychiatry.* 1999;56:407–412.

Strauss EB, Stevenson WA. Use of dehydroepiandrosterone in psychiatric practice. *J Neurol Neurosurg Psychiatry.* 1955;18:137–144.

Stuart G, Spruston N, Hausser M. *Dendrites.* 2nd ed. Oxford, UK: Oxford University Press; 2008.

Su KP, Shen WW, Huang SY. Omega-3 fatty acids as a psychotherapeutic agent for a pregnant schizophrenic patient. *Eur Neuropsychopharmacol.* 2001;11:295–299.

Sutker PB, Adams HE, eds. *Comprehensive Handbook of Psychotherapy*. New York: Kluwer; 2001.

Swanson JM, Castellanos FX. Biological Bases of ADHD – Neuroanatomy, Genetics, and Pathophysiology. In: Jensen PS, Cooper JR, eds. *Attention Deficit Hyperactivity Disorder: State of the Science, Best Practices*. Kingston, NJ: Civic Research Institute; 2002:7–20.

Swedo SE. Pediatric autoimmune neuropsychiatric disorders associated with streptococcal infections (PANDAS). *Mol Psychiatry*. 2002;7:S24–S25.

Szatmari P. Heterogeneity and the genetics of autism. *J Psychiatry Neurosci*. 1999;24:159–165.

Szatmari P. The classification of autism, Asperger's syndrome, and pervasive developmental disorder. *Can J Psychiatry*. 2000;45:731–738.

Tager Flushberg H. Understanding the language and communicative impairment in autism. In: Glidden LM, ed. *International Review of Research in Mental Retardation: Autism*. San Diego, CA: Academic Press; 2001:185–205.

Tannock R. Attention-deficit/hyperactivity disorder with anxiety disorders. In: Brown TE, ed. *Attention-Deficit Disorders and Comorbidities in Children, Adolescents, and Adults*. Washington, DC: American Psychiatric Press; 2000:125–170.

Taylor LH, Kobak KA. An open-label trial of St. John's wort (Hypericum perforatum) in obsessive–compulsive disorder. *J Clin Psychiatry*. 2000;61:575–578.

Tempesta E, Casella L, Pirrongelli C. L-acetylcarnitine in depressed elderly subjects: A crossover study vs. placebo. *Drugs Exp Clin Res*. 1987;13:417–423.

Thomas CR, Holzer CE. The continuing shortage of child and adolescent psychiatrists. *J Am Acad Child Adolesc Psychiatry*. 2006;45:1023–1031.

Thompson PM, Vidal C, Giedd JN, Gochman P, Blumenthal J, Nicolson R, Toga AW, Rapoport JL. Mapping adolescent brain change reveals dynamic wave of accelerated gray matter loss in very early-onset schizophrenia. *Proc Natl Acad Sci*. 2001;25:11,650–11,655,.

Torrioli MG, Vernacotola S, Mariotti S, Bianchi E, Calvani M, DeGaetano A, Chiurazzi P, Neri G. Double-blind, placebo-controlled study of l-acetylcarnitine for the treatment of hyperactive behavior in fragile X syndrome. *Am J Med Genet*. 1999;87:366–368.

Trebaticka J, Kopasova S, Hradecna Z, Cinovsky K. Treatment of ADHD with French maritime bark extract, Pycnogenol. *Eur Child Adolesc Psychiatry*. 2006;15:329–335.

Trice I, Haymes EM. Effects of caffeine ingestion on exercise-induced changes during high-intensity, intermittent exercise. *Int J Sport Nutr*. 1995;5:37–44.

Tsuboyama-Kasaoka N, Shozawa C, Sano K, Kamei Y, Kasaoka S, Hosokawa Y, Ezaki O. Taurine (2-aminoethanesulfonic acid) deficiency creates a vicious circle promoting obesity. *Endocrinology*. 2006;147:3276–3284.

Turkington C, Tzeel A. *Encyclopedia of Children's Health and Wellness*. New York: Facts on File; 2004.

Uebelhack R, Franke L, Schewe HJ. Inhibition of platelet MAO-B by kava pyrone-enriched extract from Piper methysticum forster (kava-kava). *Pharmacopsychiatry*. 1998;31:187–192.

Van Hiele L. L-5-hydroxytryptophan in depression: The first substitution therapy in psychiatry? *Neuropsychobiology*. 1980;6:230–240.

Veenema K, Solis C, Li R, Wang W, Maletz CV, Abratte CM, Caudill MA. Adequate intake levels of choline are sufficient for preventing elevations in serum markers of liver dysfunction in Mexican American men but are not optimal for minimizing plasma total homocysteine increases after a methionine load. *Am J Clin Nutr.* 2008;88:685–692.

Verlhurst FC, van der Ende J, Ferdinand RF, Kasius MC. The prevalence of DSM-III-R diagnoses in a national sample of Dutch adolescents. *Arch Gen Psychiatry.* 1997;54:329–336.

Vibrant Life. *How to detoxify mercury.* 2008. Retrieved May 11, 2009, from http://www.chelationtherapyonline.com/articles/p45.htm.

Viola H, Wasowski C, Levi de Stain M, Wolfman C, Silveira R, Dajas F, Medina JH, Paladini AC. Apigenin, a component of Matricaria recutita flowers, is a central benzodiazepine receptor-ligand with anxiolytic effects. *Planta Med.* 1995;61: 213–216.

Vishwakarma SL, Pal SC, Kasture VS, Kasture SB. Anxiolytic and antiemetic activity of zingiber officinale. *Phytother Res.* 2002;16:621–626.

Voigt R, Llorente A, Jensen C. A randomized, double-blind, placebo-controlled trial of docosahexaenoic acid supplementation in children with attention-deficit/hyperactivity disorder. *J Pediatr.* 2001;139:189–196.

Vorbach EU, Gortelmeyer R, Bruning J. Treatment of insomnia: effectiveness and tolerance of a valerian extract. *Psychopharmakotherapie.* 1996;3:109–115.

Wakefield AJ, Murch SH, Anthony A, Linell J, Casson DM, Malik M, Berelowitz M, Dhillon AP, Thomson MA, Harvey P, Valentine A, Davies SE, Walker-Smith JA. Ileal-lymphoid-nodular hyperplasia, non-specific colitis, and pervasive developmental disorder in children.. *Lancet.* 1998;351:637–641.

Walk A. The pre-history of child psychiatry. *Br J Psychiatry.* 1964;110:754–767.

Waller DP. *Report on kava and liver damage.* Silver Spring, MD: American Herbal Products Association; 2002.

Walsh M. *Bipolar disorders: A guide to helping children and adolescents.* Sebastopol, CA: O'Reilly & Associates, Inc; 2000.

Walsh W. Commentary on nutritional treatment of mental disorders. 2003. Retrieved April 15, 2008, from http://www.hriptc.org.

Weber W, Vander Stoep A, Mc Carthy R, Weiss N. Hypericum perforatum (St. John's wort) for attention-deficit/hyperactivity disorder in children and adolescents: A randomized controlled trial. *J Am Med Assoc.* 2008;299:2633–2641.

Weiss B, Garber J. Developmental differences in phenomenology of depression. *Dev Psychopathol.* 2003;15:403–430.

Weiss MD, Wasdell MB, Bomben MM, Rea KJ, Freeman RD. Sleep hygiene and melatonin treatment for children and adolescents with ADHD and initial insomnia. *J Am Acad Child Adolesc Psychiatry.* 2006;45:512–519.

Welfel ER, Ingersoll REMental Health Desk Reference. New York: John Wiley & Sons; 2001.

Wender PMinimal Brain Dysfunction in Children. New York: Wiley; 1971.

Wheatley D. Kava and valerian in the treatment of stress-induced insomnia.. *Phytotherapeutic Res.* 2001;15:549–551.

White SW, Oswald D, Ollendick T, Scahill L. Anxiety in children and adolescents with autism spectrum disorders. *Clin Psychol Rev.* 2009;29:216–229.

Widy-Tyszkiewicz E, Schminda R. A randomized double blind study of sedative effects of phytotherapeutic containing valerian, hops, balm and motherwort versus placebo. *Herba Polonica.* 1997;2:154–159.

Wilens TE, Biederman J, Brown S, Tanguay S, Monuteaux MC, Blake C. Psychiatric comorbidity and functioning in clinically referred preschool children and school-age youth with ADHD. *J Am Acad Child Adolesc Psychiatry*. 2002;41:262–268.

Wing L, Potter D. The epidemiology of autistic spectrum disorders: Is prevalence rising? *Dev Disabil Res Rev*. 2002;8:151–161.

Winn P. Schizophrenia research moves to the prefrontal cortex.. *Trends Neurosci*. 1994;17:265–268.

Wittenborn JR. Niacin in the long-term treatment of schizophrenia. *Arch Gen Psychiatry*. 1973;28:308–315.

Wolfman C, Viola H, Paladini A, Dajas F, Medina JH. Possible anxiolytic effects of chrysin, a central benzodiazepine receptor ligand isolated from Passiflora coerulea. *Pharmacol Biochem Behav*. 1994;47:1–4.

Wolkowitz OM, Reus VI. Dehydropiandrosterone as a neurohormone in the treatment of depression and dementia. In: Mischoulon D, Rosenbaum JF, eds. *Natural Medications for Psychiatric Disorders: Considering the Alternatives*. Philadelphia, PA: Lippincott, Williams & Wilkins; 2002:62–82.

Wolraich ML, Wilson DB, White JW. The effect of sugar on behavior or cognition in children: A meta-analysis. *J Am Med Assoc*. 1995;274:1617–1621.

Wood DR, Reimherr FW, Wender PH. Amino acid precursors for the treatment of attention-deficit disorder, residual type. *Psychopharmacol Bull*. 1985;21:146–149.

World Health Organization. *International Statistical Classification of Diseases and Related Health Problems*. 10th rev New York: United Nations University Press; 1992.

World Health Organization. *Protein and Amino Acid Requirements in Human Nutrition*. New York: United Nations University Press; 2007.

Wozniak J, Biederman J, Mick E, Waxmonsky J, Hantsoo L, Best C, Cluette-Brown JE, Laposata M. Omega-3 fatty acid monotherapy for pediatric bipolar disorder: A prospective open-label trial. *Eur Neuropsychopharmacol*. 2007;17:440–447.

Wurtman RL, Madelyn J, Growdon JH. Lecithin consumption raises serumfree choline levels. *Lancet*. 1977;2:68–69.

Xu J, Jian B, Chu R, Lu Z, Li Q, Dunlop J, Rosenzweig-Lipson S, McGonigle P, Levy RJ, Liang B. Serotonin mechanisms in heart valve disease II: The 5-HT2 receptor and its signaling pathway in aortic valve interstitial cells. *Am J Pathol*. 2002;161:2209–2218.

Yamasue H, Abe O, Suga M, Yamada H, Inoue H, Tochigi M, Rogers M, Aoki S, Kato N, Kasai K. Gender-common and -specific neuroanatomical basis of human anxiety-related personality traits. *Cereb Cortex*. 2008;18:46–52.

Yoon DY, Rippel CA, Kobets AJ, Morris CM, Lee JE, Williams PN, Bridges DD, Vandenbergh DJ, Shugart YY, Singer HS. Dopaminergic polymorphisms in Tourette syndrome: Association with the DAT gene (SLC6A3). *Am J Med Genet*. 2007;144:605–610.

Young SN. Folate and depression – a neglected problem. *J Psychiatry Neurosci*. 2007;32: 80–82.

Zanarini M, Frankenburg F. Omega-3 fatty acid treatment of women with borderline personality disorder: A double-blind, placebo-controlled pilot study. *Am J Psychiatry*. 2003;160:167–169.

Zeisel SH. Dietary influences on neurotransmission. *Adv Pediatr*. 1986;33:23–47.

Zhang CG, Kim SJ. Taurine induces anti-anxiety by activating strychnine-sensitive glycine receptor. *Ann Nutr Metab*. 2007;51:379–386.

Zhang M, Bi LF, Fang JH, Su XL, Da GL, Kuwamori T, Kagamimori S. Beneficial effects of taurine on serum lipids in overweight or obese non-diabetic subjects. *Amino Acids*. 2004;26:267–271.

Zhdanova IV, Friedman L. Melatonin for treatment of sleep and mood disorders. In: Mischoulon D, Rosenbaum JF, eds. *Natural Medications for Psychiatric Disorders: Considering the Alternatives*. Philadelphia, PA: Lippincott, Williams & Wilkins; 2002:147–171.

Zubin J, Spring B. Vulnerability: A new view of schizophrenia. *J Abnorm Psychol*. 1977;86:103–126.

Index